MELLONI'S ILLUSTRATED DICTIONARY OF THE

MUSCULOSKELETAL SYSTEM

Dedicated to three brilliant women:

my mother, Teresa Sicurro Melloni

my wife, Ida G. Dox, PhD

my daughter, June L. Melloni, PhD

MUSCULOSKELETAL SYSTEM

B. John Melloni, PhD

The Parthenon Publishing Group
International Publishers in Medicine, Science & Technology

NEW YORK   LONDON

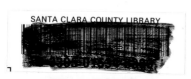

Published in the USA by
The Parthenon Publishing Group Inc.
One Blue Hill Plaza, PO Box 1564
Pearl River, New York 10965, USA

Published in the UK by
The Parthenon Publishing Group Limited
Casterton Hall, Kirkby Lonsdale
Carnforth, Lancs LA6 2LA, UK

Library of Congress Cataloging-in-Publication Data
Melloni, Biagio John.
    [Illustrated dictionary of the musculoskeletal system]
    Melloni's illustrated dictionary of the musculoskeletal system /
    by B. John Melloni.
       p.   cm
    ISBN 1-85070-667-0
    1. Musculoskeletal system -- Dictionaries. 2. Occupational therapy-
    -Dictionaries. 3. Physical therapy -- Dictionaries. I. Title.
    QM100.M44   1998
    611'.7'03 -- dc21   98–2796
                                              CIP

British Library Cataloguing in Publication Data
Melloni, Biagio John, 1929–
    Melloni's illustrated dictionary of the musculoskeletal
    system
    1.Musculoskeletal system - Outlines, syllabi, etc.
    I.Title II. Illustrated dictionary of the musculoskeletal
    system
    612.7
    ISBN 1-85070-667-0

Printed and bound by The Bath Press, Bath, UK

Preface

The aim of this book is to provide a quick and easy access to musculoskeletal information, usually found buried within anatomic textbooks. The dictionary format permits quick retrieval of this information. The book can accompany any relevant textbook and serve as handy reference.

The dictionary is heavily illustrated. It has more anatomic illustrations than most textbooks: in fact, it has more illustrations of ligaments than any anatomy textbook. The combination of single-concept illustrations and concise descriptions significantly contributes to the aim of this book.

Prolific use of illustrations reflects a conviction that the illustrations are not only essential for thorough comprehension, but that they serve as building blocks to long-term memory. Visuals are roadmaps for developing a clear, lasting framework of understanding, upon which future information can become more clearly understood. This framework of understanding, provided by well-conceived illustrations, can make a world of difference between retaining or forgetting anatomic information being studied.

When teaching gross anatomy at a school of medicine, I was constantly aware that it was rare that the fourth year medical student could pass a first year human anatomy examination. It has been shown convincingly, however, that those who have made proper use of well-conceived illustrations still possess a remarkable comprehension and retention of anatomy. The illustrations make an indelible imprint.

To help the reader identify the structures that are illustrated, the descriptive text is in color. The illustrations are generally placed either adjacent to the description or on the opposite page. Where there are numerous subentries, the illustrations may be grouped together as plates, or appear interspersed throughout the subentries.

Readers interested in commenting about this book should forward their remarks to B. John Melloni, PhD, 9308 Renshaw Dr., Bethesda, MD 20817, USA.

A special thanks is owed to the President of The Parthenon Publishing Group, Mr David G.T. Bloomer, and his Editor-in-Chief, Mr Nat Russo, for their encouraging enthusiasm and support during the development of this book.

BJM

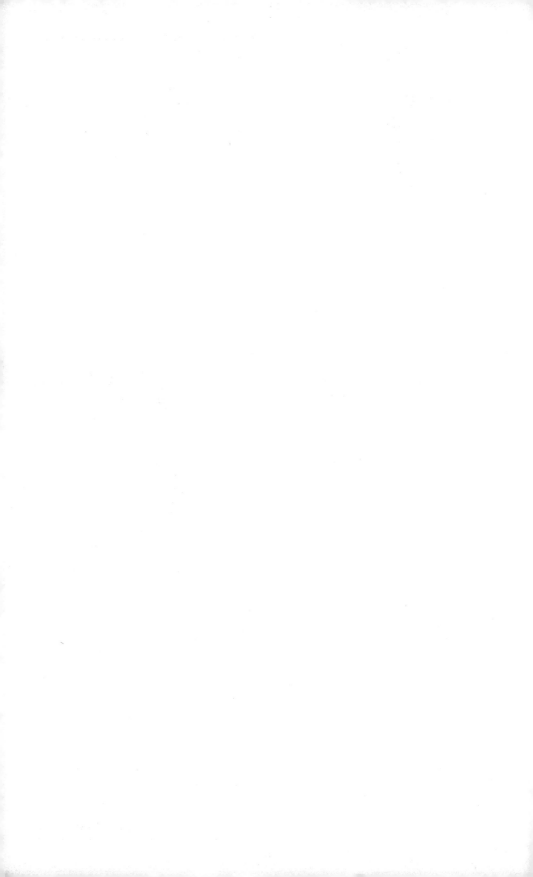

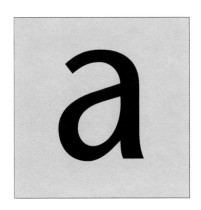

a-, an- Prefixes meaning without; not.
ab- Prefix meaning from; away from.
abapical (ab-ap'ĭ-kl) Opposite the apex.
abaxial (ab-ak'se-al) Located out of, or directed away from, the axis of the body or a part.
abdomen (ab'do-men) The part of the body below the chest and above the pelvis, containing the largest cavity of the body; divided into nine regions by imaginary planes for the purpose of identifying location of structures contained within. Abdominal contents include nerves, blood and lymph vessels, lymph nodes, and several organs: lowest part of the esophagus, stomach, intestines, liver, gallbladder, pancreas, and spleen. Popularly called belly; incorrectly called stomach.

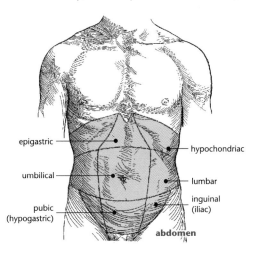

epigastric

umbilical

pubic
(hypogastric)

hypochondriac

lumbar

inguinal
(iliac)

abdomen

abdominal (ab-dom'ĭ-nal) Relating to the abdomen.
abdomino- Combining form meaning abdomen.
abdominoperineal (ab-dom-'ĭ-no-per-'ĭ-ne'al) Relating to the abdomen and perineum, used

especially to indicate surgical procedures involving those areas.
abdominothoracic (ab-dom-'ĭ-no-tho-ras'ik) Relating to the abdomen and thorax.
abducent (ab-du'sent) Drawing away; abducting.
abduct (ab-dukt') To move away from the median plane.
abduction (ab-duk'shun) Movement of a limb away from the median plane of the body or a digit away from the axial plane of a limb. Opposite of adduction.

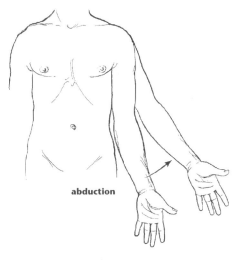

abduction

abductor (ab-duk'tor) A muscle that moves a body part away from the median plane. Opposite of adductor.
ability (ah-bil'i-te) The physical, mental, or legal competence to function.
abnormal (ab-nor'mal) Not normal; differing substantially from the usual.
abnormality (ab-nor-mal'ĭ-te) The state of being abnormal.
aboral (ab-o'ral) Directed away from the mouth.
abruption (ah-brupt'shun) A detachment or tearing away.
abterminal (ab-ter'mĭ-nal) Toward the center; denoting the direction of an electrical current in a muscle.
acampsia (ah-kamp'se-ah) Rigidity of a joint for any reason.
acanth- Combining form meaning spine; thorn.
acantha (ah-kan'thah) A spinous process.
acanthion (ah-kan'the-on) The tip of the anterior nasal spine.
acanthoid (ah-kan'thoid) Spine-shaped.
accelerator (ak-sel'er-a-tor) Anything (device, muscle, nerve, drug) that increases speed of action or function.

a-, an- ■ accelerator

accessory (ak-ses'o-re) Supplementary; having a subordinate function to a similar but more important structure.

acetabula (as-ĕ-tab'u-lah) Plural of acetabulum.

acetabular (as-ĕ-tab'u-lar) Relating to the acetabulum.

acetabulum (as-ĕ-tab'u-lum), pl. acetab'ula The cup-shaped articular depression on the lateral aspect of each hipbone into which the head of the femur fits, forming the hip joint. Also called hip socket.

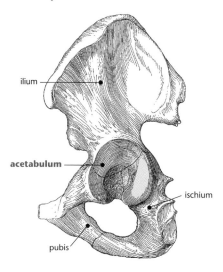

achondroplasia (ah-kon-dro-pla'ze-ah) Hereditary defect in the conversion process of cartilage into bone, resulting in dwarfism and other skeletal deformities; an autosomal dominant inheritance. Also called achondroplasty.

acro- Combining form meaning extremity; tip; an extreme.

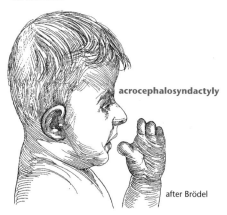

after Brödel

acroataxia (ak-ro-ah-tak'se-ah) Loss of muscular coordination of the fingers and toes.

acrocephalosyndactyly (ak-ro-sef-ah-lo-sin-dak't'ĭ-le) Any of a group of inherited conditions occurring in varying degrees of congenital malformations of the skull and digits; characterized mainly by a high-domed or peaked head, due to premature closure of the space between cranial bones, and a partial or complete webbing of fingers or toes; an autosomal dominant inheritance.

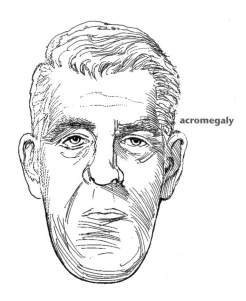

acromegaly (ak-ro-meg'ah-le) Disorder characterized by gradual overgrowth of bones in the head, face, hands and feet, with proliferation of soft tissue, especially of the hands and feet; due to over production of growth hormone (somatotropin) by the pituitary (hypophysis) after maturity.

acromial (ah-kro'me-al) Relating to the acromion.

acromioclavicular (ah-kro-me-o-klah-vik'u-lar) Anatomic term denoting a relationship to the acromion and the clavicle (bones of the shoulder joint).

acromiocoracoid (ah-kro-me-o-kor'ah-koid) See coracoacromial.

acromiohumeral (ah-kro-me-o-hu'mer-al) Anatomic term denoting a relationship to the acromion and the humerus.

acromion (ah-kro'me-on) The flattened bony process extending laterally from the spinous process of the scapula to overhang the shoulder joint; its medial surface articulates with the clavicle; it provides attachment to muscles and ligaments of the shoulder joint in addition to the trapezius and deltoid muscles; its concave underside houses the subacromial bursa. Also called acromial process.

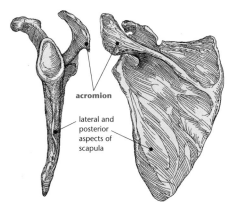

acromion

lateral and posterior aspects of scapula

acromioscapular (ah-kro-me-o-skap'u-lar) Relating to the acromion and the body of the scapula (shoulder blade).

acromiothoracic (ah-kro-me-o-tho-ras'ik) Relating to the acromion and the thorax. Also called thoracoacromial.

actin (ak'tin) A protein of muscle that, together with myosin, is responsible for muscular contraction.

actomyosin (ak-to-mi'o-sin) A contractile protein complex with a linear molecular shape composed of actin and myosin; responsible for the contraction of muscle fibers.

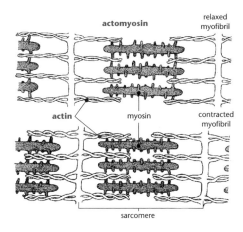

actomyosin

relaxed myofibril

actin   myosin   contracted myofibril

sarcomere

ad- Prefix meaning to or toward; adherence; increase.

-ad Suffix meaning toward the direction of (e.g., cephalad).

adducent (ah-du'sent) Bringing together; performing adduction.

adduct (ah-dukt') To draw or pull toward the median plane of the body, or the main axis of a limb (in the case of digits).

adduction (ah-duk'shun) The act of adducting or the condition of being adducted. Opposite of abduction.

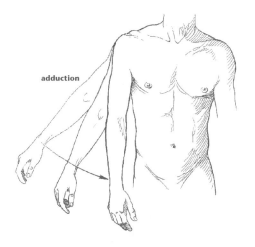

adduction

adductor (ah-duk'tor) A muscle that draws a part of the body toward the midline. Opposite of abductor.

adoral (ad-o'ral) Near or directed toward the mouth.

adsternal (ad-ster'nal) Near or toward the sternum (breastbone).

age (āj) The time elapsed since birth.

    bone a. Age as determined by x-ray studies of the degree of development in the ossification centers (epiphyses) of long bones, such as those of the extremities. Also called skeletal age.

        skeletal a. See bone age.

agonist (ag'o-nist) Denoting a muscle that initiates and maintains a particular movement, against another muscle (antagonist) that opposes such action.

alignment (ah-līn'ment) In orthopedics, the arranging of fractured bones in the normal anatomic position.

amyotonia (a-mi-o-to'ne-ah) See myatonia.

angle (ang'gl) The figure formed by two lines or planes diverging from or meeting at a common point, or the space enclosed by them.

    acromial a. The angle formed where the spine of the scapula ends and the acromion begins, forming the bony prominence at the upper back of the shoulder joint; it serves as

acromioscapular ■ **angle**

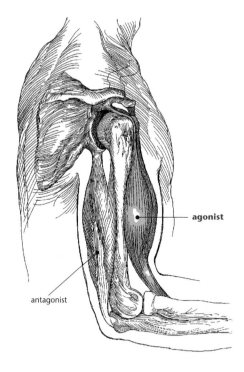

agonist

antagonist

a subcutaneous bony landmark and can be easily felt. Also called acromial angle of scapula.

acromial a. of scapula See acromial angle.

anterior a. of petrous portion of the temporal bone The anterior projection of the petrous part of the temporal bone, comprised of a medial section that articulates with the greater wing of the sphenoid bone and a lateral section that joins the squamous part of the temporal bone to form the petrosquamous suture.

Bohler's a. An angle formed by a line drawn through the anterior process and the highest point on the posterior facet of the calcaneus and a second line drawn parallel to the superior cortex of the calcaneal tuberosity. Bohler's angle is used to measure the configuration of the calcaneus; normally the angle is 25° to 40°; in displaced fractures, this angle decreases markedly.

carrying a. The angle formed by the upper arm and forearm when the forearm is fully extended and the hand supinated; the forearm is directed somewhat laterally and forming a normal angle of about 160°, determined by radiographic studies; the carrying angle disappears on full extension of the forearm.

collodiaphyseal a. The angle formed by the intersection of the long axis of the shaft of the femur with the axis of the femoral neck; it is greatest at birth, decreasing with age until adulthood when, in the male, it averages about 127°; in the adult female, the angle is less due to the obliquity of the femoral shaft and the increased breadth of the lesser pelvis. Also called angle of inclination.

costal a. See angle of rib.

costovertebral a. The angle formed at the junction of the vertebral column and the last rib on each side of the body.

epigastric a. The angle formed by the xiphoid process articulating with the body of the sternum.

ethmocranial a. The angle between the basicranial axis and the plane of the cribriform plate of the ethmoid bone. Also called ethmoid angle.

ethmoid a. See ethmocranial angle.

gnathic a. The craniometric angle between the basion-nasion and basion-prosthion lines.

gonial a. See angle of mandible.

a. of inclination See collodiaphyseal angle.

inferior a. of scapula The acute angle formed by the junction of the medial (vertebral) and lateral borders of the scapula; it usually lies over the seventh rib or seventh intercostal space and is covered dorsally by the upper border of the latissimus dorsi muscle.

infrasternal a. The angle formed at the inferior thoracic outlet by the sloping joined cartilages of the 7th to 10th ribs, which slope upwardly on each side to the xiphisternal joint. Also called subcostal angle; infrasternal angle of thorax; substernal angle.

infrasternal a. of thorax See infrasternal angle.

lateral a. of scapula The angle at the junction of the superior and lateral borders of the scapula; it bears the glenoid cavity, which articulates with the head of the humerus, forming the shoulder joint.

line a. Angle formed by the junction of any two surfaces of a tooth.

a. of Louis See sternal angle.

a. of mandible Angle formed by the lower border of the mandibular body and the lower posterior border of the mandibular ramus; eversion of the angle is often seen in the male mandible, while in the female, it is

angle ■ angle

generally seen to be incurved. Also called gonial angle.

manubriosternal a. See sternal angle.

medial a. of scapula See superior angle of scapula.

pelvivertebral a. The angle formed by the plane of the superior pelvic aperture with the general axis of the vertebral column.

point a. Angle formed by the junction of three tooth surfaces at a point.

posterior a. of rib See angle of rib.

a. of pubis See subpubic angle.

a. of rib The ridge on the outer surface of the shaft of a rib, about 5 to 6 cm outward from the tubercle, where the curvature is sharpest. Also called costal angle; posterior angle of rib.

sacrolumbar a. See sacrovertebral angle.

sacrovertebral a. The prominent angle formed by the articulation between the anterior surfaces of the 1st sacral and the 5th lumbar vertebrae. Also called sacrolumbar angle; promontory of the sacrum.

sternal a. Angle formed by the articulation of the manubrium and the body of the sternum, at the level of the sternochondral junction of the second rib; it forms a ridge on the anterior surface that can be easily felt. Also called angle of Louis; manubriosternal angle.

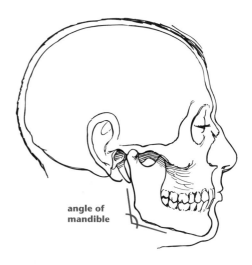

angle of mandible

subpubic a. The angle situated below the pubic symphysis at the apex of the pubic arch formed by the converging inferior rami of the pubic bones; the angle is considerably smaller in males than in females. Also called angle of pubis; subpubic arch.

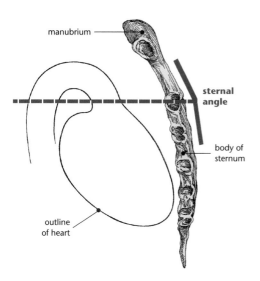

manubrium

sternal angle

body of sternum

outline of heart

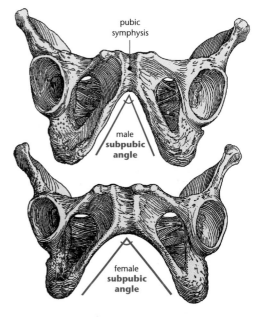

pubic symphysis

male subpubic angle

female subpubic angle

sternoclavicular a. The angle formed by the junction of the sternum and the clavicle.

subcostal a. See infrasternal angle.

substernal a. See infrasternal angle.

superior a. of scapula The angle formed at the junction of the superior and medial borders of the scapula; it is covered by muscles. Formerly called the medial angle of the scapula.

angle ■ angle

a. of torsion The angle formed by the axes of two different portions of a long bone.

    xiphoid a. The angle formed on each side of the xiphoid process at its junction with the costal cartilage of the seventh rib.

angulation (ang-gu-la'shun) An abnormal bend in an anatomic structure.

ankle (ang'kl) The part of the lower limb between the leg and the foot. See also talocrural joint, under joint.

ankylosis (ang-kĭ-lo'sis) Abnormal immobility of a joint. Popularly called frozen joint.

    bony a. See synostosis.

    false a. See fibrous ankylosis.

    fibrous a. Stiffening of a joint due to proliferation of fibrous tissue which adheres to the joint structures. Also called false ankylosis.

    true a. See synostosis.

annulus, anulus (an'u-lus) A ringlike structure.

    a. fibrosus The outer fibrocartilaginous ring surrounding the softer center of the pads between vertebrae (intervertebral disks).

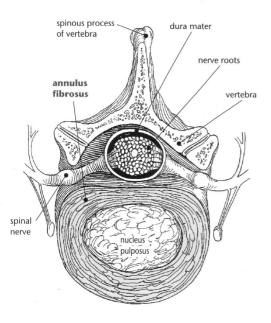

antagonist (an-tag'o-nist) Any structure or substance that opposes or counteracts the action of another structure or substance.

ante- Prefix meaning before.

antebrachium (an-te-bra'ke-um) The forearm.

antecubital (an-te-ku'bĭ-tal) In front of the elbow.

anteflexion (an-te-flek'shun) An abnormal forward bending of an organ or anatomic structure.

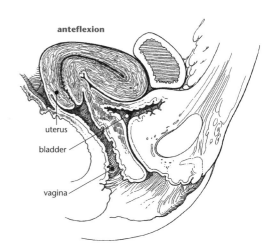

anterior (an-te're-or) Located or related to the front surface of a structure.

antero- Combining form meaning before; forward; anterior.

anterograde (an'ter-o-grād) Moving or extending forward.

anteroinferior (an-ter-o-in-fēr'e-or) In front and below.

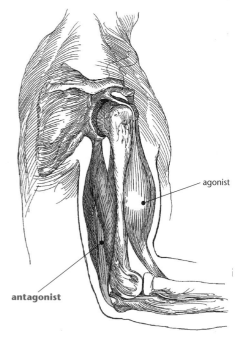

angulation ■ anteroinferior

anterolateral (an-ter-o-lat'er-al) In front and to one side of the midline.

anteromedial (an-ter-o-me'de-al) In front and toward the midline.

anteroposterior (an-ter-o-pos-tēr'e-or) In a direction from front to back.

anterosuperior (an-ter-o-su-pēr'e-or) In front and above.

antral (an'tral) Relating to an antrum.

antrotympanic (an-tro-tim-pan'ik) Relating to a cavity of the mastoid process (behind the ear) and the middle ear chamber.

antrum (an'trum) 1. A cavity within a bone. 2. The normal, enlarged portion of a hollow organ.

    mastoid a. An air-filled cavity within the mastoid process of the temporal bone, communicating anteriorly with the middle ear chamber and posterior with the mastoid air cells. Also called tympanic antrum; mastoid cavity.

    maxillary a. See maxillary sinus, under sinus.

    tympanic a. See mastoid antrum.

apatite (ap'ah-tīt) A calcium phosphate that is a constituent of bones and teeth.

aperture (ap'er-chūr) An opening.

    frontal sinus a. One of two openings in the floor of the frontal sinus leading to the nasal cavity.

    inferior a. of minor pelvis See pelvic plane of outlet, under plane.

    inferior thoracic a. See thoracic outlet, under outlet.

    sphenoid sinus a. Opening on the anterior wall of the sphenoid sinus leading to the nasal cavity.

    superior a. of minor pelvis See pelvic plane of inlet, under plane.

    superior thoracic a. See thoracic inlet, under inlet.

apex (a'peks), pl. a'pices The tip of a conical or domed structure.

    a. of head of fibula See styloid process of fibula, under process.

    orbital a. The posterior, conical portion of the eye socket (orbit).

    root a. The tip of the root of a tooth, most distal from the crown.

aponeurosis (ap-o-nu-ro'sis), pl. aponeuro'ses A broad, often thin tendinous sheet of fibrous

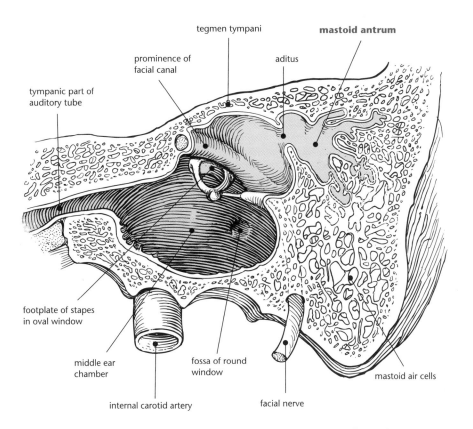

tegmen tympani

mastoid antrum

prominence of facial canal

aditus

tympanic part of auditory tube

footplate of stapes in oval window

middle ear chamber

fossa of round window

mastoid air cells

internal carotid artery

facial nerve

anterolateral ■ aponeurosis

tissue; it connects a muscle to its attachment.

epicranial a. Fibrous tissue covering the upper portion of the skull and connecting the frontal and occipital bellies of the occipitofrontal muscle. Also called galea aponeurotica; aponeurosis of occipitofrontal muscle.

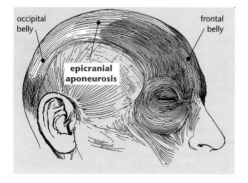

femoral a. See fascia lata, under fascia.

a. of occipitofrontal muscle See epicranial aponeurosis.

palmar a. Bundles of fibrous tissue within the palm of the hand, extending from the tendon of the long palmar muscle (palmaris longus) to the bases of the fingers. Also called palmar fascia; Dupuytren's fascia.

plantar a. The thick fibrous tissue within the sole of the foot, extending from the medial process of the calcaneal tuberosity to the bases of the toes. Also called plantar fascia.

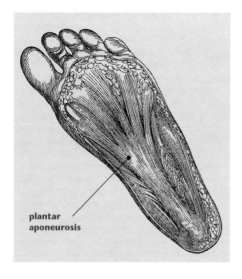

a. of occipitofrontal muscle See epicranial aponeurosis.

subscapular a. See subscapular fascia, under fascia.

aponeurotic (ap-o-nu-rot'ik) Relating to an aponeurosis.

apophyseal, apophysial (ap-o-fiz'e-al) Relating to an apophysis.

apophysis (ah-pof'ĭ-sis), pl. apoph'yses A bony outgrowth or prominence.

aqueduct (ak'we-dukt) A passage or canal.

vestibular a. A canal in the inner ear extending from the medial wall of the vestibule to the posterior surface of the petrous portion of the temporal bone; it houses the endolymphatic duct.

arch (arch) Any curved structure of the body.

costal a. The arch at the anterior lower edge of the rib cage formed by the cartilage of ribs on both sides designated 7th through 10th.

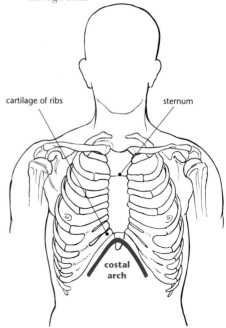

dental a. The curved contour of alveolar bone that houses maxillary and mandibular teeth.

a.'s of foot The two natural arches (longitudinal and transverse) formed by the bones of the foot. Also called plantar arches.

longitudinal a. of foot The anteroposterior curvature of the foot, formed by the seven tarsal and five metatarsal bones and the

aponeurosis ■ arch

ligaments and muscles that bind them together.

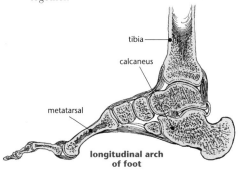

tibia
calcaneus
metatarsal

longitudinal arch of foot

plantar a.'s See arches of foot.

pubic a. The arch of the pelvis formed by the inferior pubic rami of both sides.

superciliary a. The bony ridge on the upper margin of the orbit.

transverse a. of foot The curvature of the foot formed by the proximal parts of the metatarsal bones anteriorly and the distal row of the tarsal bones posteriorly, bound together by ligaments and muscles.

vertebral a. The arch of the dorsal or posterior side of the vertebra that forms the vertebral foramen for passage of the spinal cord. Also called neural arch.

zygomatic a. The arch formed by the articulation of processes of the zygomatic and temporal bones. Also called zygoma.

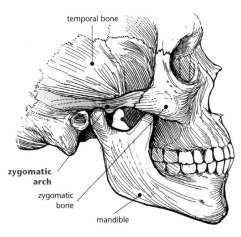

temporal bone

zygomatic arch

zygomatic bone

mandible

arthro-, arthr- Combining form meaning joint; articulation.

arthrography (ar-throg'rah-fe) The radiographic examination of a joint, usually the knee or shoulder, following injection of a water souble radiopaque material and/or air into the joint space. Arthrography outlines soft tissues (cartilage, ligaments, rotator cuff) not usually visible in ordinary x-ray images.

arthropathy (ar-throp'ah-the) Any disease of a joint.

arthroplasty (ar'thro-plas-te) Surgical restoration of joint function either by repairing damaged structures or by inserting an artificial joint.

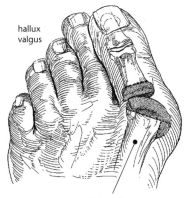

hallux valgus

metatarsal bone

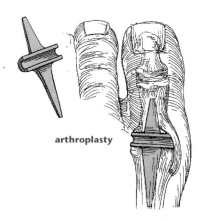

arthroplasty

arthroscopy (ar-thros'ko-pe) Visual examination of the interior of a joint (most commonly the knee) with an arthroscope after injecting sterile saline solution into the joint for better visualization; used to detect and diagnose joint disease, to monitor the progression of disease, and to perform surgery in a joint.

arthrosynovitis (ar-thro-sin-o-vi'tis) Inflammation of the synovial membrane, which surrounds a joint.

articular (ar-tik'u-lar) Relating to a joint.

articulation (ar-tik-u-la'shun) A joint between bones.

arthro-, arthr- ■ articulation

asterion (as-te're-on) A point on the surface of the skull (on either side) where three sutures (skull joints) meet; lambdoid, occipitomastoid, and parietomastoid; used in determining skull measurements.

ataxia (ah-tak'se-ah) Loss of the coordinated muscular contractions required for the execution of smooth voluntary movement. Also called incoordination.

atlantoaxial (at-lan-to-ak'se-al) Relating to the first and second cervical vertebrae (atlas and axis); e.g., the joint between the two bones.

atlanto-occipital (at-lan'to ok-sip'ĭ-tal) Relating to the first cervical vertebra (atlas) and the occipital bone (of the skull).

atlanto-odontoid (at-lan'to o-don'toid) Relating to the first cervical vertebra (atlas) and the central articulating process (dens) of the second vertebra (axis).

atlas (at'las) The first cervical vertebra; located next to the skull; articulates with the occipital bone above and the second cervical vertebra (axis) below.

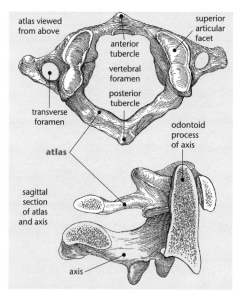

atlas viewed from above
superior articular facet
anterior tubercle
vertebral foramen
posterior tubercle
transverse foramen
atlas
odontoid process of axis
sagittal section of atlas and axis
axis

avulsion (ah-vul'shun) A tearing away of tissue or of a body part from its point of attachment.

axes (ak-sēz) Plural of axis.

axial (ak'se-al) Relating to an axis, as of a body or body part.

axilla (ak-sil'ah) The pyramidal area of the junction of the arm and the chest; it contains the axillary blood and lymph vessels, a large number of lymph nodes, brachial plexus, and muscles. Also called armpit.

axillary (ak'sĭ-lar-e) Relating to the axilla.

axis (ak'sis), pl. ax'es 1. A line, real or imaginary, used as a point of reference and about which a body or body part may rotate. 2. The second cervical vertebra.

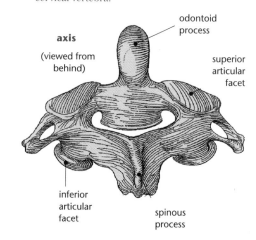

axis
(viewed from behind)
odontoid process
superior articular facet
inferior articular facet
spinous process

    long a. A line passing lengthwise through the center of a structure.

    mandibular a. A line passing through both mandibular condyles around which the mandible rotates.

    pelvic a. A hypothetical curved line passing through the center point of each of the four planes of the pelvis.

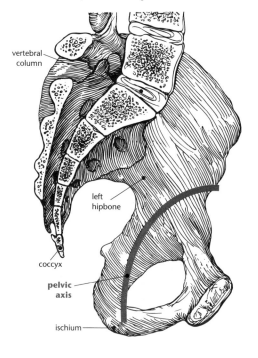

vertebral column
left hipbone
coccyx
pelvic axis
ischium

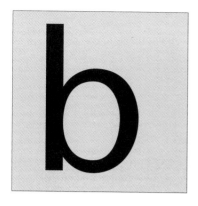

backbone (bak′bōn) The vertebral column, see under column.

band (band) 1. Any cordlike anatomic structure. 2. A distinct elongated area that traverses skeletal and cardiac muscle fibers.

    A b. One of the dark-staining zones at the center of the contraction unit (sarcomere) of skeletal and cardiac muscle, composed of overlapping thick myosin (100 Å) filaments and thin actin (50Å) filaments that traverse the sarcomere; it is bisected by the paler H band. Also called anisotropic band.

    anisotropic b. See A band.

    H b. A pale zone that bisects the A band of the contracting unit of muscle (sarcomere), representing the middle region in which the actin filaments have not penetrated; seen only in relaxed or minimally contracted muscle. Also called Hensen's line.

    I b. One of the lightly-staining zones of skeletal and cardiac muscle, composed of a collection of thin (50Å), longitudinally oriented actin filaments; it represents a region of actin filaments which do not overlap with the myosin filaments; it is bisected transversely by a thin Z band. Also called isotropic band.

    iliotibial b. See iliotibial tract, under tract.

    isotropic b. See I band.

    M b. The narrow, dark band that lies transversely across the center of the H band of the sarcomere of striated muscle myofibrils, consisting of fine strands interconnecting adjacent myosin filaments.

    oblique b. of elbow joint A poorly developed oblique band of fibers extending from the medial epicondyle of the humerus to the olecranon and coronoid processes of the ulna at the elbow joint; it forms a foramen on the medial margin of the trochlear notch.

    Z b. A dark-staining thin membrane appearing on longitudinal sections of skeletal and cardiac muscle as a dark line bisecting the I bands. It represents the demarcation of the serially repeating contracting units (sarcomeres) of striated muscle fibers. Also called Z line; zwischenscheibe band.

    zwischenscheibe b. See Z band.

basicranial (ba-se-kra′ne-al) Relating to the base of the skull.

basion (ba′se-on) A craniometric landmark; the middle point on the anterior margin of the foramen magnum, the opening at the base of the skull where the spinal cord begins.

basis (ba′sis) Latin for base; used in anatomic nomenclature.

    b. cranii The base of the skull. The internal surface is called *basis cranii interna,* the external surface, *basis cranii externa.*

belly (bel′e) The fleshy part of a muscle.

bi-, bin- Prefixes meaning two; twice.

biceps (bi′seps) A muscle with two origins.

bicipital (bi-sip′ĭ-tal) 1. Having two origins. 2. Relating to a biceps muscle.

bifurcate (bi′fur-kāt) To divide into two parts or branches.

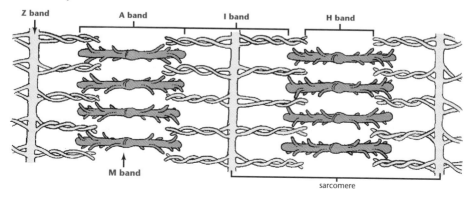

sarcomere

backbone ■ bifurcate

bifurcation (bi-fur-ka'shun) 1. A separation or branching of a structure into two parts. 2. The point at which a structure branches into two parts.

bilateral (bi-lat'er-al) Having two sides.

biparietal (bi-pah-ri'ĕ-tal) Relating to both parietal bones of the skull.

bipennate, bipenniform (bi-pen'āt, bi-pen'ĭ-form) Resembling a feather; said of a muscle with fibers arranged symmetrically along a central tendon.

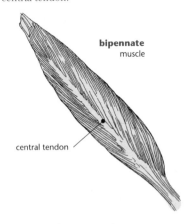

bipennate
muscle

central tendon

bitemporal (bi-tem'po-ral) Relating to both temples of temporal bones.

biventer (bi'ven-ter) Having two bellies; said of certain muscles.

bone (bōn) 1. The special mineralized connective tissue forming the skeleton of vertebrates. 2. Any of the units forming the skeleton. For individual bones, see table of bones in appendix I.

  alveolar b. The thin plate of bone forming the tooth socket.

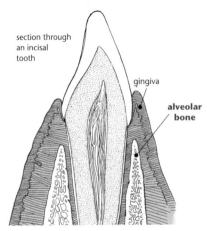

section through an incisal tooth

gingiva

alveolar bone

  ankle b. See talus, in table of bones in appendix I.

  arm b. See humerus, in table of bones in appendix I.

  back b. See vertebral column, under column.

  blade b. See scapula, in table of bones in appendix I.

  breast b. See sternum, in table of bones in appendix I.

  brittle b.'s See osteogenesis imperfecta, under osteogenesis.

  cancellous b. See trabecular bone.

  capitate b. See table of bones in appendix I.

  cartilage b. See endochondral bone.

  cranial b.'s The 21 bones forming the skull; the paired inferior nasal concha, lacrimal, maxilla, nasal, palatine, parietal, temporal, and zygomatic; and the unpaired ethmoid, frontal, occipital, sphenoid, and vomer. See individual bones, in table of bones in appendix I.

  cheek b. See zygomatic bone, in table of bones in appendix I.

  coccygeal b.'s See coccyx.

  collar b. See clavicle, in table of bones in appendix I.

  compact b. The dense, ivorylike layer of mature bone; it surrounds trabecular bone internally and is covered externally by periosteum except at the articular regions; it contains minute spaces and channels. Also called dense bone; cortical bone.

  cortical b. See compact bone.

  costal b. The bony part of the twelve pairs of ribs. See rib, in table of bones in appendix I.

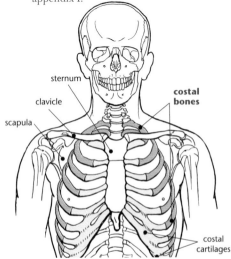

sternum

clavicle

scapula

costal bones

costal cartilages

bifurcation ■ bone

cranial b.'s The 21 bones forming the skull; the paired inferior nasal concha, lacrimal, maxilla, nasal, palatine, parietal, temporal, and zygomatic; and the unpaired ethmoid, frontal, occipital, sphenoid, and vomer. See individual bones, in table of bones in appendix I.

cribriform b. The roof of the ethmoid bone overlying its perpendicular plate and masses of air cells.

cuboid b. A bone of the foot located on the lateral side of the distal row of tarsus. See table of bones in appendix I.

cuneiform b.'s See table of bones in appendix I.

dense b. See compact bone.

ear b.'s The three auditory ossicles: malleus, incus and stapes. See individual bones in table of bones in appendix I.

elbow b. See ulna, in table of bones in appendix I.

endochondral b. Bone that develops from a cartilaginous model upon ossification. Also called cartilage bone; replacement bone.

epistropheus b. See capitate bone, in table of bones in appendix I.

ethmoid b. See table of bones in appendix I.

exercise b. A bone that has formed in a muscle or tendon resulting from continued strenuous exercise, such as one arising in the tendon of the long adductor muscle (adductor longus) from habitual horseback riding.

fabella b. See table of bones in appendix I.

facial b.'s The bones of the facial part of the skull, surrounding the nose and mouth and contributing to the orbits; they include the unpaired mandible, ethmoid, vomer, hyoid; and the paired maxilla, zygomatic, lacrimal, palatine, nasal, and the inferior nasal concha.

flank b. See ilium, in table of bones in appendix I.

flat b. Any bone of slight thickness and chiefly compact structure; generally composed of two plates arranged in a parallel direction, separated by a thin layer of trabecular bone.

forehead b. See frontal bone, in table of bones in appendix I.

funny b. The posterior, subcutaneous region of the medial epicondyle of the humerus; it is crossed by the ulnar nerve as it descends the forearm and when the nerve is jarred against the bone, it elicits a peculiar

vibrating sensation.

greater multangular b. See trapezium bone, in table of bones in appendix I.

hamate b. See table of bones in appendix I.

heel b. See calcaneus, in table of bones in appendix I.

hip b. See hipbone, in table of bones in appendix I.

inferior turbinate b. See concha, inferior nasal, in table of bones in appendix I.

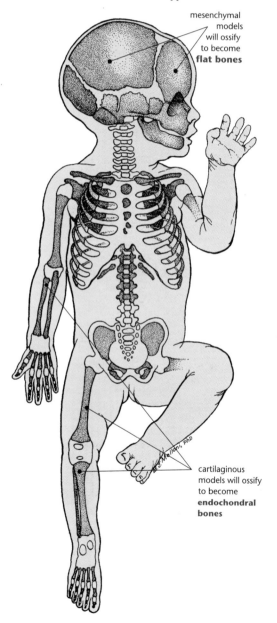

mesenchymal models will ossify to become **flat bones**

cartilaginous models will ossify to become **endochondral bones**

bone ■ bone

innominate b. See hipbone, in table of bones in appendix I.

interstitial b. The angular bone between secondary osteons, generally in the form of interstitial lamellae.

irregular b. Any bone of complex shape that cannot be classified as long, short, or flat.

ischial b. The lower posterior part of the hipbone; although a separate bone in early life, it eventually becomes fused with the ilium and pubis and contributes to the formation of the acetabulum.

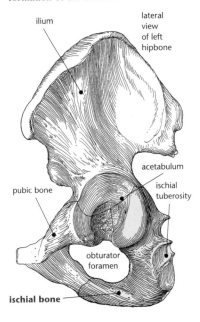

ilium

lateral view of left hipbone

acetabulum

pubic bone

ischial tuberosity

obturator foramen

ischial bone

jaw b. See mandible, in table of bones in appendix I.

lesser multangular b. See trapezoid bone, in table of bones in appendix I.

lingual b. See hyoid bone, in table of bones in appendix I.

long b. Any bone having greater length than width, consisting of a tubular shaft, which contains a medullary cavity, and two expanded ends.

lower jaw b. See mandible, in table of bones in appendix I.

lunate b. See table of bones in appendix I.

malar b. See zygomatic bone, in table of bones in appendix I.

marble b.'s See osteopetrosis.

mastoid b. An infrequently used name for the mastoid process. See under process.

maxillary b. See maxilla, in table of bones in appendix I.

membrane b. See membranous bone.

membranous b. Bone preceded by a fibro-cellular membrane, in contrast to a cartilaginous model. Facial bones develop in this manner. Also called membrane bone.

metacarpal b.'s See metacarpus, in table of bones in appendix I.

metatarsal b.'s See metatarsus, in table of bones in appendix I.

middle turbinate b. A large bony plate with curved margins projecting into the nasal cavity from the medial surface of the ethmoid bone; covered by a thick mucoperiosteum; commonly called the middle nasal concha.

nasal b. See table of bones in appendix I.

navicular b. of foot See navicular bone, in table of bones in appendix I.

navicular b. of hand See scaphoid bone, in table of bones in appendix I.

palate b. See palatine bone, in table of bones in appendix I.

perichondral b. Bone developed from a collar of osseous tissue in the perichondrium of the cartilaginous model; the outermost layer develops into periosteum while the deeper layer remains osteogenic; seen especially in the development of long bones.

petrous b. The pyramid-shaped part of the temporal bone that houses the middle ear chamber, the labyrinth of the inner ear and the second part of the internal carotid artery; it projects anteromedially and is wedged between the occipital and sphenoid bones at the base of the skull; the posterior part is contiguous with the mastoid process; it is the most dense bone of the body.

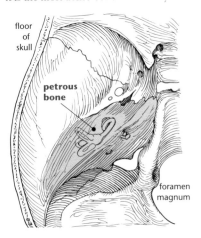

floor of skull

petrous bone

foramen magnum

bone ■ bone

pubic b. See pubis, in table of bones in appendix I.

pyramidal b. See triquetral bone, in table of bones in appendix I.

radial b. See radius, in table of bones in appendix I.

replacement b. See endochondral bone.

sacral b. See sacrum, in table of bones in appendix I.

scaphoid b. of foot See navicular bone, in table of bones in appendix I.

scroll b.'s The three thin, scroll-shaped bony laminae projecting downward and slightly medially in the nasal cavity; they include the inferior, middle, and superior conchae.

semilunar b. See lunate bone, in table of bones in appendix I.

septal b. The bony partition separating adjacent tooth sockets.

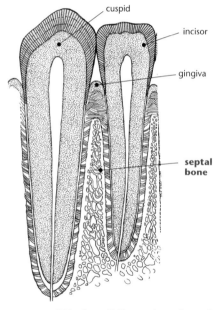

sesamoid b. A small discrete bone formed by ossification within a tendon. See also table of bones in appendix I.

shin b. See tibia, in table of bones in appendix I.

short b. A bone having the general appearance of a cube and a relatively large proportion of trabecular bone within a layer of compact bone.

sphenoid b. See table of bones in appendix I.

sphenoturbinal b. The paired pyramidal-

shaped bony structure at the anterior and lower part of the sphenoid bone that forms part of the roof of the nasal cavity.

splint b. See fibula, in table of bones in appendix I.

spoke b. See radius, in table of bones in appendix I.

spongy b. See trabecular bone.

squamous b. The thin, upper portion of the temporal bone forming part of the lateral wall of the cranium.

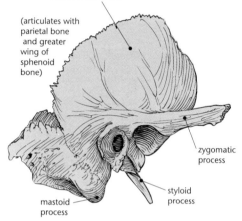

squamous bone

(articulates with parietal bone and greater wing of sphenoid bone)

zygomatic process

styloid process

mastoid process

stirrup b. See stapes, in table of bones in table I.

superior turbinate b. The portion of the ethmoid bone that projects medially into the nasal cavity; scroll-shaped, with a thick covering of mucoperiosteum, it is commonly called the superior nasal concha.

supreme turbinate b. The small portion of the ethmoid bone that projects medially into the posterosuperior part of the nasal cavity; it is the smallest bony projection from the medial surface of the ethmoid bone; covered by a thick olfactory epithelium, it is commonly called the supreme nasal concha.

sutural b. See table of bones in appendix I.

tail b.'s See coccyx.

thigh b. See femur, in table of bones in appendix I.

trabecular b. The inner meshwork of bony intercommunications separated by numerous large spaces filled with vascular tissue, fat, and bone marrow; the interior of a mature bone, it receives nutriment from the marrow and is surrounded by an outer layer of compact bone. Also called cancellous bone; spongy bone.

bone ■ bone

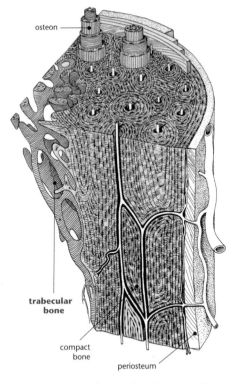

osteon

trabecular
bone

compact
bone

periosteum

bregma (breg'mah) A craniometric point situated on the upper surface of the skull at the junction of three bones: frontal and the two parietal bones.

brim (brim) The upper border or edge of a hollow structure.

 pelvic b. The circumference of the oblique plane dividing the major and minor pelves.

bronchotracheal (brong-ko-tra'ke-al) Relating to the bronchi and to the trachea. Also called tracheobronchial.

bunion (bun'yun) An abnormal bony protrusion at the junction of the big toe and the foot (1st metatarsal head), with inflamed bursa, and callosity formation; associated with an outward displacement of the big toe (hallux valgus).

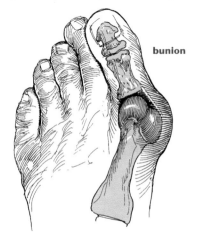

bunion

 triangular b. See triquetral bone, in table of bones in appendix I.

 turbinate b.'s The four bony projections into the nasal cavity; they include the inferior turbinate bone, middle turbinate bone (not a separate bone), superior turbinate bone (not a separate bone) and the supreme turbinate bone (not a separate bone).

 tympanic b. The tympanic part of the temporal bone that forms part of the innermost walls of the external auditory canal to which is attached the tympanic membrane (eardrum).

 unciform b. See hamate bone, in table of bones in appendix I.

 upper jaw b. See maxilla, in table of bones in appendix I.

 vomer b. See table of bones in appendix I.

 wormian b.'s See sutural bones, in table of bones in appendix I.

 xiphoid b. See xiphoid process, under process.

brachial (bra'ke-al) Relating to the arm.

brachium (bra'ke-um) 1. The arm. 2. Any armlike structure.

braincase (brān'kās) The cranial part of the skull enclosing the brain; the facial bones are not included.

 tailor's b. See bunionette.

bunionette (bun-yun-et') Enlargement of the lateral aspect of the head of the little toe (5th metatarsal head) with bursitis over the bony prominence. Also called tailor's bunion.

bursa (ber'sah), pl. bur'sae A closed, flattened sac of synovial membrane containing a viscid fluid; usually present over bony prominences, between and beneath tendons, and between certain movable structures; it serves to facilitate movement by diminishing friction and by creating discontinuity between tissues, thus allowing complete freedom of movement.

 Achilles b. See bursa of calcaneal tendon.

 b. of acromion A small subcutaneous bursa located at the shoulder between the upper surface of the acromion and the overlying skin.

 adventitious b. An abnormal bursa or cyst developed as a result of continued irritation.

 anserine b. A bursa located at the medial side of the knee joint between the tibial

brachial ■ bursa

(medial) collateral ligament and the tendon insertions of the semitendinous, gracilis and sartorius muscles. Also called tibial intertendinous bursa.

b. of biceps brachii muscle See bicipitoradial bursa.

b. of biceps femoris See bursa of biceps muscle of thigh.

b. of biceps muscle of arm See bicipitoradial bursa.

b. of biceps muscle of thigh Either of two subtendinous bursae: *Lower b. of biceps muscle of thigh*, a small bursa between the tendon of the biceps muscle of thigh (biceps femoris) and the fibular (lateral) collateral ligament of the knee joint. Also called lower bursa of biceps femoris. *Upper b. of biceps of thigh*, a small bursa, under the tendon of origin of the long head of the biceps muscle of the thigh (biceps femoris) at the ischial tuberosity of the hipbone. Also called upper bursa of biceps femoris.

bicipitoradial b. A small bursa interposed between the tendon of the biceps muscle of the arm (biceps brachii) and the front part of the tuberosity of the radius. Also called bursa of biceps brachii muscle; bursa of biceps muscle of arm.

b. of big toe A bursa interposed between the lateral side of the base of the 1st metatarsal bone of the foot and the medial side of the adjoining shaft of the 2nd metatarsal bone.

b. of calcaneal tendon A large bursa located at the heel, between the calcaneal tendon (Achilles tendon) and the back of the calcaneus (heel bone). Also called bursa of tendo calcaneus; Achilles bursa; retrocalcaneal bursa; subtendinous bursa of calcaneal tendon.

Calori's b. A bursa interposed between the aortic arch and the trachea.

communicating b. A bursa whose synovial membrane is continuous with that of the articular cavity of a joint.

b. of coracobrachial muscle An occasional bursa of the upper arm located between the tendons of the coracobrachial and subscapular muscles.

deep trochanteric b. See trochanteric bursa of greater gluteal muscle (gluteus maximus).

b. of extensor carpi radialis brevis muscle See bursa of short radial extensor muscle of wrist.

b. of fibular collateral ligament A bursa interposed between the lateral part of the knee joint capsule and the fibular (lateral) collateral ligament, which it partially envelopes; it keeps the ligament away from the capsule.

Fleischmann's b. A bursa near the frenulum of the tongue interposed between the floor of the mouth and the genioglossus muscle.

b. of gastrocnemius muscle Either of two subtendinous bursae: *Lateral b. of gastrocnemius muscle*, a bursa located under the tendon of origin of the lateral head of the gastrocnemius muscle. *Medial b. of gastrocnemius muscle*, a bursa located under the tendon of origin of the medial head of the gastrocnemius muscle; it is often connected with the semimembranous bursa (of clinical importance because when distended with fluid, it is the usual cause of a popliteal cyst); it is occasionally connected to the knee joint.

gluteofemoral b. A bursa interposed between the tendon of the greater gluteal muscle (gluteus maximus) and the tendon of the lateral vastus muscle (vastus lateralis).

b. of greater pectoral muscle A bursa between the tendons of insertion of the greater pectoral muscle (pectoralis major) and the latissimus dorsi muscle on the upper anterior aspect of the humerus. Also called bursa of pectoralis major muscle.

b. of greater psoas tendon See iliopectineal bursa.

iliac b. A large subtendinous bursa lying deep to the tendon of the iliac muscle just above the hip joint; sometimes in communication with the cavity of the hip joint.

iliopectineal b. A large bursa on the anterior surface of the hip joint capsule, interposed between the robust tendon of the iliopsoas muscle and the articular capsule overlying the iliopubic eminence of the hipbone; it frequently communicates with the capsule of the hip joint. Also called bursa of greater psoas tendon; bursa of psoas major muscle.

b. of iliotibial tract A bursa interposed between the lateral part of the knee joint capsule and the iliotibial tract just above where it fuses with the patella retinaculum and capsule.

infrahyoid b. A small bursa between the hyoid bone and the upper part of the thyrohyoid membrane.

infrapatellar b. Either of two bursae of the

bursa ■ bursa

BURSAE

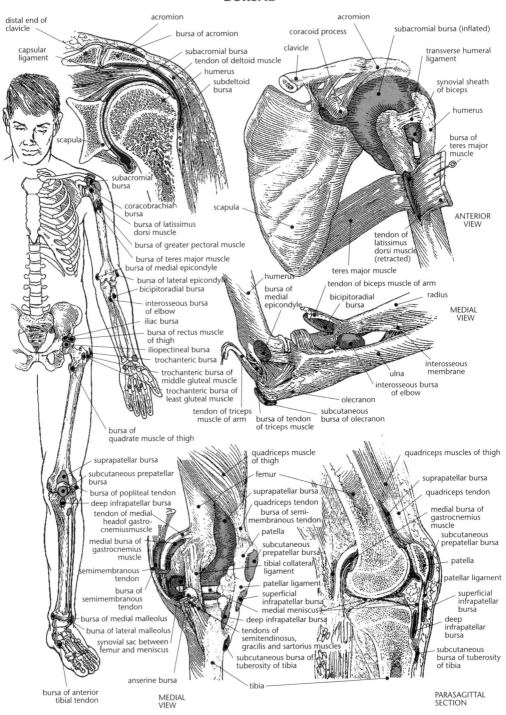

bursa ■ bursa

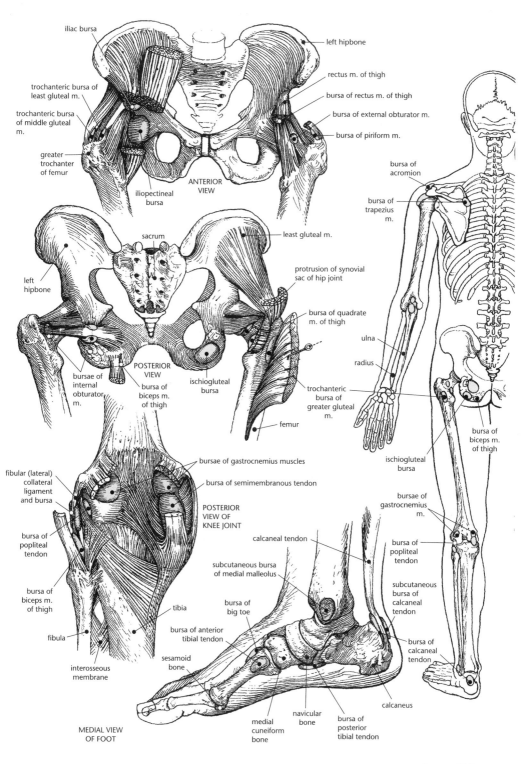

iliac bursa

left hipbone

trochanteric bursa of least gluteal m.

rectus m. of thigh

bursa of rectus m. of thigh

trochanteric bursa of middle gluteal m.

bursa of external obturator m.

bursa of piriform m.

greater trochanter of femur

ANTERIOR VIEW

iliopectineal bursa

bursa of acromion

bursa of trapezius m.

sacrum

least gluteal m.

left hipbone

protrusion of synovial sac of hip joint

bursa of quadrate m. of thigh

ulna

radius

POSTERIOR VIEW

bursae of internal obturator m.

bursa of biceps m. of thigh

ischiogluteal bursa

trochanteric bursa of greater gluteal m.

femur

ischiogluteal bursa

bursa of biceps m. of thigh

bursae of gastrocnemius muscles

bursa of semimembranous tendon

fibular (lateral) collateral ligament and bursa

POSTERIOR VIEW OF KNEE JOINT

bursae of gastrocnemius m.

bursa of popliteal tendon

calcaneal tendon

bursa of popliteal tendon

subcutaneous bursa of medial malleolus

subcutaneous bursa of calcaneal tendon

bursa of biceps m. of thigh

tibia

bursa of big toe

fibula

bursa of anterior tibial tendon

bursa of calcaneal tendon

interosseous membrane

sesamoid bone

calcaneus

MEDIAL VIEW OF FOOT

medial cuneiform bone

navicular bone

bursa of posterior tibial tendon

bursa ■ **bursa**

knee: *Deep infrapatellar b.*, a subtendinous bursa located just below the kneecap (patella) between the lower part of the patellar ligament (just above its insertion) and the upper part of the front of the tibia. *Superficial infrapatellar b.*, a subcutaneous bursa situated between the patellar ligament and the overlying skin.

b. of infraspinous muscle A small synovial bursa interposed between the tendon of the infraspinous muscle (infraspinatus) and the capsule of the shoulder joint.

interligamentous b. A bursa located between ligaments.

interosseous b. of elbow An occasional bursa interposed between the tendon of the biceps muscle of the arm (biceps brachii) and the depression of the anterior ulna and its covering muscles between the supinator crest and tuberosity. Also called interosseous cubital bursa.

interosseous cubital b. See interosseous bursa of elbow.

ischial b. of gluteus maximus muscle See ischiogluteal bursa.

ischiogluteal b. A large bursa separating the greater gluteal muscle (gluteus maximus) from the ischial tuberosity; chronic ischiogluteal bursitis is caused by prolonged sitting on hard surfaces and is commonly known as weaver's bottom. Also called ischial bursa of gluteus maximus muscle.

b. of laryngeal prominence A small subcutaneous bursa found occasionally between the prominence of the thyroid cartilage (Adam's apple) and the overlying skin.

b. of lateral epicondyle A small subcutaneous bursa at the elbow occasionally found between the bony prominence of the lateral epicondyle of the humerus and the overlying skin.

b. of lateral malleolus A subcutaneous bursa at the ankle between the lateral malleolus of the fibula and the overlying skin.

b. of latissimus dorsi muscle An elongated bursa in front of the tendon of the latissimus dorsi muscle at the intertubecular sulcus of the humerus in the upper part of the arm.

b. of medial epicondyle A small subcutaneous bursa at the elbow found occasionally between the bony prominence of the medial epicondyle of the humerus and the overlying skin.

b. of medial malleolus A subcutaneous bursa at the ankle between the medial malleolus of the tibia and the overlying skin.

b. of obturator muscle Either of three bursae of the hip: *External b. of obturator muscle,* a bursa interposed between the tendon of the external obturator muscle and the hip joint capsule and femoral neck; it communicates with the synovial cavity of the hip joint; *Internal b. of obturator muscle,* a) a well-developed sciatic bursa partially encircling the tendon of the internal obturator muscle as it emerges from the lesser sciatic notch of the hipbone; b) a bursa between the tendon of the internal obturator muscle and the femur.

b. of olecranon A subcutaneous bursa between the olecranon process of the ulna and the overlying skin of the elbow.

b. of pectoralis major muscle See bursa of greater pectoral muscle.

b. of piriform muscle A small bursa under the tendons of the piriform muscle and the superior gemellus muscle at their insertion on the greater trochanter of the femur.

b. of popliteal tendon A bursal extension of the synovial cavity of the knee joint, between the lateral condyle of the femur and the tendon of the popliteal muscle. Also called subpopliteal recess.

prepatellar b. Either of three bursae of the knee: *Subcutaneous prepatellar b.*, a large superficial bursa between the lower part of the front of the patella (kneecap) and the overlying skin; chronic irritation causes housemaid's knee (prepatellar bursitis); *Subfascial prepatellar b.*, an occasional bursa between the deep fascia and the tendinous fibers in front of the patella; *Subtendinous prepatellar b.*, an occasional bursa between the patella and the tendinous fibers to its front.

b. of psoas major muscle See iliopectineal bursa.

b. of quadrate muscle of thigh A bursa located between the front of the quadrate muscle of the thigh (quadratus femoris) and the lesser trochanter of the femur. Also called bursa of quadratus femoris muscle.

b. of quadratus femoris muscle See bursa of quadrate muscle of thigh.

quadrate b. See suprapatellar bursa.

quadriceps b. See suprapatellar bursa.

radial b. See synovial sheath of flexor pollicis longus, under sheath.

radiohumeral b. A bursa located at the elbow, over the radiohumeral joint, between the extensor muscle of the fingers (extensor digitorum) and the supinator muscle.

b. of rectus muscle of thigh A small bursa between the tendon of origin of the rectus muscle of the thigh (rectus femoris) and the margin of the acetabulum.

retrocalcaneal b. See bursa of calcaneal tendon.

retrohyoid b. A bursa interposed between the back of the body of the hyoid bone and the upper part of the thyrohyoid membrane.

sciatic b. See bursa of obturator muscle, internal.

b. of semimembranous tendon A bursa located on the medial side of the knee, between the flattened tendon of the semimembranous muscle and the medial head of the gastrocnemius muscle.

b. of short radial extensor muscle of wrist A small bursa between the base of the third metacarpal bone and the tendon of the short radial extensor muscle of the wrist (extensor carpi radialis brevis). Also called bursa of extensor carpi radialis brevis muscle.

subacromial b. A large bursa, approximately the size of a U.S. fifty-cent piece, near the capsule of the shoulder joint, situated between the acromion and the tendons of the supraspinous and infraspinous muscles.

subcoracoid b. See bursa of subscapular muscle.

subcutaneous b. A bursa located between the skin and an underlying superficial structure.

subcutaneous calcaneal b. A subcutaneous bursa between the skin on the sole of the foot and the calcaneus (heel bone).

subcutaneous prepatellar b. See prepatellar bursa.

subdeltoid b. An extension of the subacromial bursa, which lies between the deltoid muscle and the greater tubercle of the humerus; it facilitates the movement of the deltoid muscle over the shoulder joint capsule.

subfascial b. A bursa located between a layer of fascia and bone.

subfascial prepatellar b. See prepatellar bursa.

submuscular b. A bursa located between muscle and bone, tendon or ligament.

b. of subscapular muscle A large subtendinous bursa located between the tendon of the subscapular muscle and the glenoid border of the anterior surface of the neck of the scapula; it communicates with the cavity of the shoulder joint. Also called subcoracoid bursa.

subtendinous b. A bursa located between tendons and bone, tendons and ligaments, or between one tendon and another.

subtendinous b. of calcaneal tendon See bursa of calcaneal tendon.

subtendinous prepatellar b. See prepatellar bursa.

subtendinous b. of triceps brachii muscle See bursa of tendon of triceps muscle.

b. of superior oblique muscle of eyeball A synovial sheath encircling the tendon of the superior oblique muscle of the eyeball as it passes through the cartilaginous pulley (trochlea) at the superomedial angle of the orbit. Also called synovial trochlear bursa; synovial sheath of superior oblique muscle.

suprapatellar b. An anterior extension of the synovial sac of the knee joint, between the femur and the tendon of the quadriceps muscle of the thigh (quadriceps femoris). Also called quadriceps bursa; quadrate bursa; suprapatellar synovial pouch.

synovial b. A closed sac formed by the synovial membrane and moistened by a small amount of viscid fluid (similar to the white part of an egg) that facilitates movement; located where structures rub together or are subject to pressure; may by subcutaneous, submuscular, subtendinous, or subfascial in location.

synovial trochlear b. See bursa of superior oblique muscle of eyeball.

b. of tendo calcaneus See bursa of calcaneal tendon.

b. of tendon of triceps muscle A bursa interposed between the tendon of the triceps muscle of the arm (triceps brachii) and the distal end of the posterior humerus and the blunt end of the posterior projection of the elbow (olecranon process of the ulna). Also called subtendinous bursa of the triceps brachii muscle.

b. of tensor muscle of soft palate A small bursa partly surrounding the tendon of the tensor muscle of soft palate (tensor veli palatini) as it turns around the medial pterygoid hamulus of the sphenoid bone.

b. of teres major muscle A synovial sac between the tendons of the teres major and latissimus dorsi muscles.

tibial intertendinous b. See anserine bursa.

b. of tibial tendon Either of two bursae of the foot: *Anterior b. of tibial tendon*, a small

bursa ■ bursa

bursa seen under the tendon of the anterior tibial muscle, at the medial surface of the proximal part of the first metatarsal bone; *Posterior b. of tibial tendon,* a small bursa interposed between the tendon of the posterior tibial muscle and the calcaneonavicular ligament on the sole of the foot.

b. of trapezius muscle A subtendinous bursa interposed between the tendinous part of the trapezius muscle and the medial end of the spine of the scapula.

trochanteric b. A subcutaneous bursa between the greater trochanter of the upper femur and the overlying skin.

trochanteric b. of gluteus medius muscle See trochanteric bursa of middle gluteal muscle.

trochanteric b. of gluteus maximus muscle See trochanteric bursa of greater gluteal muscle.

trochanteric b. of gluteus minimus muscle See trochanteric bursa of least gluteal muscle.

trochanteric b. of greater gluteal muscle A bursa, often double, that separates the tendon of the greater gluteal muscle (gluteus maximus) from the posterolateral surface of the greater trochanter of the femur, over which it glides. Also called deep trochanteric bursa; trochanteric bursa of gluteus maximus muscle.

trochanteric b. of least gluteal muscle A bursa between the tendon of the least gluteal muscle (gluteal minimus) and the medial part of the anterior surface of the greater trochanter of the femur. Also called trochanteric bursa of gluteus minimus muscle.

trochanteric b. of middle gluteal muscle A bursa interposed between the tendon of the middle gluteal muscle (gluteus medius) and the lateral surface of the greater trochanter of the femur. Also called trochanteric bursa of gluteus medius muscle.

b. of tuberosity of tibia A subcutaneous bursa located between the tuberosity of the tibia and the overlying skin of the knee.

ulnar b. The complex synovial covering for the eight digital flexor tendons of the medial four fingers as they pass through the carpal tunnel, commencing about several centimeters proximal to the flexor retinaculum and terminating about the middle of the palm, except for the sheath on the tendons for the little finger, which

continues to the terminal phalanx; the superficial digital flexor tendons are folded into it superficially while the deep digital tendons are folded into the sac more deeply. Also called common synovial flexor sheath.

bursitis (ber-si'tis) Inflammation of a thin-walled sac (bursa) surrounding muscles and tendons over bony prominences; may be caused by injury, repeated trauma, or associated with a systemic disorder.

Achilles b. See retrocalcaneal bursitis.

ischial b. Bursitis of the ischiogluteal bursa at the buttocks, between the greater gluteus muscle (gluteus maximus) and the ischial tuberosity of the hipbone. Also called tailor's bottom; weaver's bottom.

olecranon b. Bursitis at the tip of the elbow. Also called miner's elbow; student's elbow.

prepatellar b. Inflammation of the bursa situated in front of the patella (kneecap). Also called housemaid's knee.

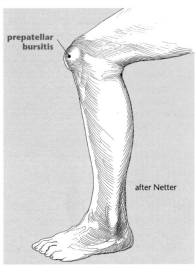

prepatellar bursitis

after Netter

retrocalcaneal b. Inflammation of the bursa lying at the back of the heel, between the skin and the Achilles (calcaneal) tendon at the site of its insertion to the bone. Also called Achilles bursitis.

subacromial b. Pain and tenderness of the shoulder caused by bursitis of the subacromial bursa at the shoulder joint, accompanied by tears and calcification; may also involve the subdeltoid bursa (located under the deltoid muscle).

buttocks (but'oks) The protuberances formed by the gluteus muscles.

bursa ■ buttocks

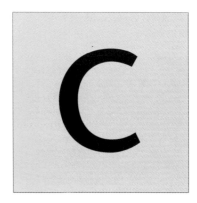

cage (kāj) 1. Any box or enclosure. 2. An anatomic structure resembling an enclosure.

    rib c. See thoracic cage.

    thoracic c. The bones and musculature of the chest; it contains the thoracic organs and functions during respiration. Commonly called rib cage.

calcaneal, calcanean (kal-ka'ne-al, kal-ka'ne-an) Relating to the calcaneus (heel bone).

calcaneonavicular (kal-ka-ne-o-nah-vik'u-lar) Relating to the calcaneus and the navicular bone of the foot.

calcaneus (kal-ka'ne-us) See table of bones in appendix I.

calcar (kal'kar) A bony projection; a spur.

    c. femorale A thin vertical plate of bone within the femur, arising from the compact wall of the shaft near the upper end of the linea aspera and projecting to the trabecular substance of the femoral neck, which it strengthens.

calf (kaf), pl. calves The fleshy mass at the back of the human leg, formed by the bellies of the gastrocnemius and soleus muscles.

calisthenics (kal-is-then'iks) A system of light exercises for improving muscle tone and posture.

calvaria (kal-va're-ah), pl. calva'riae The upper, domelike part of the skull (cranium), composed of the upper portions of the frontal, parietal, and occipital bones; it encloses and protects the brain. Also called roof of skull.

calvarium (kal-va're-um) Term used incorrectly for calvaria.

canal (kah-nal') A tubular structure; a channel; a relatively narrow passage or conduit.

    adductor c. A tunnel through the aponeurosis of the great adductor muscle (adductor magnus) in the middle third of the thigh; it communicates with the popliteal

fossa situated at the back of the knee; it transmits the femoral vessels and the saphenous nerve. Also called Hunter's canal.

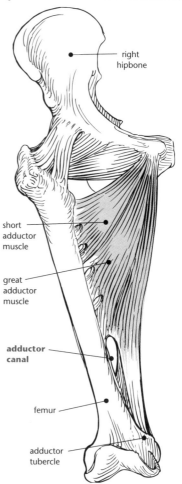

right hipbone

short adductor muscle

great adductor muscle

adductor canal

femur

adductor tubercle

    Alcock's c. See pudendal canal.

    alveolar c.'s of maxilla Two or three small dental canals in the maxilla for passage of the alveolar vessels and nerves to the maxillary posterior dentition.

    anterior condyloid c. See hypoglossal canal.

    auditory c.'s Either of two canals of the ear: *External*, see external auditory canal; *Internal*, see internal auditory canal.

    bony semicircular c.'s See semicircular canals.

    carotid c. A curved passage through the petrous part of the temporal bone of the skull, occupied by the internal carotid artery and its plexus of sympathetic nerves and veins; it opens into the cranial cavity.

cage ■ canal

cartilage c.'s Canals in cartilage that accommodate the ramifications of the perichondrial artery and vein which perfuse cartilage undergoing vascularization and ossification.

caudal c. See sacral canal.

central c.'s of cochlea See longitudinal canals of modiolus.

cochlear c. See cochlear duct, under duct.

diploic c. A channel in the trabecular (diploë) tissue of certain cranial bones providing passage for the diploic veins; absent at birth, it begins to develop at the age of about 2 years.

ethmoidal c.'s Anterior and posterior minute bony canals situated between the frontoethmoidal suture and open on the medial wall of the orbit; they conduct the anterior and posterior ethmoidal nerves and vessels.

external auditory c. The passage that extends from the concha of the external ear (auricle) to the eardrum (tympanic membrane); in the adult, it is approximately 25 mm in length on its superoposterior wall and 6 mm longer on its anteroinferior wall, due to the obliquely directed eardrum. Also called external auditory meatus.

facial c. The canal through the petrous part of the temporal bone that begins at the internal auditory canal and exits at the stylomastoid foramen on the bottom surface of the skull; it conducts the facial nerve.

frontonasal c. A bony canal that permits the frontal sinus to communicate with the nasal cavity.

greater palatine c. A canal formed at the roof of the mouth between the posterior surface of the maxilla and the perpendicular plate of the palatine bone; it transmits the descending palatine artery and the large (anterior) palatine nerve.

haversian c.'s Canals at the center of concentrically arranged thin plates of bony tissue (osteons) in compact bone; the canals contain nerves, capillaries and postcapillary venules. Also called haversian spaces.

Hunter's c. See adductor canal.

hypoglossal c. A canal piercing the lateral part of the skull at the front of the condyle of the occipital bone; it transmits the hypoglossal nerve and a branch of the meningeal artery. Also called anterior condyloid canal.

incisive c. of mandible One of the two terminal branches of the mandibular canal that originates near the roots of the premolar teeth and continues anteriorly to just below the sockets of the cuspid and incisor teeth; it conducts the inferior alveolar

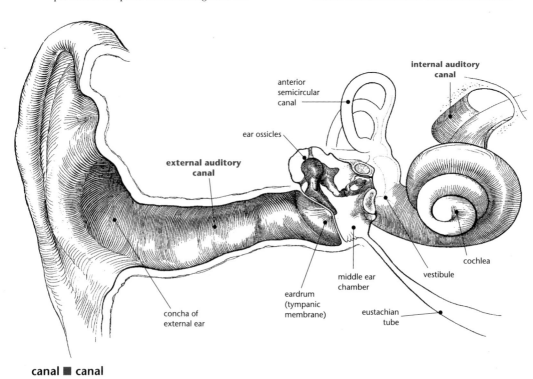

internal auditory canal

anterior semicircular canal

ear ossicles

external auditory canal

cochlea

vestibule

middle ear chamber

eardrum (tympanic membrane)

concha of external ear

eustachian tube

canal ■ canal

nerve and vessels to the roots of the anterior teeth.

incisive c. of maxilla One of two canals leading from the nasal cavity, on either side of the midline, and opening through the hard palate, just behind the central incisor tooth; through it pass the terminal branches of the greater palatine artery and the nasopalatine nerve.

inferior dental c. See mandibular canal.

infraorbital c. A canal running between the floor of the orbit and the roof of the maxillary sinus, connecting the infraorbital foramen on the surface of the body of the maxilla (just above the canine fossa) to the infraorbital groove; it transmits the infraorbital nerve (continuation of the maxillary nerve) and the infraorbital vessels.

inguinal c. An obliquely directed passage through the layers of the lower abdominal wall on either side, through which pass the spermatic cord in the male and the round ligament of the uterus in the female.

internal auditory c. A transverse canal through the petrous part of the temporal bone of the skull, about 1 cm in length, extending from the cranial cavity to the medial wall of the inner ear; it provides passage for the vestibulocochlear (8th cranial) nerve, the motor and sensory roots of the facial (7th cranial) nerve and the labyrinthine blood vessels. Also called internal auditory meatus.

longitudinal c.'s of modiolus Short longitudinal canals in the modiolus of the inner ear that transmit the cochlear nerves and vessels. Also called central canal of cochlea.

mandibular c. A canal that traverses the ramus and body of the mandible, from the mandibular foramen to the area of the premolar teeth where it divides into mental and incisive canals; it runs horizontally below the tooth sockets with which it communicates by small canals; it contains the inferior alveolar vessels and nerves, from which terminal branches reach the mandibular teeth. Also called inferior dental canal.

mental c. One of the two terminal branches of the mandibular canal that originates near the roots of the premolar teeth and approaches the mental foramen on the lateral side of the mandible.

nasolacrimal c. A canal, slightly more than one centimeter long in the adult, that communicates with the lacrimal groove in

the orbit above and the inferior meatus of the nose below; it passes medial to the maxillary sinus and transmits the nasolacrimal duct.

obturator c. of pubic bone See obturator groove, under groove.

optic c. A short canal through the sphenoid bone at the apex of the orbit through which pass the optic nerve and ophthalmic artery from the cranial cavity to the orbit. Also called optic foramen.

palatovaginal c. A narrow canal situated in the roof of the nasal cavity between the undersurface of the vaginal process of the sphenoid bone and the sphenoid process of the palatine bone; it extends from the pterygopalatine fossa to the nasal cavity and transmits the pharyngeal branch of the maxillary artery and pharyngeal nerve from the pterygopalatine ganglion.

pterygoid c. A canal running through the root of the pterygoid process of the sphenoid bone; it conducts the nerve, artery, and vein of the pterygoid canal.

pudendal c. A fibrous tunnel formed by the splitting of the obturator fascia that lines the lateral wall of the ischiorectal fossa; it transmits the internal pudendal vessels and nerves. Also called Alcock's canal.

pulp c. See root canal.

root c. The portion of the pulp cavity within a tooth, leading from the pulp

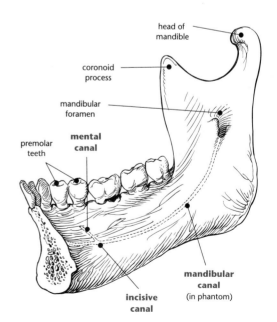

head of mandible

coronoid process

mandibular foramen

premolar teeth

mental canal

mandibular canal (in phantom)

incisive canal

chamber to the apical foramen at the tip of the root; it transmits blood vessels and sensory nerves into the pulp chamber. Also called pulp canal.

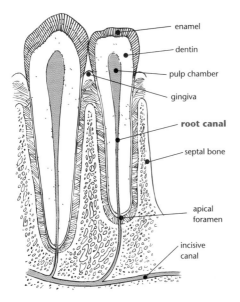

- enamel
- dentin
- pulp chamber
- gingiva
- **root canal**
- septal bone
- apical foramen
- incisive canal

sacral c. The part of the vertebral canal from the first sacral vertebra to the lower end of the sacrum (sacral hiatus); it is triangular in transverse section and contains a collection of spinal roots (cauda equina), the terminal filament (filum terminale) of the spinal cord and the spinal membranes (meninges). Also called caudal canal.

semicircular c.'s Three canals (anterior, lateral, posterior) of the bony labyrinth of the inner ear in which the membranous semicircular ducts are enclosed; each canal, 0.8 mm in diameter, presents a dilatation at one end (ampulla) while the other end opens into an oval cavity (vestibule) within the temporal bone. Also called bony semicircular canals.

spinal c. See vertebral canal.

c. for tensor tympani muscle A small canal in the petrous part of the temporal bone, above and parallel to the osseous part of the auditory tube; it opens between the petrous and squamous parts of the temporal bone and ends just above the oval window where the tendon of the tensor tympani muscle bends laterally to attach to the malleus.

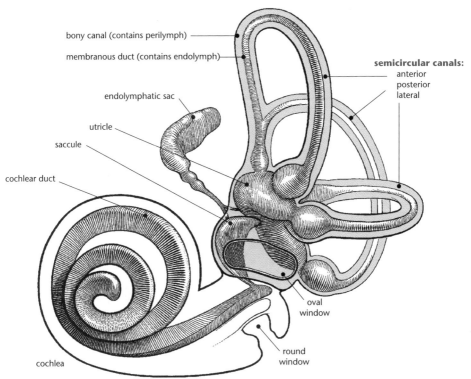

- bony canal (contains perilymph)
- membranous duct (contains endolymph)
- **semicircular canals:**
  - anterior
  - posterior
  - lateral
- endolymphatic sac
- utricle
- saccule
- cochlear duct
- oval window
- round window
- cochlea

canal ■ canal

tympanic c. of cochlea See scala tympani, under scala.

vertebral c. The canal formed by the foramina of successive vertebrae; it is large and triangular in the cervical and lumbar regions, small and circular in the thoracic region, and small and triangular in the sacral region; it encloses the spinal cord, the meninges, and associated vessels. Also called spinal canal.

vestibular c. of cochlea See scala vestibuli, under scala.

Volkmann's c.'s Small oblique and transverse channels in compact bone linking the larger haversian canals with each other and with the medullary cavity, spaces in trabecular (spongy) bone, and the surface of the bone; they permit the trasmission of blood vessels and nerves throughout the bone.

canalicular (kan-ah-lik'u-lar) Relating to a small canal (canaliculus).

canaliculi (kan-ah-lik'u-li) Plural of canaliculus.

canaliculus (kan-ah-lik'u-lus), pl. canalic'uli A small channel or canal.

    c. of cochlea The small canal in the petrous part of the temporal bone that serves as a communication between the scala tympani of the inner ear and the subarachnoid space; it extends from the bottom of the cochlea to the front of the jugular fossa; it accommodates the perilymphatic duct and a small vein that empties into the inferior petrosal sinus.

    bone canaliculi Minute branching passages in compact bone connecting adjacent lacunae with one another into a system of cavities and with the central haversian canal; contain cytoplasmic processes of osteocytes (bone cells).

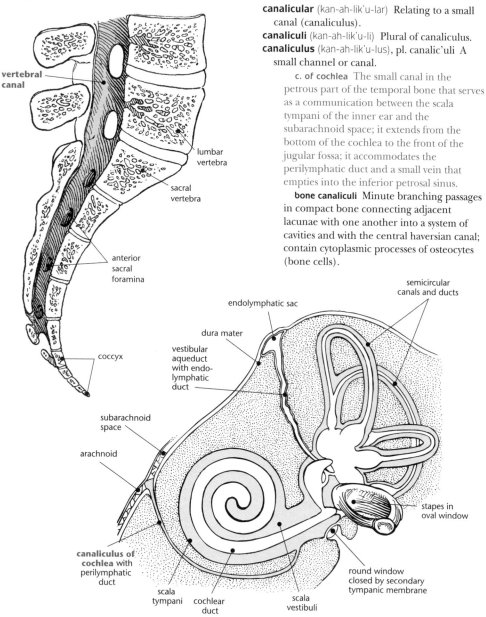

vertebral canal

lumbar vertebra

sacral vertebra

anterior sacral foramina

coccyx

semicircular canals and ducts

endolymphatic sac

dura mater

vestibular aqueduct with endo-lymphatic duct

subarachnoid space

arachnoid

stapes in oval window

canaliculus of cochlea with perilymphatic duct

scala tympani   cochlear duct

scala vestibuli

round window closed by secondary tympanic membrane

canal ▪ canal

anterior c. for the chorda tympani nerve A small bony canal at the medial end of the petrotympanic fissure, through which the chorda tympani nerve leaves the middle ear chamber as it travels to the tongue.

inferior tympanic c. A minute bony canal passing from the inferior surface of the petrous part of the temporal bone (between the jugular fossa and the carotid canal) to the floor of the middle ear chamber; it houses the tympanic nerve which arises from the inferior ganglion of the glossopharyngeal nerve and enters the chamber to form the tympanic ganglia and a tympanic plexus overlying the promontory.

mastoid c. The small canal beginning in the lateral part of the jugular fossa of the skull and passing through the mastoid process to exit at the tympanomastoid fissure; it accommodates the auricular branch of the vagus nerve.

posterior c. for the chorda tympani nerve A small bony canal leading from the facial canal about 6 mm before its termination, located between the posterior and lateral walls of the middle ear chamber (tympanic cavity) just behind the tympanic membrane; it allows the chorda tympani nerve and a branch of the stylomastoid artery to enter the middle ear chamber.

cancellous (kan'sĕ-lus) Honeycomb-like, particularly of reticular bony tissue.

canine (ka'nīn) Popular term for cuspid.

cap (kap) Any structure that resembles or serves as a cover.

enamel c. In embryology, the caplike structure covering the enamel organ of a developing tooth.

knee c. Kneecap; see patella.

capitate (kap'ĭ-tāt) Possessing a rounded extremity; head-shaped.

capitulum (kah-pit'u-lum) A small rounded eminence or articular end of a bone by which it articulates with another bone.

c. humeri The small rounded eminence of the humeral condyle, located on the lateral half of the distal end of the humerus between the trochlea and the lateral epicondyle; it articulates with the head of the radius at the elbow joint.

capsule (kap'sūl) A saclike structure enveloping an organ or a part.

articular c. A double-layered sac enclosing the cavity of a synovial joint, formed by an outer fibrous membrane and an inner synovial membrane; it permits movements of the joint. Also called joint capsule; synovial capsule.

articular c. of ankle joint The capsule that surrounds the ankle joint, extending from the distal tibia and malleoli, downward to the talus; it is strengthened on each side by strong collateral ligaments.

articular c. of elbow joint The thin capsule investing the elbow joint; posteriorly, the fibers extend from the humerus just behind the capitulum, to the lower part of the rim of the olecranon process, and the back of the medial epicondyle; anteriorly, it is attached from the front of the humerus and medial epicondyle to the anterior area of the coronoid process of the ulna and to the annular ligament around the head of the radius; inferomedially, it is attached to the olecranon; laterally, it blends into the radio-ulnar joint underlying the annular ligament.

articular c. of hip joint The strong and dense, but lax capsular ligamentous sac attached from the margin of the acetabulum of the hip joint and edge of the obturator foramen to the base of the neck and intertrochanteric line of the femur.

articular c. of humerus See articular capsule of shoulder joint.

articular c. of knee joint A complex, strong, thin sac enclosing the knee joint; posteriorly, the fibers extend from the margins of the femoral condyles and posterior margin of the intercondylar fossa, down to the posterior margins of the tibial condyles and the backside of the intercondylar area; medially, the fibers extend from the femoral to tibial condyles; laterally, the fibers extend from the femur down to the lateral condyle of the tibia and head of the fibula; anteriorly, the fibers

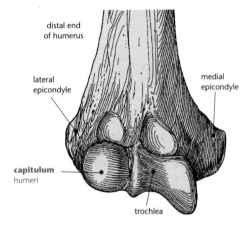

distal end of humerus

lateral epicondyle

medial epicondyle

capitulum humeri

trochlea

blend with the expansions from the lateral and medial vastus muscles and are attached to the margins of the patella, patellar ligament, and condyles of the tibia. The capsule is strengthened by strong bands (e.g., the iliotibial tract, fibular (lateral) collateral ligament, expansions of the sartorius and semimembranous muscles, oblique popliteal ligament) and fuses with other strong bands (e.g., tibial (medial) collateral ligament).

articular c. of shoulder joint The lax capsular ligamentous sac attached to the circumference of the glenoid cavity of the scapula and to the anatomic neck of the humerus. Also called articular capsule of humerus.

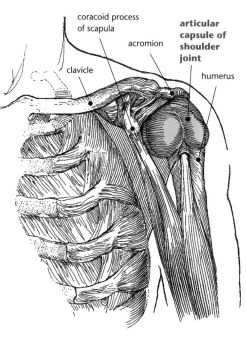

coracoid process of scapula
acromion
clavicle
articular capsule of shoulder joint
humerus

joint c. See articular capsule.
synovial c. See articular capsule.
capsulorrhaphy (kap-su-lor'ah-fe) Suture of a tear in the enveloping capsule of a joint.
capsulotomy (kap-su-lot'o-me) The procedure of cutting into a capsule, as of the articular capsule.
caput (kap'ut) 1. The head. 2. The expanded extremity of a structure.
    c. costae See head of rib, under head.
    c. femoris See head of femur, under head.
    c. fibulae See head of fibula, under head.
    c. humeri See head of humerus, under head.

    c. mallei See head of malleus, under head.
    c. mandibulae See head of mandible, under head.
    c. metacarpalis See head of metacarpus, under head.
    c. metatarsalis See head of metatarsus, under head.
    c. phalangis See head of phalanx, under head.
    c. radii See head of radius, under head.
    c. stapedis See head of stapes, under head.
    c. tali See head of talus, under head.
    c. ulnae See head of ulna, under head.
carina (kah-ri'nah) Any ridgelike structure, as the central ridge formed by the bifurcation of the trachea.
caroticotympanic (kah-rot-ĭ-ko-tim-pan'ik) Relating to the bony carotid canal in the skull or internal carotid artery and the middle ear chamber (tympanic cavity) or the tympanic membrane.
carpal (kar'pal) Relating to the carpus or to the wrist.
carpocarpal (kar-po-kar'pal) Relating to the articulation between the proximal and distal rows of the carpus.
carpophalangeal (kar-po-fah-lan'je-al) Relating to the carpus and the phalanges.
carpus (kar'pus) The wrist, between the distal end of the forearm and the proximal end of the hand; the eight bones of the wrist and associated structures. See also carpal bones, in table of bones in appendix I.

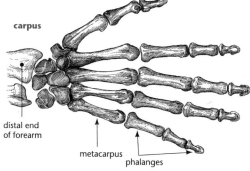

carpus
distal end of forearm
metacarpus
phalanges

cartilage (kar'tĭ-lij) A firm, slightly elastic connective tissue present throughout the body; e.g., in articular surfaces of bones, in the ear, auditory (eustachian) tube, nose, larynx, air passages (trachea and bronchi), etc.; it consists of specialized cells (chondrocytes) embedded in a ground substance (matrix), which is permeated by collagenous fibers; it has no nerve or blood supply of its own. The different

capsulorrhaphy ■ cartilage

types of cartilage include hyaline, cellular, and white and yellow fibrocartilage. Cartilage constitutes the major portion of the fetal skeleton.

accessory c.'s of nose See minor alar cartilages.

articular c. A type of hyaline cartilage covering most of the articular surfaces of bones in a synovial joint.

arytenoid c. One of two triangular cartilages in the posterior larynx, between the cricoid and corniculate cartilages.

c. of auditory tube A cartilaginous tube about 24 mm in length (in the average adult), comprising the inner two-third segment of the auditory (eustachian) tube, which connects the middle ear chamber with the nasal part of the pharynx; it is shaped like an inverted gutter and consists of a broad medial lamina and a narrow lateral lamina. Also called cartilage of eustachian tube.

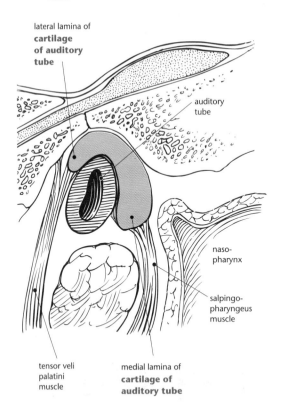

lateral lamina of **cartilage of auditory tube**

auditory tube

naso-pharynx

salpingo-pharyngeus muscle

tensor veli palatini muscle

medial lamina of **cartilage of auditory tube**

auricular c. A single plate of elastic fibrocartilage forming the framework of the ear (auricle), except for the lobe; it is

continuous with the cartilage of the external auditory canal.

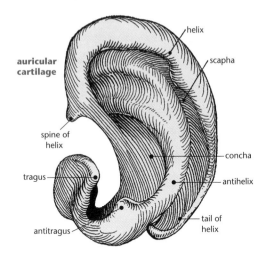

auricular cartilage

helix

scapha

spine of helix

concha

tragus

antihelix

antitragus

tail of helix

costal c. One of 24 bars of hyaline cartilage at the anterior end of each rib, serving to extend the rib anteriorly and contribute to the elasticity of the chest wall. Also called costicartilage.

elastic c. Cartilage composed of matrix permeated with elastic fibers, as in the cartilage of the ear, auditory tube, and epiglottis. Also called yellow elastic cartilage; yellow fibrocartilage.

epiphyseal c. The layer of cartilage between the shaft and the epiphysis of a long bone; present during bone development, after which it ossifies as growth in length ceases. Also called growth cartilage; epiphyseal plate; growth plate; epiphyseal disk.

c. of eustachian tube See cartilage of auditory tube.

c. of external auditory canal The trough-shaped cartilage forming the lateral third of the external auditory canal; it is incomplete above and firmly joins the margins of the medial two-thirds of the bony canal completing the passage from the concha of the ear to the tympanic membrane.

external semilunar c. of knee joint See lateral meniscus of knee joint, under meniscus.

fetal c. A fibrous cartilage that forms most of the temporary skeletal tissue of a fetus; eventually much of it is replaced by bone.

greater alar c. See major (lower) alar cartilage.

cartilage ■ cartilage

growth c. See epiphyseal cartilage.

hyaline c. A semielastic bluish-white, transparent cartilage with a homogeneous glassy appearance; it is usually covered with a membrane (perichondrium) except when coating the articular ends of bones; it possesses considerable elasticity.

interarticular c. See articular disk, under disk.

internal semilunar c. of knee joint See medial meniscus of knee joint, under meniscus.

intervertebral c.'s See intervertebral disks, under disk.

c. of larynx The major constituent of the framework of the larynx, comprised of the single thyroid, cricoid, and epiglottis, and the paired arytenoid, corniculate, and cuneiform cartilages.

cartilages of larynx

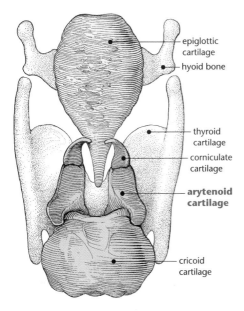

- epiglottic cartilage
- hyoid bone
- thyroid cartilage
- corniculate cartilage
- **arytenoid cartilage**
- cricoid cartilage

lateral (upper) nasal c. The triangular cartilage positioned on either side of the nose between the nasal bone above and the major alar cartilage below; anteriorly, it is partly fused to the cartilage of the nasal septum.

lesser alar c.'s See minor alar cartilages.

loose c. A cartilage that has been damaged and torn; a common athletic injury, usually involving the semilunar cartilages of the knee (menisci).

major (lower) alar c. The thin flexible cartilaginous plate on either side of the nose just below the lateral nasal cartilage; it curves around and supports the anterior part of the nostril and its medial margin attaches to the opposite cartilage and to the bottom of the anterior border of the cartilage of the nasal septum. Also called greater alar cartilage.

minor alar c.'s Two to four small cartilaginous plates in the fibrous membrane that joins the back of the major alar cartilage to the frontal process of the maxilla. Also called lesser alar cartilages; accessory cartilages of nose.

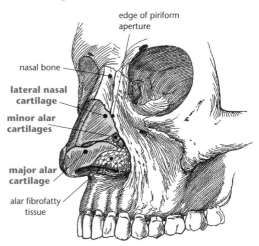

- edge of piriform aperture
- nasal bone
- **lateral nasal cartilage**
- **minor alar cartilages**
- **major alar cartilage**
- alar fibrofatty tissue

c. of nasal septum The thin cartilaginous plate that forms the anterior nasal septum; it is wedged in the nasal cavity between the vomer, the perpendicular plate of the ethmoid, and the nasal bones; it is relatively quadrilateral in shape and completes the separation of the nasal cavities.

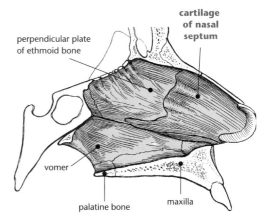

- **cartilage of nasal septum**
- perpendicular plate of ethmoid bone
- vomer
- palatine bone
- maxilla

cartilage ■ cartilage

ossifying c. Temporary cartilage that eventually ossifies during normal development.

permanent c. Cartilage that persists and is not replaced by bone.

semilunar c.'s of knee See lateral meniscus and medial meniscus, under meniscus.

synarthrodial c. Cartilage in a fibrous joint, an articulation without a joint cavity.

thyroid c. The largest of the cartilages of the larynx, consisting of two flat laminae or plates that fuse anteriorly, forming the laryngeal prominence (Adam's apple).

tracheal c.'s The 16 to 20 hyaline cartilages extending the length of the trachea; they are horseshoe-shaped and form approximately two-thirds of the anterior circumference of the trachea; behind, a fibrous membrane joins the free ends of each cartilage, forming a ring. Also called tracheal rings.

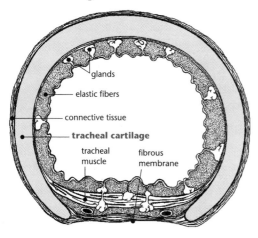

vomeronasal c. The narrow strip of cartilage situated along the lower edge of the cartilage of the nasal septum, attached to the maxilla anteriorly, and to the vomer posteriorly.

xiphoid c. See xiphoid process, under process.

yellow elastic c. See elastic cartilage.

cartilaginous (kar-tĭ-laj'ĭ-nus) Relating to cartilage.

cartilagotropic (kar-tĭ-lag-o-trop'ik) Having the affinity for turning into cartilage; a substance conducive to the growth of cartilage cells.

cauda (kaw'dah) A tapering tail-like anatomic structure.

caudal (kaw'dal) Relating to the part of the body opposite or away from the head; toward the tail

end of the long axis of the body. Also called inferior.

caudocephalad (kaw-do-sef'ah-lad) In a direction from the lower part of the body toward the head.

cavity (kav'ĭ-te) A hollow space within the body, often designating a potential space between layers of tissue or membranes.

abdominal c. The body cavity between the diaphragm above and the pelvis below.

axillary c. The armpit.

bony c. of nose The bony skeleton of the nasal cavity on either side of the nasal septum, extending from the base of the skull downward to the roof of the mouth and from the nostrils in front to the posterior nasal apertures in back; it communicates with the pharynx and the frontal, ethmoidal, maxillary, and sphenoidal sinuses. Also called nasal cavity.

cranial c. The space within the skull, enclosed by the cranial bones; it contains the brain, cranial nerves and blood vessels, and the meninges. Also called intracranial cavity.

glenoid c. The depression on the lateral angle of the scapula for articulation with the head of the humerus, forming the shoulder joint; it is covered with articular cartilage. Also called glenoid fossa.

intracranial c. See cranial cavity.

marrow c. See medullary cavity.

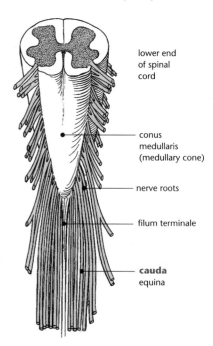

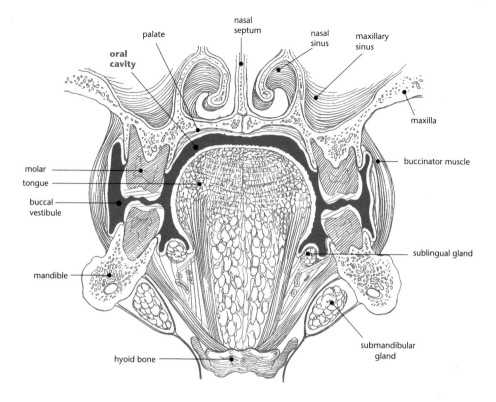

Labels on the figure:
- oral cavity
- palate
- nasal septum
- nasal sinus
- maxillary sinus
- maxilla
- buccinator muscle
- molar
- tongue
- buccal vestibule
- sublingual gland
- mandible
- submandibular gland
- hyoid bone

mastoid c. See mastoid antrum, under antrum.

medullary c. The large, trabecular space within the shaft of a long bone; it is surrounded by compact bone and contains the bone marrow. Also called marrow cavity; medullary space.

middle ear c. See tympanic cavity.

nasal c. See bony cavity of nose.

oral c. The cavity of the mouth, divided into two parts: a) an outer, smaller part, the slit-like vestibule bounded one side by the teeth and gums and on the other side by the lips and cheeks; b) an inner, larger part, the oral cavity proper, internal to the teeth; posteriorly, at the region of the palatoglossal folds, it is continuous with the oropharynx.

orbital c. See orbit.

pelvic c. The short, wide, curved space within the bony framework of the minor pelvis, between the pelvic brim and the pelvic floor (pelvic diaphragm); it contains the pelvic colon, rectum, bladder, and some organs of reproduction.

pulp c. The central space within a tooth, including the space within its crown (crown cavity) and its root (root cavity); it contains pulp, blood and lymphatic vessels, and nerves.

sigmoid c. of ulna See radial notch of ulna, under notch.

thoracic c. The space between the neck and the respiratory diaphragm.

tympanic c. A small irregular space of the middle ear in the temporal bone of the skull; it communicates anteriorly with the nasopharynx through the auditory (eustachian) tube and posteriorly with air cells of the mastoid process. It contains a chain of tiny articulated bones (ossicles) for transmission of sound vibrations across the cavity. Also called middle ear cavity; middle ear chamber. See also middle ear, under ear.

visceral c. One of the three major cavities of the body: cranial, thoracic, and abdominal.

cell (sel) 1. The smallest unit of living organisms capable of independent functioning, composed of a nucleus and organelle-containing cytoplasm within a semipermeable plasma membrane. 2. An anatomic, small hollow cavity or somewhat closed compartment.

cavity ■ cell

air c. An air-containing space, such as those found in the ethmoid bone and mastoid process.

body c. See somatic cell.

bone c. See osteocyte.

cardiac muscle c. A muscle cell (myocyte) about 80 μm in length, usually with a single contrally placed nucleus; it exhibits a spontaneous rhythm of contraction and relaxation; each cardiac muscle cell is partially divided at its ends to form an interlacing network with adjacent cells; conspicuous cross striations (intercalated disks) that mark the junctions between the ends of the cells are evident as well as striations similar to those of the skeletal muscle cells.

cartilage c. See chondrocyte.

ethmoid air c.'s The small, honeycomblike accessory nasal air sinuses in the labyrinth of the ethmoid bone, designated on the basis of their openings into the nasal cavity, as anterior, middle, and posterior, and collectively called the ethmoid sinus; they lie between the upper part of the nasal cavity and the orbits and vary in number from four to fifteen on each side.

germ c. See sex cell.

involuntary muscle c. See non-striated muscle cell.

mastoid air c.'s The numerous interconnecting air spaces, lined with mucous membrane, in the mastoid process of the petrous part of the temporal bone; they communicate with the middle ear chamber (tympanic cavity) through the mastoid antrum and the aditus; they vary considerably in number and size, with those most distant from the antrum often the largest.

muscle c. An elongated, specialized contractile cell.

non-striated muscle c. A fusiform muscle cell (myocyte) with a single centrally placed nucleus; it varies in length from 25 μm to 450 μm; usually arranged in small fasciculi. Also called smooth muscle cell; involuntary muscle cell.

osseous c. See osteocyte.

osteochondrogenic c. A young cell of the inner layer of periosteum, capable of developing into a primitive bone cell (osteoblast) or a primitive cartilage cell (chrondroblast).

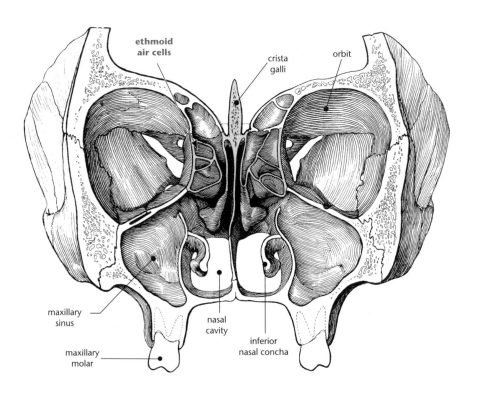

ethmoid air cells

crista galli

orbit

maxillary sinus

nasal cavity

inferior nasal concha

maxillary molar

cell ■ cell

palatine air c. An air sinus situated in the orbital process of the palatine bone; it usually represents an extension from the neighboring ethmoid air cells.

petrosal air c.'s Air sinuses in the petrosal part of the temporal bone, often extending to the petrosal apex.

satellite c.'s of skeletal muscle Elongated spindle-shaped muscle cells derived from myoblasts (primitive muscle cells); they occupy shallow depressions on the surface of the sarcolemma, between the muscle and the basal lamina; thought to contribute to limited regeneration of muscle by fusing with adjacent myofibrils.

sex c. An ovum or a spermatozoon. Also called germ cell.

skeletal muscle c. An elongated muscle cell (myocyte) up to 25 cm in length in long muscles, with hundreds of nuclei; it contains contractile myofibrils, across which run transverse striations, enclosed in a cell membrane or sarcolemma.

smooth muscle c. See non-striated muscle cell.

somatic c. An uncommitted or undifferentiated cell of an organism, other than a germ cell.

synovial c. A specialized connective tissue cell embedded in an intercellular matrix that lines the nonarticulating parts of synovial joints, synovial bursae, and synovial tendon sheaths; it contributes to synovial fluid production and absorption, and the removal of unwanted substances from joint cavities.

tendon c.'s Elongated fibroelastic cells that produce the collagenous fibers of tendinous tissue and remain embedded, usually in rows, between the primary bundles of the resultant tendon. Also called tendon corpuscle.

cementoblast (sĕ-men'to-blast) A mesodermal cell with a large central nucleus that plays an active role in forming the layer of cementum on the root of a tooth. When the cementoblast becomes completely embedded or trapped in the forming cementum, it becomes known as a cementocyte.

cementoclast (sĕ-men'to-klast) The bone cell involved with the progressive resorption of the cementum on the root of a tooth, as seen during the replacement of the deciduous dentition.

cementocyte (sĕ-men'to-sīt) An osteocyte-like cell with numerous processes, embedded or trapped, in a lacuna in the cementum of a tooth.

cementum (sĕ-men'tum) A specialized, bonelike tissue surrounding the root of a tooth; it offers attachment to the periodontal ligament.

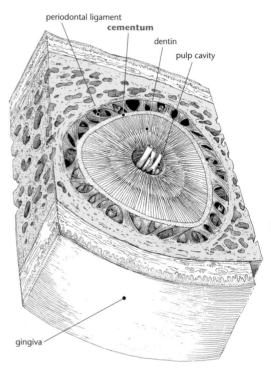

periodontal ligament
cementum
dentin
pulp cavity
gingiva

center (sen'ter) 1. The middle part of an organ or structure. 2. A point or region at which a process begins.

basioccipital c. The ossification center of the cartilaginous model of the occipital bone of the skull that eventually develops into its basilar part; it generally appears during the second month of fetal development.

basisphenoid c. Four ossification centers of the cartilaginous model of the sphenoid bone of the skull that consolidate and fuse during fetal development.

Béclard's ossification c. The secondary ossification center in the epiphyseal cartilage at the distal end of the femur; it appears from about the last month of intrauterine development onwards into the late teens.

chondrification c. Embryonic mesenchymal cells clustered at a site where cartilage is first laid down.

condylar c. An ossification center on each of the lateral parts of the preformed cartilage of the occipital bone, below the highest nuchal line; it appears around the seventh week of fetal life and shortly thereafter

cementoblast ■ **center**

unite to form a single bone. Also called exoccipital center.

exoccipital c. See condylar center.

interparietal c. Each of two centers of ossification on each side of the median plane of the occipital bone, above the highest nuchal line; the ossifications occur within a membrane of fibrous tissue at about the second month of fetal life to form the upper squamous part of the occipital bone.

Kerckring's c. An occasional independent ossification center in the cartilage model of the occipital bone, situated between the suboccipital center and the posterior margin of the foramen magnum; it unites with the rest of the occipital bone before birth.

ossification c. Any region in a tissue or structure where bone begins to form.

phrenic c. See central tendon of diaphragm, under tendon.

primary ossification c. An ossification center that develops before birth, usually in the shaft of long bones, which continues to grow after birth, until physical maturity.

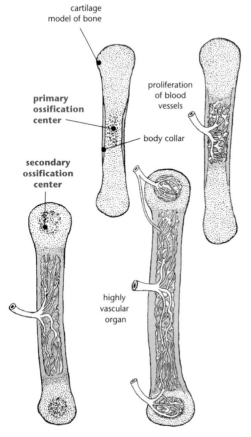

cartilage model of bone

primary ossification center

proliferation of blood vessels

body collar

secondary ossification center

highly vascular organ

secondary ossification c. An ossification center that develops in the epiphyses of long bones, most often occurring after birth to form the architecture of the proximal and distal ends of the long bones. Bone growth is terminated when the secondary ossification center fuses with the primary ossification center.

tendinous c. See central tendon of diaphragm, under tendon.

centi- Combining form meaning one hundredth (10^{-2}).

centimeter (sen'tĭ-me-ter) (cm) A unit of length; one hundredth of a meter.

centrad (sen'trad) Toward the middle or center.

centric (sen'trik) 1. Situated at the center. 2. The position of the lower jaw when the condyles are bilaterally balanced, as during a forceful bite.

centrifugal (sen-trif'u-gal) Tending to move away from the center or from the axis.

centripetal (sen-trip'e-tal) Tending to move toward the center or toward the axis.

centrum (sen'trum) The center of any anatomic structure.

cephalad (sef'a-lad) Directed toward the head.

cephalic (sĕ-fal'ik) Relating to the head.

cephalo-, cephal- Combining forms meaning head.

cephalocaudal (sef-ah-lo-kaw'dal) Relating to the long axis of the body, from cephalic (head) to the caudal end (tail).

cephalometry (sef-ah-lom'ĕ-tre) Measurement of the head.

ultrasonic c. Measurement of the fetal head by means of ultrasonic methods.

-ceptor Suffix meaning receiver (e.g., proprioceptor)

cerebrospinal (ser-ĕ-bro-spi'nal) Relating to the brain and the spinal cord.

cervico- Combining form meaning neck.

cervicobrachial (ser-vĭ-ko-bra'ke-al) Relating to the neck and the arm.

cervicodorsal (ser-vĭ-ko-dor'sal) Relating to the neck and the back.

cervicomuscular (ser-vĭ-ko-mus'ku-lar) Relating to the muscles of the neck.

cervico-occipital (ser'vĭ-ko ok-sip'ĭ-tal) Relating to the neck and the lower back of the head.

cervix (ser'viks) Any constricted, necklike part of an organ or structure.

dental c. See neck of tooth, under neck.

chain (chān) A series of linked bones.

ossicular c. The three small movable auditory bones in the middle ear chamber (tympanic cavity) that extends in a chainlike fashion from the tympanic membrane

center ■ chain

(eardrum) to the oval window.

chamber (cham'ber) An enclosed space or cavity.

>**middle ear c.** See middle ear cavity, under cavity.

>**pulp c.** The expansion of the pulp cavity of a tooth at the coronal end of the cavity, above the gum line; it accommodates the main part of the pulp.

>**utriculosaccular c.** The vestibule of the inner ear containing a dorsal utricle, a ventral saccule, and a narrow communication, the utriculosaccular duct.

charley horse (char'le hors) Popular name of painful stiffness of muscles, especially of the leg, following injury or excessive activity.

cheekbone (chek'bōn) See zygomatic bone, in table of bones in appendix I.

chest (chest) The thorax.

>**barrel c.** A short, rounded chest with expanded, almost horizontal ribs; seen in persons with advanced emphysema.

>**flail c.** Condition in which part of the chest moves independently, usually caused by fractures of the sternum or the ribs, or both.

>**funnel c.** Backward displacement of the sternum, especially its lower portion, which creates a depression of the chest. Also called pectus excavatum.

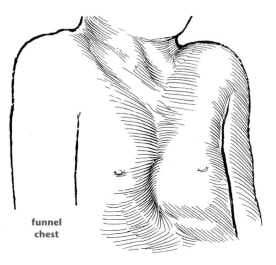

funnel chest

>**keeled c.** Protrusion of the sternum with flattening of the rib cage on either side, giving the chest the appearance of the keel of a boat. Also called pectus carinatum; pigeon breast.

>**phthinoid c.** A long, narrow chest with ribs directed in a more oblique direction than normal.

chiasm, chiasma (ki'azm, ki-as'mah) The crossing of two structures, such as tendons or nerves.

>**tendinous c. of fingers** The point at which the tendons of the deep flexor muscle of the fingers slip through the openings in the flattened tendons of the superficial flexor muscle of the fingers, to insert onto the proximal part of the distal phalanx of the medial four fingers.

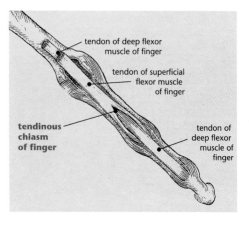

tendon of deep flexor muscle of finger

tendon of superficial flexor muscle of finger

tendinous chiasm of finger

tendon of deep flexor muscle of finger

>**tendinous c. of toes** The point at which the tendons of the long flexor muscle of the toes slip through the openings into the flattened tendons of the short flexor muscle of the toes, to insert onto the proximal part of the distal phalanx of the lateral four toes.

chin (chin) The anterior protuberance of the lower jaw.

choana (ko'a-nah), pl. cho'anae Any funnel-shaped opening, cavity, or hollow. Also called posterior naris.

>**bony c.** The bones forming the infrastructure of the two posterior openings between the nasal cavity and the nasopharynx; they include the base of the skull above, the medial pterygoid plate on the lateral wall, the horizontal plate of the palatine bone below, separated from each other medially, by the posterior border of the nasal septum.

chondral (kon'dral) Relating to cartilage; cartilaginous.

chondrification (kon-dri-fi-ka'shun) The process of forming cartilage or converting into cartilage.

chondro- chondrio- Combining forms meaning cartilage.

chondroblast (kon'dro-blast) A cell that forms cartilage.

chamber ■ chondroblast

chondroclast (kon'dro-klast) A large multinucleated cell concerned with cartilage absorption.

chondrocostal (kon-dro-kos'tal) Relating to the cartilage of the ribs.

chondrocranium (kon-dro-kra'ne-um) The cartilaginous skull of the fetus.

chondrocyte (kon'dro-sīt) A mature cartilage cell occupying a small space (lacuna) within the cartilage matrix; it is occasionally multinucleated and generally increases in size with age. Also called cartilage cell; cartilage corpuscle.

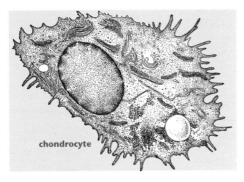

chondrocyte

chondroepiphyseal (kon-dro-ep-ĭ-fiz'e-al) Relating to the epiphyseal cartilages.

chondrolysis (kon-drol'ĭ-sis) Dissolution of cartilage, especially articular cartilage.

chondro-osseous (kon'dro os'e-us) Composed of both cartilage and bone.

chondroseptum (kon-dro-sep'tum) The part of the nasal septum made of cartilage.

chondrosternal (kon-dro-ster'nal) Relating to the rib cartilages and the sternum.

cingulum (sin'gu-lum) The V- or W-shaped enamel ridge on the lingual surface of incisor teeth.

circum- Prefix meaning around, surrounding.

circumflex (ser'kum-fleks) Arched.

circumscribed (ser'kum-skrībd) Confined within boundaries or to a limited area.

clamp (klamp) An instrument for compressing a part or tissue, usually to maintain it in a desired position or to control hemorrhage.

   bone c. A clamp used to stabilize a fractured bone in a desired position during orthopedic treatment. Also called bone-holding clamp.

   bone-holding c. See bone clamp.

-clasia, -clasis Combining forms meaning disintegration, breaking up (e.g., osteoclasis).

classification (klas-sĭ-fĭ-ka'shun) A systematic grouping according to established criteria.

   Angle's c. Classification of dental malocclusion based on the anteroposterior (mesiodistal) position of upper and lower permanent molars.

   c. of bones A classification of bones based on several criteria, including: *Developmental origin,* developed either by the ossification of a preformed cartilaginous model or by the transformation of condensed mesenchyme; *Characteristics of cut surface,* either trabecular or compact; *Regions of long bones,* either diaphysis, metaphysis, or epiphysis; *Appearance of collagen fibers,* either irregular collagen network or regular parallel collagen network; *Microstructure,* either lamellar or non-lamellar; *Architecture of lamellae,* either circumferential, osteonic, or interstitial; *Types of osteon,* either primary or secondary.

   Caldwell-Moloy c. Classification of the female pelvis based on anteroposterior and transverse dimensions of the pelvic inlet, as gynecoid, android, anthropoid, and platypelloid.

   c. of pelves A classification of the various types of maternal pelves predicated on the shape and the dimensions, to assess the obstetric and fetal outcome of the pregnancy.

classification of pelves (♀)

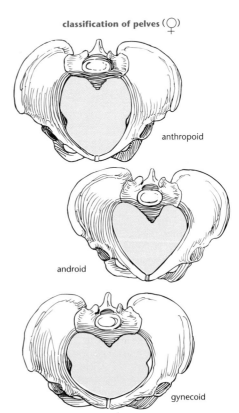

anthropoid

android

gynecoid

Salter-Harris c. Classification of fractures through the end of a growing bone involving the growth plate; grouped into: *Type I,* transverse fracture of the growth plate; *Type II,* fracture of the growth plate and adjacent portion (metaphysis) of the bone shaft; *Type III,* fracture of the growth plate and the end (epiphysis) of the bone; *Type IV,* fracture along the long axis of the bone and crossing the growth plate; *Type V,* a crush or compacting fracture of the growth plate.

c. of synovial joints Classification of synovial joints based on the geometric form of the articular surface and the gross movement permitted; includes: *Simple synovial joint,* one with only two articulating surfaces; *Compound synovial joint,* one with more than one pair of articulating surfaces; *Complex synovial joint,* one possessing an intracapsular disk or meniscus; *Uni-axial synovial joint,* one that is severely limited to rotation about a single axis; *Bi-axial synovial joint,* one capable of independent movement around two axes; *Tri-axial synovial joint,* one capable of independent movement around three axes.

wrist fracture c. Classification of fractures of the distal ends of the radius and ulna, at the wrist; grouped into: *I,* fracture pattern; *II,* fracture extent; *III,* angulation; *IV,* displacement.

-clast Combining form meaning something that destroys (e.g., osteoclast).

claudication (klaw-dĭ-ka'shun) Limping, often accompanied by pain.

intermittent c. Cramplike pain of the leg muscles, usually of the calf, brought on by walking and disappearing with rest; caused by insufficient blood supply to muscle fibers due to narrowing of the arteries.

clavicle (klav'ĭ-kl) The S-shaped subcutaneous long bone at the upper part of the chest on either side, extending from the root of the neck to the point of the shoulder and articulating with the clavicular notch of the sternum and the medial side of the acromion of the scapula; it consists of a thick layer of compact bone enveloping trabecular bone, which does not possess a medullary cavity. In women, the acromial end is slightly below the level of the sternal end, while in men, the ends are generally level. Also called collarbone.

clavicular (klah-vik'u-lar) Relating to the clavicle (collarbone).

clavipectoral (klav-ĭ-pek'to-ral) Relating to the clavicle and the pectoral region of the chest.

clawfoot (klaw'fut) A foot deformity marked by abnormally high longtudinal arch and a turning under of the toes. Also called pes cavus.

cleft (kleft) A groove or slit.

interdigital c. One of the spaces located between any two fingers or toes.

middle-ear c. The narrow cleft in the petrous part of the temporal bone consisting of the auditory (eustachian) tube, the middle ear chamber, the mastoid antrum and the mastoid air cells; the structures are contiguous and allow the free circulation of air. Also called tubotympanic cleft.

tubotympanic c. See middle-ear cleft.

cleidal (kli'dal) Relating to the clavicle.

cleidocostal (kli-do-kos'tal) See costoclavicular.

-cleisis Suffix meaning closure (e.g., otocleisis).

clidal (kli'dal) Relating to the clavicle.

clido-, clid- Combining forms meaning clavicle.

clidocostal (kli-do-kos'tal) Relating to the clavicles and ribs.

clinoid (kli'noid) Resembling a bed; said of certain anatomic structures (e.g., the clinoid process of the sphenoid bone).

clivus (kli'vus) The sloped area within the base of the skull, from the front of the foramen magnum to the dorsum sellae, formed by the basilar part of the occipital bone and the posterior part of the body of the sphenoid bone; it supports the pons and the medulla oblongata.

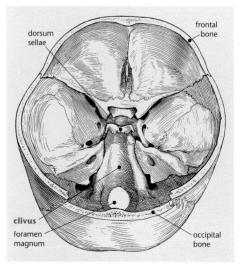

clubfoot (klub'fut) See talipes equinovarus, under talipes.

coaptation (ko-ap-ta'shun) The approximation of two surfaces, such as the margins of a broken bone.

coat (kōt) An enveloping sheath lining an organ or structure; an investing layer of tissue.

    conjoint longitudinal c. of anal canal The blending at the anorectal junction of the pubococcygeal fibers of the levator ani muscle with the longitudinally directed muscle coat of the rectum; it is situated between the internal and external anal sphincters.

    muscular c. Any of the middle coats of muscle in the walls of tubular structures or hollow organs (e.g., the uterine tube) that usually consists of an inner layer of circular muscle fibers and an outer layer of longitudinal muscle fibers.

coccygeal (kok-sij'e-al) Relating to the coccyx.

coccyx (kok'siks), pl. coc'cyges The three to four fused rudimentary vertebrae that form the lower end of the vertebral column; it articulates with the sacrum above by two facets, and the free end below tapers downward and anteriorly, so that its pelvic surface faces up and forward. Also called coccygeal bones; tail bones.

cochlea (kok'le-ah) The spiral bony channel of the inner ear that turns two and three-quarters times through dense bone at the base of the skull; it is divided lengthwise into three fluid-filled spaces: the scala vestibuli and scala tympani (filled with perilymph) and, between them, the cochlear duct (filled with endo-lymph), which contains the essential organ of hearing (spiral organ of Corti) and the terminal fibers of the cochlear nerve. The cochlea measures about 5 mm from base to apex; its base is about 9 mm wide.

cochlear (kok'le-ar) Relating to the cochlea.

cochleovestibular (kok-le-o-ves-tib'u-lar) Relating to the cochlea and the vestibule of the inner ear.

collar (kol'ăr) An anatomic structure that surrounds another.

    perichondral bony c. The periosteal bone that envelops the cartilaginous shaft of immature long bones.

    periosteal bone c. Thick periosteum that envelops the middle of the diaphysis of immature long bones.

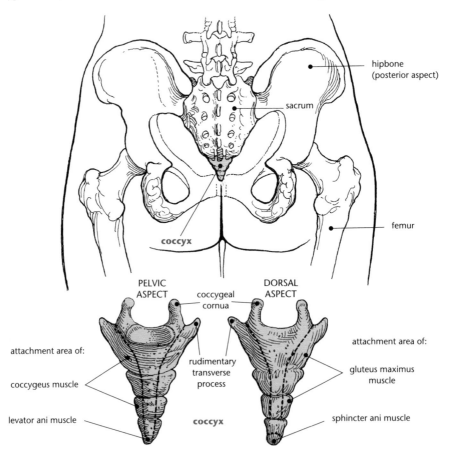

hipbone (posterior aspect)

sacrum

femur

coccyx

PELVIC ASPECT

DORSAL ASPECT

coccygeal cornua

attachment area of:

coccygeus muscle

levator ani muscle

rudimentary transverse process

coccyx

attachment area of:

gluteus maximus muscle

sphincter ani muscle

coat ■ collar

collarbone (kol'ăr-bōn) See clavicle, in table of bones.

collateral (kŏ-lat'er-al) Secondary or alternate.

collum (kol'lum) The neck or constricted necklike part of an organ or structure.

    c. anatomicum humeri See anatomic neck of humerus, under neck.

    c. chirurgicum humeri See surgical neck of humerus, under neck.

    c. ostae See neck of rib, under neck.

    c. femoris See neck of femur, under neck.

    c. mallei See neck of malleus, under neck.

    c. mandibulae See neck of mandible, under neck.

    c. radii See neck of radius, under neck.

    c. scapulae See neck of scapula, under neck.

column (kol'um) A cylindrical, pillar-shaped structure.

    spinal c. See vertebral column.

    vertebral c. The arrangement of a series of vertebrae, from just below the skull through the coccyx, that encloses and provides flexible support to the spinal cord and nerve roots; the opposed surfaces of the adjacent vertebral bodies are firmly bound to each other by fibrocartilaginous disks and ligaments, forming a contiguous, flexible supporting pillar; it is divided into cervical, thoracic, lumbar, sacral, and coccygeal regions. Also called backbone; spinal column; spine. See also table of bones in appendix I.

comminuted (kom'ĭ-nūt-ed) Broken into several small pieces, such as multiple fractures of a bone.

comminution (kom-ĭ-nu'shun) 1. The process of breaking into small pieces. 2. The condition of being broken into small pieces or fragments.

compact (kom-pakt') Compressed; having a dense structure, such as compact bone.

compartment (kom-part'ment) One of the sections into which an area is subdivided; a small space within a large area.

    intracellular c. The space within a tissue occupied by a formative cell, such as the chondrocyte within cartilaginous tissue.

    muscular c. A compartment between the inguinal ligament and the hipbone through which passes the iliopsoas muscle, thereby allowing attachment to the lesser trochanter of the femur.

con- Prefix meaning with; together; in association.

concameration (kon-kam-er-a'shun) A group of interconnecting cavities.

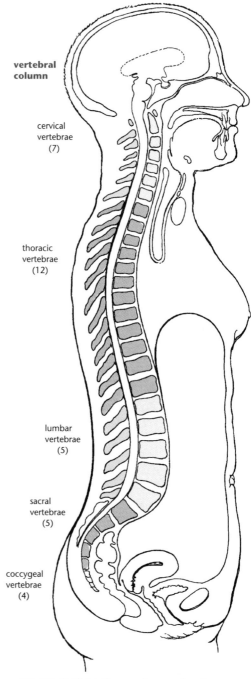

vertebral column

cervical vertebrae (7)

thoracic vertebrae (12)

lumbar vertebrae (5)

sacral vertebrae (5)

coccygeal vertebrae (4)

concave (kon'kāv) Haing a depressed surface.

concavity (kon-kav'i-te) A depression.

concentric (kon-sen'trik) Having a common center.

concha (kon'kah), pl. con'chae A shell-shaped structure.

collarbone ■ concha

c. of ear The deep hollow of the external ear between the antihelix, posteriorly, and the tragus, anteriorly.

inferior c. a) A thin, curved bony plate on the lateral wall of the nasal cavity; it articulates with the maxilla and the ethmoid, palatine, and lacrimal bones; its lacrimal process helps to form the canal for the nasolacrimal duct; b) The thick, highly vascular mucoperiosteum covering the above bone. Also called inferior turbinate.

middle c. a) A thin, curved bony plate projecting on the lateral wall of the nasal cavity; it is part of the ethmoid bone and separates the superior meatus from the middle meatus; b) The thick, highly vascular mucoperiosteum covering the above bone. Also called middle turbinate.

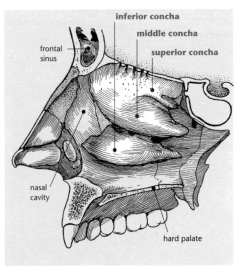

sphenoid c. A paired, thin, cone-shaped bony plate forming part of the roof of the nasal cavity. Also called sphenoid turbinate.

superior c. a) The upper, thin, bony plate projecting from the medial surface of the ethmoidal labyrinth into the nasal cavity above and behind the middle concha; b) The mucoperiosteum covering the above bone. Also called superior turbinate.

conduction (kon-duk'shun) The transmission of a form of energy through tissue, air or material.

air c. Transmission of sound waves to the inner ear through the external auditory canal and structures of the middle ear chamber.

bone c. Transmission of sound waves to the inner ear through the bones of the skull. Also called osteotympanic conduction.

osteotympanic c. See bone conduction.

condylar (kon'dĭ-lar) Relating to a condyle.

condylarthrosis (kon-dil-ar-thro'sis) A joint composed of an ovoid surface (condyle) fitting into an elliptical cavity.

condyle (kon-dĭl) A knoblike prominence at the end of a bone by means of which it articulates with another bone.

c. of humerus A modified condyle at the distal end of the humerus consisting of articular and near-articular portions; the articular portion is divided by a shallow groove into a lateral capitulum (articulates with the head of the radius), and a medial trochlea (articulates with the trochlear notch of the ulna), and adjoins with the proximal ends of the radius and ulna to form the elbow joint; the non-articular portion consists of the lateral and medial epicondyles.

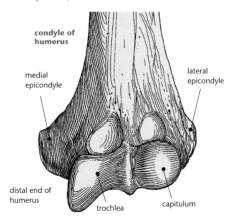

internal c. of femur See medial condyle of femur.

internal c. of tibia See medial condyle of tibia.

lateral c. of femur A mass of bone, partly covered by articular cartilage, at the lateral side of the distal femur, that articulates with the tibia; united anteriorly with the medial condyle to accommodate articulation with the patella and separated posteriorly with the medial condyle by a deep gap, the intercondylar fossa. Also called external condyle of femur.

lateral c. of humerus See lateral epicondyle, under epicondyle.

lateral c. of tibia A bone mass at the lateral side of the proximal tibia covered by a nearly circular cartilage (meniscus) on its upper surface for articulation with the lateral

conduction ■ condyle

condyle of the femur; its posterolateral side has a small circular facet for articulation with the proximal fibula; its medial border projects upward to form the lateral intercondylar tubercle.

mandibular c. The articular process of the ramus of the mandible; the flattened posterior process of the mandible, expanded above to form the head that articulates with the mandibular fossa of the temporal bone.

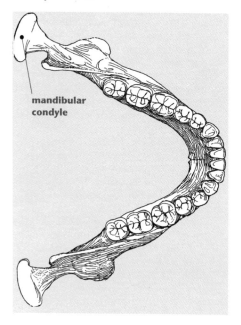

mandibular condyle

medial c. of femur A mass of bone, partly covered by articular cartilage, at the medial side of the distal femur, that articulates with the tibia; united anteriorly with the lateral condyle to accommodate articulation with the patella and separated posteriorly with the lateral condyle by a deep gap, the intercondylar fossa. Also called internal condyle of femur.

medial c. of humerus See medial epicondyle, under epicondyle.

medial c. of tibia A bone mass at the medial side of the proximal tibia covered by an oval cartilage (meniscus) on its upper surface for articulation with the medial condyle of the femur; its lateral border projects upward to form the medial intercondylar tubercle. Also called internal condyle of tibia.

occipital c. One of two oval or kidney-shaped condyles on either side of the foramen magnum of the occipital bone for articulation with the superior facets of the first cervical vertebra (atlas).

confluence of sinuses (kon'floo-ens of si'nus-es) The dilated posterior part of the superior sagittal sinus, lodged within the back of the skull, at the internal protuberance of the occipital bone; it receives venous blood from the occipital sinus and straight sinus and is drained out of the skull by the two transverse sinuses.

conjoined (kon'joined) Joined together peripherally so as to maintain some separate identity, as a conjoined tendon in which two distinct muscles are united by sharing a common tendon of insertion.

contract (kon-tract') To compress or shorten, as a muscle.

contractile (kon-trac'til) Capable of contracting.

contractility (kon-trak-til'i-te) The ability to shorten, said of a muscle.

conjugate (kon'ju-gāt) See diameter.

constriction (kon-strik'shun) A stricture; a shortening, as in muscle contraction; the condition of being constricted.

constrictor (kon-strik'tor) Anything that narrows or squeezes a part or canal, as a muscle that contracts to narrow an opening; a sphincter.

contiguous (kon-tig'u-us) Sharing an edge or margin; adjacent without being in contact.

contra- A prefix meaning opposed, against, opposite.

contractile (kon-trak'til) Capable of being drawn together in response to an appropriate stimulus; tending to contract when stimulated.

contractility (kon-trak-til'i-te) Capable of being able to draw together or shorten in response to an appropriate stimulus.

contraction (kon-trak'shun) A reversible shortening or increase of tension, as a normally functioning muscle.

aerobic c. Muscular contraction sustained by energy from the oxidation of carbohydrates and fat.

anaerobic c. Muscular contraction sustained by energy from the breakdown of glycogen (glycogenolysis).

Braxton-Hicks c.'s Short, relatively painless muscle contractions of the pregnant uterus, usually beginning at irregular intervals during early pregnancy and becoming more frequent and rhythmic as pregnancy advances, especially during the last two weeks of gestation, when they may be mistaken for labor pains; they occasionally occur without pregnancy, as in the response of soft tumors of

confluence of sinuses ■ contraction

the uterine wall.

cardiac c. The contraction of cardiac muscles that results in the expulsion of blood from the heart chambers.

isokinetic c. Contraction of a muscle characterized by a constant force sustained throughout the range of the muscle's activity.

isometric c. Contraction of a muscle devoid of appreciable shortening of its length from origin to insertion.

isotonic c. Contraction of a muscle in which the distance between origin and insertion diminishes, while the force at the tendon remains somewhat constant.

lengthening c. Contraction of a muscle by an external force that results in its progressive lengthening.

myotactic c. Contraction of a muscle brought on by a sharp tap to its tendon, as with a percussion hammer (plexor).

postural c. The state of muscular contraction and tension that sustains the posture of the body.

tetanic c. Sustained muscular contraction devoid of rest period intervals.

tonic c. A slowly occurring muscular contraction with a protracted phase of relaxation.

twitch c. A contraction of a muscle lasting only a brief time that results from a single stimulation of its motor nerve; it may be repetitive.

contracture (kon-trak'tūr) Permanent contraction of a muscle due to tonic spasm, atrophy, or development of fibrous tissue within the muscle or its tendon.

flexion c. The inability of a joint to extend fully.

ischemic c. Contraction of a muscle resulting from interference with the circulation from external pressure, as by a tight bandage.

Volkmann's c. Tissue degeneration and contracture of muscle due to deprivation of blood supply, usually occurring in the finger following a severe injury or improper use of a tourniquet.

contrafissure (kon-trah-fish'ūr) Contrecoup; an injury to bone occurring on the surface opposite to the site of impact.

contralateral (kon-trah-lat'er-al) Relating to the opposite side.

convex (kon'veks) An outwardly curved surface.

coracoacromial (kor-ah-ko-ah-kro'me-al) Relating to the coracoid and acromial processes of the scapula. Also called acromiocoracoid.

coracobrachial (kor-ah-ko-bra'ke-al) Relating to the coracobrachial muscle; also relating to the coracoid process of the scapula and the arm.

coracoclavicular (kor-ah-ko-klah-vik'u-lar) Relating to the coracoid process of the scapula and the clavicle.

coracohumeral (kor-ah-ko-hu'mer-al) Relating to the coracoid process of the scapula and the humerus.

coracoid (ko'rah-koid) Shaped like a crow's beak; denoting the thick, curved process (coracoid process) at the upper border of the scapula.

cornu (kor'nu), pl. cor'nua Any horn-shaped anatomic structure. Also called horn.

coccygeal cornua Bilateral extensions from the back of the upper part of the first coccygeal vertebra; they articulate with the cornua of the sacrum. Also called coccygeal horns.

greater c. of hyoid bone Either of the two slender bony projections passing backward and upward from each end of the body of the hyoid bone; it ends in a tubercle and can be felt when the throat is grasped between the finger and thumb just above the thyroid cartilage. Also called greater horn of hyoid bone.

inferior c. of thyroid cartilage The short, downward extension of the posterior border of the thyroid cartilage containing a facet on its medial surface for articulation with the side of the cricoid cartilage (cricothyroid joint). Also called inferior horn of thyroid cartilage.

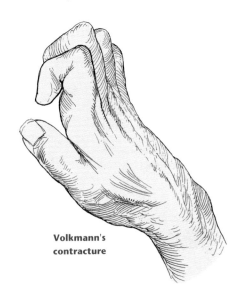

Volkmann's contracture

lesser c. of hyoid bone Either of two small conical eminences connected by fibrous tissue to both sides of the hyoid bone at the angle of junction between the body and greater cornu. Also called lesser horn of hyoid bone.

sacral cornua Bilateral processes extending downward from the arch of the fifth or last sacral vertebra; they articulate with the cornua of the coccyx. Also called sacral horns; coccygeal eminences.

superior c. of thyroid cartilage The long, upward extension of the posterior border of the thyroid cartilage, ending in a conical extremity, to which is attached the lateral thyrohyoid ligament. Also called superior horn of thyroid cartilage.

coronal (ko-rō′nal) Relating to a vertical plane at right angles to the median plane; positioned in the direction of the coronal suture, the arched articulation between the frontal bone of the skull and the two parietal bones.

coronion (ko-ro′ne-on) A craniometric point situated at the tip of the coronoid process of the lower jaw.

coronoid (kor′o-noid) 1. Shaped like a crow's beak; said of processes of certain bones. 2. Crown-shaped.

corpuscle (kor′pus-l) A cell in the body, either one capable of moving freely or restricted to a particular structure.

bone c. See osteocyte.

cartilage c. See chondrocyte.

Golgi c. See Golgi tendon organ, under organ.

tendon c.'s See tendon cells, under cell.

corrugator (kor′u-ga-tor) 1. Anything that causes wrinkling. 2. The small superciliary corrugator muscle on the medial portion of the supraorbital margin that when contracted, produces vertical wrinkles or furrows of the skin; it is commonly called frowning muscle. See also table of muscles in appendix II.

cortex (kor′teks), pl. cor′tices The outer investing layer of an organ such as a bone; distinguished from the inner medullary substance. Also

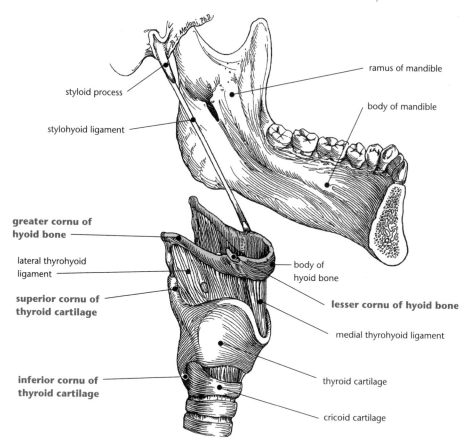

styloid process

stylohyoid ligament

ramus of mandible

body of mandible

greater cornu of hyoid bone

lateral thyrohyoid ligament

superior cornu of thyroid cartilage

body of hyoid bone

lesser cornu of hyoid bone

medial thyrohyoid ligament

inferior cornu of thyroid cartilage

thyroid cartilage

cricoid cartilage

coronal ■ cortex

called cortical layer.

cortical (kor'tĭ-kal) Relating to the cortex.

cortico- A combining form meaning cortex.

corticomedullary (kor-tĭ-ko-med'u-lār-e) Relating to the cortex and the medulla of an organ or structure, as of a bone.

costa (kos'tah), pl. cos'tae Latin for rib.

costal (kos'tal) Relating to a rib.

costicartilage (kos'tĭ-kar'tĭ-lij) See costal cartilage, under cartilage.

costo- Combining form meaning rib.

costochondral (kos-to-kon'dral) Relating to a rib and its cartilage.

costoclavicular (kos-to-klah-vik'u-lar) Relating to the ribs and the clavicle. Also called cleidocostal.

costocoracoid (kos-to-kor'ah-koid) Relating to the ribs and the coracoid process of the scapula.

costophrenic (kos-to-fren'ik) Relating to the ribs and the diaphragm.

costoscapular (kos-to-skap'u-lar) Relating to the ribs and the scapula.

costosternal (kos-to-ster'nal) Relating to the ribs and the sternum.

costovertebral (kos-to-ver'tĕ-bral) Relating to the ribs and the thoracic vertebrae.

cotyloid (kot'i-loid) acetabular.

coxa (kok'sah) The hip joint.

    c. magna The hip joint in which the head of the femur is excessively broad.

    c. valga A deformity of the neck of the femur, characterized by an increased angle (>135°) between it and the shaft of the bone.

    c. vara A deformity of the neck of the femur, characterized by a decreased angle (<135°) between it and the shaft of the bone.

coxitis (kok-si'tis) Inflammation of the hip joint.

coxofemoral (kok-so-fem'o-ral) 1. Relating to the hipbone and the femur. 2. Relating to the hip and the thigh.

cramp (kramp) A painful spasm of variable duration, due to involuntary muscular contraction, with subsequent slow relaxation and slow reduction in pain.

cranial (kra'ne-al) 1. Relating to the cranium, i.e., the part of the skull containing the brain. 2. Relating to the head.

cranio-, crani- Combining forms meaning the cranium.

craniofacial (kra-ne-o-fa'shal) Relating to the skull and the face.

craniomandibular (kra-ne-o-man-dib'u-lar) Relating to the skull and the lower jaw.

craniometry (kra-ne-om'e-tre) Measurement of the distances between standard (craniometric) points on the skull, and the study of their proportions.

craniospinal (kra-ne-o-spi'nal) Relating to the skull and the vertebral column. Also called craniovertebral.

craniovertebral (kra-ne-o-ver'te-bral) See craniospinal.

cranium (kra'ne-um) The skull; in general, the bones of the head; in particular, the bones enclosing the brain, excluding the bones of the face.

cremaster (kre-mas'ter) In males, the muscle that suspends the testicle in the scrotum; upon contraction, e.g., in cold weather, it elevates the testicle toward the warm body. In females, the muscle that encircles the round ligament.

crepitis (krep'ĭ-tus) The grating sound elicited by friction of the ends of a broken bone or motion of arthritic joints.

crest (krest) A bony ridge or linear elevation.

    alveolar c. The margin of the alveolar bone socket surrounding a tooth.

    anterior c. of fibula The anterolateral crest of the shaft of the fibula extending from the head of the bone down to an inch or two above the level of the lateral malleolus, where it divides into two ridges; the anterior intermuscular septum of the leg is attached to its upper three-fourths.

    anterior intertrochanteric c. See trochanteric crest.

    anterior lacrimal c. The crest that forms the anterior boundary of the lacrimal fossa.

    anterior c. of tibia The shin; the subcutaneous crest on the anteromedial surface of the shaft of the tibia; it extends from the tibial tuberosity to the medial malleolus and affords attachment to the deep fascia of the leg.

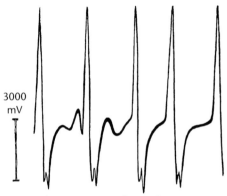

3000 mV

electromyogram of **muscle cramp**

basilar c. of occipital bone See pharyngeal spine, under spine.

buccinator c. A ridge passing from the base of the anterior border of the coronoid process of the lower jaw to the region near the molars, affording attachment to the buccinator muscle.

conchal c. A horizontal ridge just above the inferior meatus of the nasal cavity; it articulates with the inferior nasal concha.

deltoid c. See deltoid tuberosity of humerus, under tuberosity.

ethmoidal c. of maxilla A horizontal ridge located on the medial side of the frontal process of the maxilla; it articulates with the nasal concha of the ethmoid bone.

frontal c. The median sagittal ridge on the internal surface of the frontal bone projecting inward to the anterior cranial fossa; it extends from the foramen cecum to the sulcus for the superior sagittal sinus; it gives attachment to the falx cerebri.

gluteal c. See gluteal tuberosity of femur, under tuberosity.

c. of greater tubercle of humerus A downward extension of the greater tubercle of the humerus, forming the lateral edge of the intertubercular groove (sulcus); it affords attachment to the greater pectoral muscle (pectoralis major).

c. of head of rib A transverse crest or ridge separating the two articular facets on the head of most of the ribs; the lower, larger facet articulates with the upper side of the body of the vertebra, the crest of the head is attached to the intervertebral disk and the upper, smaller facet articulates with the lower side of the body of the above vertebra. Also called interarticular ridge of head of rib.

iliac c. The crest of the ilium; the thickened, curved, upper and outer border of the wing of the ilium; its anterior and posterior extremities are named anterior and posterior superior iliac spines; the highest point of the crest is on the level with the fourth lumbar vertebra and with the umbilicus.

iliopectineal c. of pelvis A crest on the inner (medial) surface of either hipbone, extending obliquely from the sacroiliac joint to the iliopectineal crest of pubis anteriorly; posteriorly, it is continuous with the promontory of the sacrum; it marks the plane separating the false (major) pelvis from the true (minor) pelvis; the brim of the true pelvis. Also called terminal line of pelvis; arcuate line of pelvis; iliopectineal line.

incisor c. The front part of the nasal crest of maxilla that rises as it passes forward to form a sharp spine (anterior nasal spine).

infratemporal c. A transverse crest on the lateral surface of the greater wing of the sphenoid bone dividing the temporal (upper) from the infratemporal (lower) surface.

intertrochanteric c. See trochanteric crest.

lateral supracondylar c. of humerus See lateral supracondylar ridge of humerus, under ridge.

c. of lesser tubercle of humerus A downward extension of the lesser tubercle of the humerus, forming the medial edge of the intertubercular groove (sulcus).

medial c. of fibula The long, sharp crest on the posteromedial surface of the shaft of the fibula; it affords attachment to the deep fascia of the leg, which separates the posterior tibia muscle from the long flexor muscle of the big toe (flexor hallucis longus) and the long flexor muscle of the toes (flexor digitorum longus).

medial supracondylar c. of humerus See medial supracondylar ridge of humerus, under ridge.

median nuchal c. See occipital crest, external.

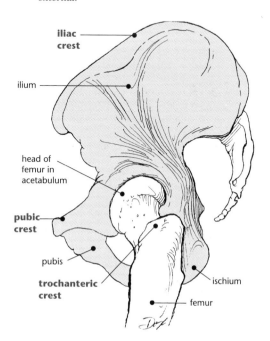

iliac crest

ilium

head of femur in acetabulum

pubic crest

pubis

trochanteric crest

ischium

femur

crest ■ crest

47

nasal c. of maxilla The ridge along the middle of the nasal cavity floor, which, along with the ridge of the opposite maxilla, forms a groove for the articulation of the vomer; it makes a minor contribution to the formation of the nasal septum.

nasal c. of palatine bone A thick ridge along the medial border of the horizontal plate of the palatine bone; it articulates with the back portion of the vomer and makes a minor contribution to the nasal septum.

c. of neck of rib A sharp crest on the upper border of the neck of a rib; it affords attachment to the anterior costotransverse ligament.

obturator c. The inferior border of the crest extending from the tubercle of the pubic bone to the acetabular notch, forming the anterior part of the circumference at the obturator foramen and affording attachment to the obturator membrane and the pubofemoral ligament of the hip joint.

occipital c.'s *External occipital c.*, a vertical ridge on the external occipital bone extending from the external occipital protuberance toward the anterior margin of the foramen magnum; it accommodates the attachment of the nuchal ligament. Also called median nuchal crest. *Internal occipital c.*, the cross-shaped bony elevation on the internal surface of the occipital bone of the skull, at the intersection of sinus ridges; it accommodates the attachment of the falx cerebelli.

palatine c. A transverse, curved crest on the inferior surface of the horizontal plate of the palatine bone, near the posterior border of the bony plate.

pectineal c. of femur A crest on the posterior surface of the shaft of the femur, from the underside of the lesser trochanter to the top of the linea aspera; it affords attachment to the pectineus muscle. Also called pectineal line of femur.

posterior lacrimal c. The crest that forms the posterior boundary of the lacrimal fossa.

pubic c. The roughened free upper anterior border of the body of the pubic bone.

sacral c. Either one of the five rows of highly irregular ridges on the dorsal surface of the sacrum: *Intermediate sacral c.*, one of two rows of four small tubercles seen medial to the dorsal sacral foramina, which represents the fusion of contiguous articular processes of the sacral vertebrae; *Lateral*

sacral c., one of two interrupted ridges lying on either side, lateral to the dorsal sacral foramina, formed by the fused transverse processes of the sacral vertebrae. The four tips on each crest are called transverse tubercles. Also called lateral mass of sacrum; lateral part of sacrum. *Median sacral c.*, a raised interrupted ridge in the median plane of the dorsal sacrum; it is formed by the fusion of the spines of the upper four sacral vertebrae and bears four prominent spinous tubercles.

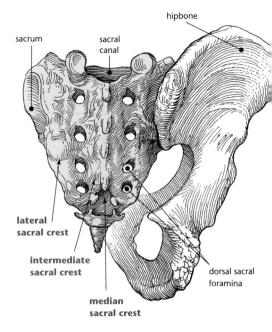

sacrum / sacral canal / hipbone / lateral sacral crest / intermediate sacral crest / median sacral crest / dorsal sacral foramina

sphenoid c. A triangular crest in the median plane of the anterior surface of the body of the sphenoid bone; its anterior surface articulates with the perpendicular plate of the ethmoid bone to form a small part of the nasal septum.

c. of spine of scapula The posterior border of the spine of the scapula; it continues laterally to the acromion and provides attachment to the supraspinous, infraspinous, deltoid, and trapezius muscles.

spiral c. The serrated edge of the delicate bony spiral lamina of the cochlea, which winds around a central core approximately two turns and three-quarters.

supinator c. A strong lateral ridge forming the posterior margin of the supinator fossa, just below the radial notch of the ulna; it represents the proximal part of the interosseous border and affords attachment to the supinator muscle. Also called supinator ridge.

supramastoid c. A thick, curved ridge extending backward and upward from the root of the zygomatic process of the temporal bone; it affords attachment to the temporal fascia overlying the temporal muscle.

temporal c. of frontal bone A crest on the posterior edge of the zygomatic process of the frontal bone that extends upward and backward to divide into superior and inferior lines that traverse the parietal bone.

trochanteric c. A prominent ridge between the greater and lesser trochanters of the femur, marking the junction of the neck and shaft of the bone. Also called intertrochanteric crest; anterior intertrochanteric crest; intertrochanteric ridge.

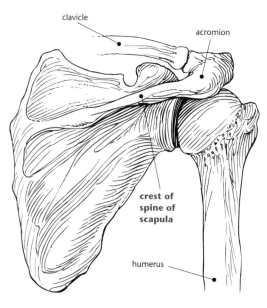

clavicle
acromion
crest of spine of scapula
humerus

cribriform (krib'rĭ-form) Having many small perforations; sievelike.

crista (kris'ta), pl. cris'tae A ridge or a protruding structure.

c. galli A perpendicular bony ridge on the upper surface of the ethmoid bone in the midline of the anterior cranial fossa at the base of the skull, projecting above the level of the cribriform plate; it serves as a point of attachment for the fold of cranial dura mater (the falx cerebri) that separates the cerbral hemispheres.

c. terminalis A muscular band in the wall of the right atrium of the heart; it separates the atrium proper from the sinus (sinus venarum) that receives blood from the superior vena cava and the inferior vena cava.

cross section (kros sek'shun) A two-dimensional section formed by a plane cutting through an anatomic structure, usually at right angles to an axis.

cross striations (kros stri-a'shuns) Transverse bands or lines as seen in longitudinal sections of striated muscle fibers.

cruciate (kroo'she-āt) Resembling the shape of a cross.

crura (kroo'rah) Plural of crus.

crural (krōōr'al) Relating to the leg, thigh, or to a crus.

crus (krus), pl. cru'ra 1. In anatomic nomenclature, the leg; the region between the knee joint and ankle joint. 2. Any elongated process or leglike structure.

common osseous c. The short bony canal of the inner ear formed by the union of the upper end of the posterior semicircular canal with the anterior semicircular canal; it accommodates the common membranous

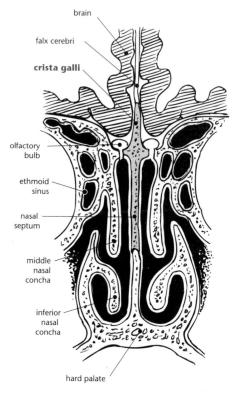

brain
falx cerebri
crista galli
olfactory bulb
ethmoid sinus
nasal septum
middle nasal concha
inferior nasal concha
hard palate

cribriform ■ crus

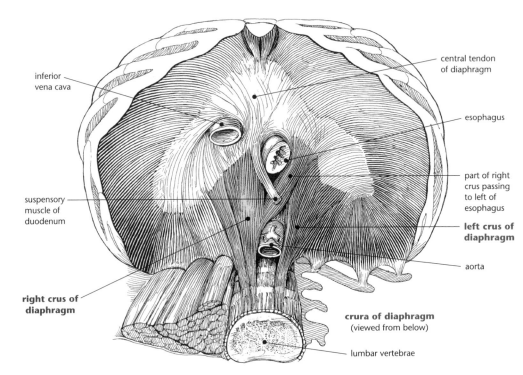

central tendon of diaphragm

inferior vena cava

esophagus

part of right crus passing to left of esophagus

suspensory muscle of duodenum

left crus of diaphragm

aorta

right crus of diaphragm

crura of diaphragm (viewed from below)

lumbar vertebrae

crus, which is about one-fourth the diameter of the canal. Also called crus commune.

c. commune See common osseous crus.

crura of diaphragm Two fibromuscular bands that encircle the aorta and connect the respiratory diaphragm to the lumbar vertebrae: *Left crus of diaphragm,* the fibromuscular origin of the left side of the respiratory diaphragm arising from the upper two or three lumbar vertebral bodies. *Right crus of diaphragm,* the fibromuscular origin of the right side of the respiratory diaphragm arising from the first three or four lumbar vertebral bodies; during its course, it separates to accommodate for the passage of the esophagus from the thoracic cavity to the abdominal cavity.

c. of incus Either of two crura of the incus (middle ear ossicle): *Long c. of incus,* the process coming off the body of the incus, directed downward; at its lower end it articulates with the head of the stapes. Also called long process of incus. *Short crus of incus,* a conical process coming off the body of the incus, directed backward; it is attached by a ligament to the posterior wall of the middle ear chamber. Also called short process of incus.

c. of inguinal ring Either of two bands forming the margins of the superficial inguinal ring: *Lateral c. of inguinal ring,* a curved band forming the lateral margin of the superficial inguinal ring, composed of fibers of the inguinal ligament; *Medial c. of inguinal ring,* a thin, flat band forming the medial margin of the superficial inguinal ring, composed of the aponeurosis of the external abdominal oblique muscle.

c. ossea The bony labyrinth of the inner ear.

c. of stapes Either of two crura of the stapes (innermost ear ossicle): *Anterior c. of*

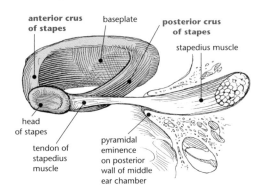

anterior crus of stapes   baseplate   **posterior crus of stapes**

stapedius muscle

head of stapes

tendon of stapedius muscle

pyramidal eminence on posterior wall of middle ear chamber

crus ■ crus

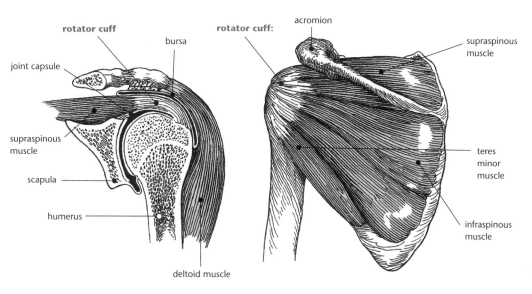

stapes, the anterior crus that extends from the neck of the stapes to the baseplate; it is the shorter and less curved of the two crura. *Posterior c. of stapes*, the posterior crus that extends from the neck of the stapes to the baseplate; it is the longer, larger, and more curved of the two crura.

crypt (kript) A small blind pocket or recess.
  synovial c. A pouchlike expansion of the synovial membrane beyond the joint capsule.
cubital (ku'bĭ-tal) Relating to the forearm, the ulna, or the elbow.
cubitocarpal (ku-bĭ-to-kar'pal) See radiocarpal.
cubitoradial (ku-bĭ-to-ra'de-al) Relating to the ulna and the radius.
cubitus (ku'bĭ-tus) The elbow.
cuboid (ku'boid) Shaped like a cube.
cuboidal (ku-boi'dal) Relating to the cuboid bone of the foot.
cuboideonavicular (ku-boi-de-o-nav-ik'u-lar) See cubonavicular.
cubonavicular (ku-bo-nav-ik'u-lar) Relating to the cuboid and navicular bones of the foot.
cuff (kuf) A bandlike structure encircling a part of the body.
  musculotendinous c. See rotator cuff.
  rotator c. A structure reinforcing the shoulder joint, formed by the tendons of four muscles (supraspinous, infraspinous, teres minor, subscapular); it covers, and

blends with, the upper portion of the joint capsule and provides active support for the joint in motion. Also called musculotendinous cuff.
cuneiform (ku-ne'ĭ-form) Wedge-shaped.
  c. bones Any of the three foot bones shaped like a wedge and located in the front row of tarsal bones: *Intermediate c. bone*, the smallest of the three wedge-shaped tarsal bones, situated, back-to-front, between the navicular bone and the metatarsal of the second toe; *Lateral c. bone*, the wedge-shaped tarsal bone, situated, back-to-front, between the navicular bone and the metatarsal of the third toe; *Medial c. bone*, the largest of the three wedge-shaped tarsal bones, situated, back-to-front, between the navicular bone and the metatarsal of the big toe. See also table of bones in appendix I.
cuspid (kus'pid) The single-cusped tooth between the lateral incisor and the first premolar (bicuspid).
-cyte A combining form meaning cell (e.g., osteocyte).
cyto- A combining form meaning cell (e.g., cytoplasm).
cytology (si-tol'o-je) The branch of biology dealing with the study of the formation, structure, function, and pathology of the cell; cellular biology.

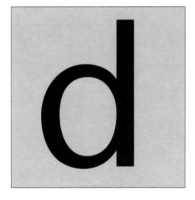

dacryon (dak're-on) A cranial point where the lacrimal, frontal, and maxillary bones meet on the medial aspect of the ocular orbit.

dactylo- Combining form meaning digit, usually a finger.

dactyloid (dak'tĭl-oid) An anatomic structure resembling a finger.

dartos (dar'tos) Greek for flayed.

    d. muliebris A thin layer of smooth (nonstriated) muscle beneath the skin of the labia majora and continuous with the superficial fascia of the groin and perineum.

    d. muscle of scrotum A thin subcutaneous layer of smooth (nonstriated) muscle fibers enclosing the scrotum and continuous with the superficial fascia of the groin and perineum; it contributes to the formation of the sagittal septum of the scrotum separating the two cavities for the testes and is responsible for the characteristic folds (rugae) on the surface of the scrotum.

decalcification (de-kal-sĭ-fi-ka'shun) The loss of calcium from bones or teeth.

deciduous (de-sid'uous) Temporary; not permanent (e.g., the primary dentition).

decussate (de-kus'āt) 1. Crossing in the form of the letter X. 2. To intersect.

defatigation (de-fat-ĭ-ga'shun) Extreme fatigue of muscular tissue to an unhealthy degree; exhaustion.

deformity (de-for'mĭ-te) A structural or functional deviation from normal; a distortion of any anatomic part; malformation.

    boutonnière d. A finger deformity in which the proximal interphalangeal joint is flexed and the distal joint is hyperextended, due to damage to the middle strand of the extensor tendon to the middle phalanx. Also called buttonhole deformity.

    buttonhole d. See boutonniere deformity.

    gunstock d. A forearm inclined toward the midline of the body instead of away from it, seen in the anatomic position (extended forearm with palm facing forward); due to lateral angulation of the elbow joint usually the result of a fracture at the elbow.

    Ilfeld-Holder d. A prominent winging of the scapula resulting in limitations in raising the arm.

    Madelung's d. A distal radioulnar subluxation, with deviation of the hand, usually due to an overgrowth of the distal ulna or undergrowth of the distal radius.

    silver fork d. The deformity seen in Colles' fracture in which the deformity of the distal forearm and wrist resembles the curve of the back of a fork.

    swan-neck d. Finger deformity occurring as a frequent complication of mallet finger, but is also seen associated with other conditions; consists of hyperextension of the proximal interphalangeal joint and flexion of the distal interphalangeal joint.

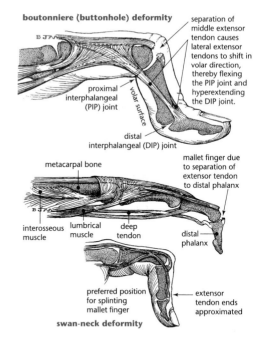

boutonniere (buttonhole) deformity — separation of middle extensor tendon causes lateral extensor tendons to shift in volar direction, thereby flexing the PIP joint and hyperextending the DIP joint.

proximal interphalangeal (PIP) joint — volar surface

distal interphalangeal (DIP) joint

mallet finger due to separation of extensor tendon to distal phalanx

metacarpal bone

interosseous muscle — lumbrical muscle — deep tendon — distal phalanx

preferred position for splinting mallet finger — extensor tendon ends approximated

swan-neck deformity

degeneration (de-jen-er-a'shun) 1. Any deterioration or process of worsening. 2. The process of deterioration of tissues with corresponding functional impairment as a result of injury or disease; the process may advance to an irreversible stage and eventually cause death of the tissues (necrosis).

dacryon ■ degeneration

fascicular d. Neurogenic atrophy; degeneration of bundles of muscle fibers due to diseases of the lower motor neurons, such as amyotrophic (progressive) lateral sclerosis (Lou Gehrig disease).

hyaline d. A cellular change in which the cytoplasm becomes glossy and homogeneous; may be due to viral inclusions or to injury that causes coagulation of proteins.

Zenker's d. A severe form of hyaline degeneration affecting the cytoplasm of striated muscle cells, which becomes clumped, homogeneous, and waxy; seen in severe infections.

deltoid (del'toid) Triangular.

d. muscle A large, thick triangular muscle covering the shoulder region; it is attached at its base above to the lateral third of the clavicle, the acromion and the lower edge of the spine of the scapula; the apex of the muscle is attached to the deltoid tuberosity near the middle of the shaft of the humerus. See also table of muscles in appendix II.

deltopectoral (del-to-pek'to-ral) Relating to the deltoid muscle and the greater pectoral muscle (pectoralis major).

demi- Prefix meaning half; lesser.

demifacet (dem-e-fas'et) A part, usually one half, of an articular surface of a bone (e.g., on a thoracic vertebra for articulation with a rib).

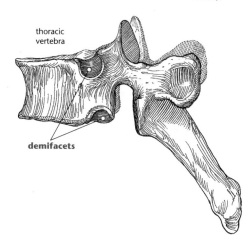

thoracic vertebra

demifacets

inferior d. for head of rib of vertebra See inferior costal facet of vertebra, under facet.

superior d. for head of rib of vertebra See superior costal facet of vertebra, under facet.

demipenniform (dem-e-pen'ĭ-form) See unipennate.

dens (dens), pl. den'tes 1. Latin for tooth. 2. See odontoid process, under process.

density (den'sĭ-te) The state of compactness; the quantity of matter per unit volume, expressed in grams per cubic centimeter.

bone d. In clinical practice, the amount of mineral per square centimeter of bone; usually measured by photon absorptiometry or by x-ray computed tomography. Actual bone density is expressed in grams per milliliter.

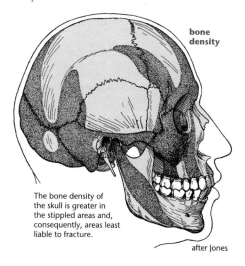

bone density

The bone density of the skull is greater in the stippled areas and, consequently, areas least liable to fracture.

after Jones

dentin (den'tin) The hard tissue forming the main substance of teeth; it surrounds the tooth pulp and is covered by enamel in the crown and by cementum in the root; permeated by tubules that contain odontoblast processes; it is softer than enamel but harder than bone. Also spelled dentine.

functional d. See secondary regular dentin.

mantle d. The outer part of the dentin abutting the enamel or cementum; it consists of mostly coarse fibers.

primary d. Dentin formed during the physiologic development of the tooth, before its eruption; it is separated from the secondary dentin by a line of demarcation.

reparative d. See secondary irregular dentin.

secondary irregular d. Highly irregular protective barrier of dentin formed by the cells of the pulp in response to severe pulp irritation from expanding caries, cavity preparation, or injury. Also called reparative dentin.

secondary regular d. Dentin formed by the cells of the pulp in response to the normal

deltoid ■ dentin

wearing down of the tooth (attrition). Also called functional dentin.

dentition (den-tish'un) The arrangement of the natural teeth in the mouth; the teeth, considered collectively, in the dental arch.

    deciduous d. The set of 20 teeth that erupts between six and 26 months of age and is replaced by permanent dentition in children from six to 12 years of age. Also called primary dentition.

    delayed d. Eruption of the first deciduous tooth after 13 months of age or eruption of the first permanent tooth after seven years of age. Also called retarded dentition.

    mandibular d. Dentition of the lower jaw.

    maxillary d. Dentition of the upper jaw.

    mixed d. Dentition composed of erupted permanent and deciduous teeth, as seen in children between six and 12 years of age. Also called transitional dentition.

    permanent d. The set of 32 teeth that begins to appear at about six years of age, when the first permanent molars erupt, to about 18 years of age, when the third molars erupt. Also called secondary dentition.

primary d. See deciduous dentition.

retarded d. See delayed dentition.

secondary d. See permanent dentition.

transitional d. See mixed dentition.

desmectasis (des-mek'tah-sis) The excessive extension or stretching of a ligament.

desmo-, desm- Combining forms meaning ligament.

detrusor (de-troo'sor) Denoting a muscle that effects an expulsion or pushing out of something (e.g., the detrusor muscle of the bladder). See also table of muscles in appendix II.

diameter (di-am'e-ter) 1. A straight line passing through the center of any circular anatomic structure or space; frequently used to specify certain dimensions of the female pelvis and fetal head. 2. The distance along such a line. 3. The thickness or width of any structure or opening.

    anteroposterior d. The distance between two points located on the anterior and posterior aspects of the structure measured.

    anteroposterior d. of pelvic inlet The distance between the midpoints of the upper rim of the pubic symphysis and the sacral promontory; in the average adult female, it is approximately 112 mm in length, while in the average adult male it measures about 100 mm.

    anteroposterior d. of pelvic outlet The distance between the midpoint of the lower rim of the pubic symphysis and the tip of the

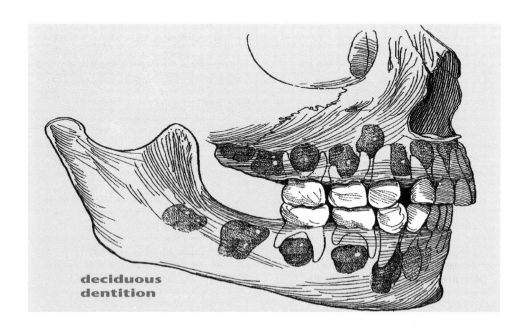

deciduous dentition

coccyx. Sometimes the sacrococcygeal junction is used for the posterior point; in the average adult female, it is approximately 125 mm in length, as compared to about 80 mm in the adult male pelvis.

biparietal d. The transverse distance between the two parietal eminences of the skull, representing the maximal cranial breadth.

bisacromial d. The distance between the acromia, the outermost points of the shoulder.

bisiliac d. The distance between the two most distant parts of the iliac crests.

bispinous d. See interspinous diameter.

bitemporal d. The distance between the two temporal sutures of the fetal skull at term, usually around 8.0 cm.

bituberous d. See transverse diameter of pelvic outlet.

conjugate d. The distance between two specified opposite parts on the periphery of the pelvic inlet, such as the anteroposterior distance from the sacral promontory to the upper edge of the pubic symphysis (true conjugate); or the anteroposterior distance from the sacral promontory to the lower edge of the pubic symphysis (false conjugate).

fronto-occipital d. See occipitofrontal diameter.

interspinous d. The transverse pelvic diameter between the two ischial spines. Also called bispinous diameter.

intertuberous d. See transverse diameter of pelvic outlet.

mento-occipital d. See occipitomental diameter.

oblique d.'s of pelvis a) Of the inlet: the distance from one sacroiliac joint to the opposite junction of the ischial and pubic rami (iliopubic eminence); in the average adult female, it is approximately 125 mm in length, as compared to about 120 mm in the adult male pelvis. b) Of the midpoint of the sacrotuberous ligament to the junction of the ischial and pubic rami (iliopubic eminence); in the average adult female, it is approximately 118 mm in length, as compared to about 100 mm in the adult male pelvis.

occipitofrontal d. The diameter of the skull from the frontal bone between the eyebrows (glabella) to the external occipital protuberance (furthest point at occiput); it represents the maximal cranial diameter. The greatest circumference of the head corresponds to the plane of the occipitofrontal diameter. Also called fronto-occipital diameter.

occipitomental d. The distance of a skull from the chin to the most prominent portion of the occipital bone (external occipital protuberance). Also called mento-occipital diameter.

posterior sagittal d. of midpelvis A right-angled diameter extending posteriorly from the midpoint on the interspinous diameter and a point on the sacrum on the same plane.

posterior sagittal d. of pelvic outlet A right-angled diameter extending posteriorly from the midpoint on the transverse diameter of the pelvic outlet to the sacrococcygeal junction.

suboccipitobregmatic d. The diameter of a fetal skull at term from the middle of the anterior fontanel to the under surface of the occipital bone, just where it joins the neck. The smallest circumference of the fetal head corresponds to the plane of the suboccipitobregmatic diameter.

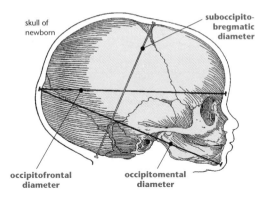

skull of newborn · suboccipito-bregmatic diameter · occipitofrontal diameter · occipitomental diameter

d. transversa pelvis See transverse diameter of pelvic inlet.

transverse d. of pelvic inlet The maximum distance between opposite sides of the pelvic brim; i.e., between the iliopectineal crests of the pelvis; in the average adult female, it is approximately 131 mm in length, while in the average adult male it measures about 125 mm. Also called intertuberous diameter.

transverse d. of pelvic outlet The distance between the lower border of the medial surface of the two ischial tuberosities; in the average adult female, it measures approximately 118 mm in length, as compared to about 85 mm in the adult male pelvis. Also called bituberous diameter.

diameter ■ diameter

diaphragm (di'ah-fram) 1. A dome-shaped, musculofibrous partition separating the thoracic cavity from the abdominal cavity, and functioning in such activities as respiration, defecation, and parturition; its periphery consists of muscular fibers attached to the circumference of the thoracic outlet, namely to the back of the xiphoid process, to the internal surface of the lower six ribs and their cartilages, to the arcuate ligaments and to the lower lumbar vertebrae; they converge into a central tendon, a thin but strong aponeurosis situated near the center of the dome, immediately below the pericardium of the heart, with which it is partly blended. A number of apertures appear in the diaphragm including the aortic, the esophageal, and the vena caval, plus a number of smaller openings. The elevation of the diaphragm on the right side is positioned noticeably higher than on the left side. Also called thoracoabdominal diaphragm. 2. Any membranous partition that divides or separates structures.

   pelvic d. The part of the pelvic floor formed by the paired levator ani and coccygeal muscles and their fasciae.
      thoracoabdominal d. See diaphragm (1).
      urogenital d. A deep and strong

musculomembranous partition stretched across the anterior half of the pelvic outlet between the ischiopubic rami; it is composed of the sphincter muscle of the membranous urethra, the right and left deep transverse muscle of the perineum (transversus perinei profundus) and fascia. In the female, it is primarily pierced by the urethra and vagina; in the male, by the membranous urethra and the ducts of the bulbourethral (Cowper's) glands.

diaphyseal (di-ah-fiz'e-al) Relating to the shaft of a long bone (diaphysis).

diaphysis (di-af'ĭ-sis), pl. diaph'yses The shaft of a long bone, consisting of an elongated cylinder of compact bone enveloping a medullary cavity.

diapophysis (di-ah-pof'ĭ-sis) The upper articular surface of a transverse vertebral process.

diarthric (di-ar'thrik) Relating to two joints.

diarthrodial (di-ar-thro'dĭ-al) Relating to a synovial joint.

diarthrosis (di-ar-thro'sis) See synovial joint, under joint.

diastasis (di-as'tah-sis) Abnormal separation of two normally joined structures.

   d. recti Separation of the two abdominal rectus muscles along the midline, sometimes occurring in pregnancy or abdominal surgery.

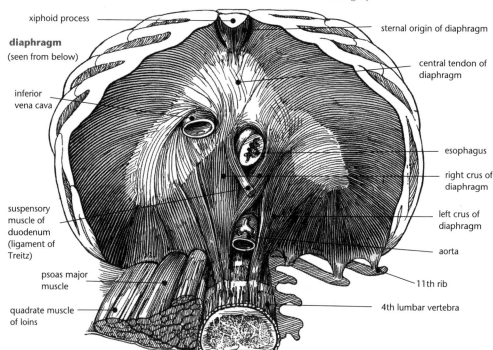

xiphoid process

diaphragm
(seen from below)

inferior
vena cava

suspensory
muscle of
duodenum
(ligament of
Treitz)

psoas major
muscle

quadrate muscle
of loins

sternal origin of diaphragm

central tendon of
diaphragm

esophagus

right crus of
diaphragm

left crus of
diaphragm

aorta

11th rib

4th lumbar vertebra

diaphragm ■ diastasis

digastric (di-gas'trik) Having two muscle bellies (fleshy parts of a muscle), as the digastric muscle, situated below the body of the mandible, in which two muscle bellies are united end-to-end by an intermediate rounded tendon; it stretches from the mastoid process of the temporal bone to the chin of the mandible.

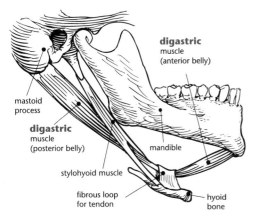

digastric muscle (anterior belly)

mastoid process

digastric muscle (posterior belly)

mandible

stylohyoid muscle

fibrous loop for tendon

hyoid bone

digit (dij'it) A finger or toe.

digital (dij'ĭ-tal) Relating to a finger or a toe.

digitate (dij'ĭ-tāt) Having processes resembling fingers, such as the anterior serratus muscle.

digitation (dij-ĭ-ta'shun) A fingerlike process, such as the intercalated disk of cardiac muscle.

digitofibular (dij-ĭ-to-fib'u-lar) Relating to the fibular (lateral) side of the toes.

digitometatarsal (dij-ĭ-to-met-ah-tar'sal) Relating to the toes and the metatarsus.

digitoradial (dij-ĭ-to-ra'de-al) Relating to the radial (lateral) side of the fingers.

digitotibial (dij-ĭ-to-tib'e-al) Relating to the tibial (medial) side of the toes.

digitoulnar (dij-ĭ-to-ul'nar) Relating to the ulnar (medial) side of the fingers.

dimple (dim'pl) A shallow depression on the skin surface, often due to an underlying bone or a developmental defect.

    coccygeal d. A dimple over the coccyx caused by a fibrous tissue stretching from the tip of the coccyx to the overlying skin. Also called postanal dimple.

    postanal d. See coccygeal dimple.

    posterior superior iliac spine d. A dimple in the skin overlying the posterior superior iliac spine of the hipbone on either side.

diploë (dip'lo-e) The trabecular bone substance that lies between the outer and inner tables of most cranial bones; it contains red bone marrow in its interspaces.

disc (disk) See disk.

discus (dis'kus), pl. dis'ci Latin for disk.

disimpaction (dis-im-pak'shun) Separation of an impacted bone fracture.

disinsertion (dis-in-ser'shun) The separation or rupture of a tendon from its insertion into a bone.

disk (disk) Any platelike structure, usually circular in form. Also spelled disc.

    acromioclavicular d. A fibrocartilaginous disk that partially separates the articular surfaces of the joint between the lateral end of the clavicle and the medial margin of the acromion of the scapula.

    articular d. A circular fibrocartilaginous pad present in some synovial joints and attached to the joint capsule; it serves to reduce friction between the articulating surfaces of the bones. Also called interarticular cartilage.

    articular d. of distal radioulnar articulation See radioulnar disk.

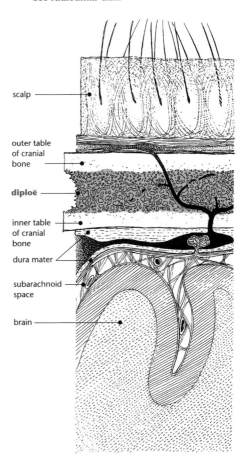

scalp

outer table of cranial bone

diploë

inner table of cranial bone

dura mater

subarachnoid space

brain

digastric ■ disk

articular d. of sternoclavicular articulation
See sternoclavicular disk.

articular d. of temporomandibular joint See
temporomandibular articular disk.

epiphyseal d. See epiphyseal cartilage,
under cartilage.

herniated intervertebral d. The posterior
rupture of the inner portion (nucleus
pulposus) of an intervertebral disk through
disruption of the confining fibrous ring
(annulus fibrosus), often causing pressure on
the nerve roots with resulting pain;
occurring most commonly in the lower back.
Also called ruptured disk; prolapsed disk;
slipped disk.

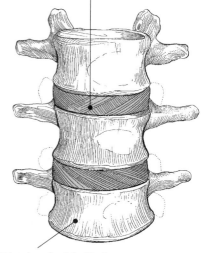

intervertebral disk

anterior view of vertebral body

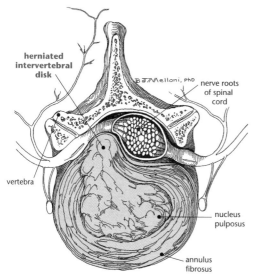

herniated
intervertebral
disk

B.J.Melloni, PhD

nerve roots
of spinal
cord

vertebra

nucleus
pulposus

annulus
fibrosus

intercalated d. A specialized region of cell
membrane and dense adjacent cytoplasm
that marks the junctions between the ends of
cardiac muscle cells, presenting an elaborate,
zigzagged, interdigitated region for
attachment to neighboring cells; it contains
numerous desmosomes that serve as
intercellular bridges and many tight (gap)
junctions that permit intercellular spread of
the excitatory impulse over the muscle;
because of the relative unimpeded flow of
electric current between cells, excitation,
and therefore contraction, quickly
disseminates within the heart.

interpubic d. A midline plate of
fibrocartilage interposed between the pubic
bones at the symphysis; anteriorly, the disk is
strengthened by several superimposed layers
of fibers. Also called interpubic
fibrocartilaginous lamina.

intervertebral d.'s The fibrocartilaginous
pads interposed between the bodies of
adjacent vertebrae, from the axis (second
cervical vertebra) to the sacrum, consisting
of a jellylike center (nucleus pulposus)
surrounded by a fibrous ring (annulus
fibrosus). They act as elastic buffers to absorb
the daily mechanical shocks sustained by the
spinal column. The disks are lacking between
the atlas (first cervical vertebra) and the axis
(second cervical vertebra), and between the
atlas and the lower part of the skull
(occiput). Also called intervertebral
cartilages; intervertebral fibrocartilages.

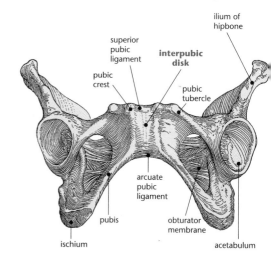

ilium of
hipbone

superior
pubic
ligament

**interpubic
disk**

pubic
crest

pubic
tubercle

arcuate
pubic
ligament

pubis

obturator
membrane

ischium

acetabulum

disk ■ disk

mandibular d. See temporomandibular articular disk.

epiphyseal d. See epiphyseal cartilage, under cartilage.

prolapsed d. See herniated intervertebral disk.

radioulnar d. A triangular articulating disk that holds together the distal (lower) ends of the radius and ulna; the fibrocartilaginous tissue is attached by its broad apex to the styloid process and distal head of the ulna and by its base to the radius; the circumference of the disk is connected to the ligaments of the wrist joint. Also called articular disk of distal radioulnar articulation.

ruptured d. See herniated intervertebral disk.

sacrococcygeal d. A thin disk of fibrocartilage interposed between the apex of the sacrum and the base of the coccyx; the joint is strengthened by ventral, dorsal, and lateral sacrococcygeal ligaments.

slipped disk See herniated intervertebral disk.

sternoclavicular d. A nearly circular articular disk, interposed between the articulating surfaces of the sternal (medial) end of the clavicle and the manubrium of the sternum; its circumference is attached to the articular surface of the clavicle, the cartilage of the first rib and by the articular capsule of the sternoclavicular joint. Also called articular disk of sternoclavicular articulation.

temporomandibular articular d. A somewhat oval disk of fibrocartilage that completely divides the temporomandibular joint into two separate cavities; the lower surface of the disk, in contact with the head of the mandible, is concave in shape, while the upper surface, in contact with the articular fossa and articular tubercle of the temporal bone, is concavoconvex in shape; the circumference of the disk is connected to the articular capsule. Also called articular disk of temporomandibular joint; mandibular disk; temporomandibular membrane.

dislocate (dis'lo-kat) To shift from the usual or normal position, especially to displace a bone from its joint; to luxate.

dislocation (dis-lo-ka'shun) Displacement of a body part from its normal location, especially of a bone from its joint or socket. Also called luxation.

anterior shoulder d. A common dislocation of the shoulder joint marked by the head of the humerus displaced anteriorly out of the glenoid cavity.

Bell-Dally d. A nontraumatic dislocation of the atlas (first cervical vertebra).

Bennett's d. The displacement of the thumb joint between the trapezium bone and the first metacarpal bone.

closed d. Dislocation of a bone occurring without an external wound. Also called simple dislocation.

complete d. A dislocation in which the joint surfaces are entirely separated.

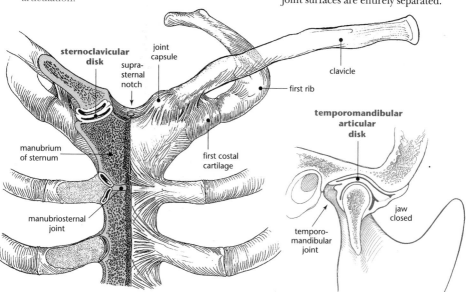

disk ■ dislocation

complicated d. A dislocation with injury sustained to other important nearby structures.

compound d. See open dislocation.

congenital d. A dislocation existing at birth.

congenital d. of hip Congenital dislocation of the femur in a newborn, marked by backward slippage out of the acetabulum of the hipbone, often due to laxity of surrounding ligaments; more commonly occurs in female newborns.

fracture d. One in which the joint of a luxated bone is fractured.

frank d. A dislocation at a joint that is clinically quite evident.

gamekeeper's d. A dislocation of the thumb joint between the first metacarpal bone and the proximal phalanx.

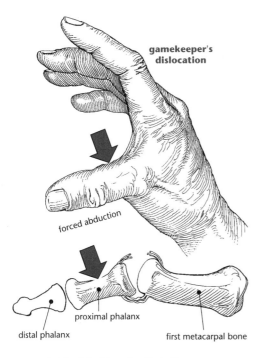

gamekeeper's dislocation

forced abduction

proximal phalanx

distal phalanx

first metacarpal bone

habitual d. A luxation that often recurs after reduction. Also called recurrent dislocation.

incomplete d. An incomplete dislocation of a joint with joint surfaces remaining in partial contact. Also called subluxation; partial dislocation.

Lisfranc's d. Dislocation of the foot joint between the tarsus and the metatarsus.

Kienböck's d. A dislocation of the lunate

bone of the wrist, situated in the proximal carpal row.

Nelaton's d. A severe dislocation of the ankle joint, marked by the talus forcibly wedged between the distal ends of the tibia and the fibula; often accompanied by a fracture.

open d. Dislocation of a bone occurring in conjunction with an open wound. Also called compound dislocation.

partial d. See incomplete dislocation.

pathologic d. Dislocation resulting from a disorder of the joint, its constituent bones, or as a complication of another disease.

posterior shoulder d. An uncommon dislocation of the shoulder joint marked by the head of the humerus displaced posteriorly out of the glenoid cavity.

recent d. A dislocation immediately after the causative injury, prior to the development of complicating inflammation.

recurrent d. See habitual dislocation.

simple d. See closed dislocation.

Smith's d. Backward displacement of the metatarsals and medial cuneiform bone due to an extreme extension injury of the foot.

subclavicular d. Dislocation of the shoulder joint whereby the misplaced head of the humerus lies just below the clavicle.

subcoracoid d. Dislocation of the shoulder joint whereby the misplaced head of the humerus lies just below the coracoid process of the scapula.

subglenoid d. Anterior dislocation of the shoulder joint whereby the misplaced head of the humerus lies beneath the glenoid cavity of the scapula.

subspinous d. Posterior displacement of the shoulder joint whereby the misplaced head of the humerus lies in the subspinous fossa below the spine of the scapula.

vertebral d. Dislocation of any intervertebral disk or vertebra.

voluntary d. Dislocation that can be voluntarily performed, usually without much discomfort.

distad (dis'tad) Toward the periphery.

distal (dis'tal) Farthest from a point of reference.

dolicho- Combining form meaning long.

dolichopelvic (dol-ĭ-ko-pel'vik) Having a long narrow pelvis.

dorsad (dor'sad) In the direction of the back; toward the dorsal surface.

dorsal (dor'sal) Relating to the back of the body or to the posterior part of an anatomic structure.

dislocation ■ dorsal

dorsiflexion (dor-sī-flek'shun) Flexion or bending upward and backward, as of the foot or toes.

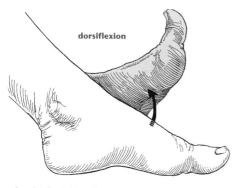

dorsiflexion

dorsispinal (dor-sī-spi'nal) Relating to the back of the body and the vertebral column.

dorso- Combining form meaning the back (posterior) of a structure or of the body.

dorsolumbar (dor-so-lum'bar) Relating to the back of the body between the ribs and the iliac crest; the lumbar region of the back.

dorsoradial (dor-so-ra'de-al) Relating to the radial (outside) border and the back of the forearm or hand.

dorsoscapular (dor-so-skap'u-lar) Relating to the dorsal (posterior) surface of the scapula.

dorsum (dor'sum) The back of the body; the upper or posterior surface of a part (e.g., the top of the foot or the back of a hand).

    d. sellae The part of the sphenoid bone of the skull forming the posterior boundary of the sella turcica.

duct (dukt) A channel or tube, usually for conveying fluid to another part of the body.

    cochlear d. A spirally arranged membranous tube ($2^3/_4$ turns in humans) within the bony canal of the cochlear of the inner ear; it is triangular in transverse section, houses the spiral organ of Corti, and is filled with endolymph; its apex is closed and its base communicates with the saccule by way of the ductus reuniens. Also called scala media; cochlear canal.

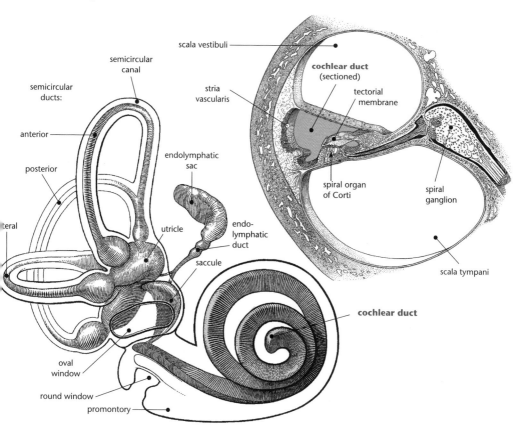

scala vestibuli
semicircular canal
semicircular ducts:
stria vascularis
cochlear duct (sectioned)
tectorial membrane
anterior
posterior
endolymphatic sac
spiral organ of Corti
spiral ganglion
lateral
utricle
endolymphatic duct
saccule
scala tympani
cochlear duct
oval window
round window
promontory

frontonasal d. A fine bony channel in the lateral wall of the nasal cavity that drains the frontal sinus into the middle meatus of the nasal cavity.

nasolacrimal d. A small canal, about 2 cm in length in the adult, which conveys tears from the lacrimal sac to the front part of the inferior nasal meatus.

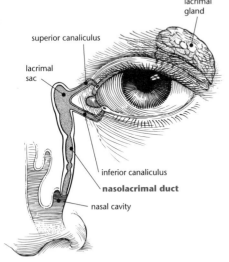

lacrimal gland

superior canaliculus

lacrimal sac

inferior canaliculus

nasolacrimal duct

nasal cavity

perilymphatic d. A minute canal connecting the perilymphatic space of the cochlea with the subarachnoid space. Also called cochlear aqueduct.

dysarthrosis (dis-ar-thro'sis) 1. Malformation of a joint. 2. A false joint.

dyschondrogenesis (dis-kon-dro-jen'ĕ-sis) Defective formation of cartilage.

dysostosis (dis-os-to'sis) Faulty formation of bone, often due to defective ossification of fetal cartilage.

cleidocranial d. An autosomal dominant inheritance marked by partial or complete absence of the clavicles (collarbones) and delay in ossification of the skull, often with underdeveloped facial bones, and defective teeth. Also called cleidocranial dysplasia.

craniofacial d. An autosomal dominant inheritance characterized by a wide skull, widely separated eyes, undersized upper jaw, beaked nose, and exophthalmos.

mandibulofacial d. Abnormalities of the palpebral fissures, lower jaw, zygomatic (cheek) bones, and lower lids, associated with malposition of teeth, low-set malformed ears, and high cleft palate.

dysplasia (dis-pla'se-ah) In pathology, abnormality of cell growth in which some cells in a tissue

have some of the characteristics of malignancy but not enough for a diagnosis of an early cancer; unlike cancer (which is irreversible), dysplastic tissue may sometimes reverse spontaneously to normal.

chondroectodermal d. A disorder inherited as an autosomal recessive trait characterized by short limbs with normal trunk, more than ten fingers (polydactyly), and abnormal development of teeth and nails; frequently associated with heart defects.

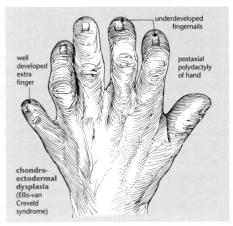

underdeveloped fingernails

well developed extra finger

postaxial polydactyly of hand

chondro-ectodermal dysplasia (Ellis-van Creveld syndrome)

cleidocranial d. See cleidocranial dysostosis, under dysostosis.

dentin d. Hereditary abnormality of dentin formation marked by disarrangement of dentin tubules by masses of collagenous matrix, poorly developed tooth roots with varying amounts of pulpal obliteration; the pulp chamber is filled with an abnormal dentin; inherited as an autosomal dominant trait.

epiphyseal d. Faulty ossification of the epiphyses which interferes with bone development and results in decreased stature.

fibrous d. of bone A benign, progressive condition marked by localized replacement of bone by proliferating fibrous tissue.

dyssynergia (dis-sin-er'je-ah) Disturbance of muscular coordination.

detrusor-sphincter d. Disturbance of the normal coordination between bladder muscles during voiding efforts, i.e., between contraction of the detrusor muscle and relaxation of the urinary sphincter; instead, sphincter spasm occurs simultaneously with bladder contraction.

dystonia (dis-to'ne-ah) Abnormality of muscle tone.

dysarthrosis ■ dystonia

cervical d. Asymmetric muscle spasms of the neck, causing turning or tilting movements and sustained abnormal postures of the head; may be accompanied by moderate head tremor and musculoskeletal pain. Spontaneous remission may occur. Also called spasmodic torticollis.

focal d. Dystonia usually affecting one area of the body; it occasionally affects two contiguous ones.

generalized d. A rare disorder that usually begins in childhood with a gait abnormality or with torticollis (wryneck), resulting in sustained, often bizarre postures. Also called torsion dystonia.

occupational d. A focal dystonia marked by spasm of limited muscles precipitated by voluntary muscle contractions while performing skilled movements, such as writing or playing a musical instrument (writer's cramp, musician's cramp).

oromandibular d. Neurological disorder marked by continuous, bilateral, asynchronous spasms of muscles of the face, lower jaw, pharynx, tongue and, in some severe cases, the neck, larynx, and respiratory system.

torsion d. See generalized dystonia.

dystrophin (dis-tro'fin) Protein present in normal muscle bound to the muscle membrane; it helps to maintain the integrity of the muscle fiber; in its absence, the muscle fiber degenerates, as seen in Duchenne muscular dystrophy.

dystrophy (dis'tro-fe) Disorder caused by faulty nutrition or by lesions of the pituitary (hypophysis) and/or other parts of the brain.

Becker's muscular d. Genetic disorder similar to Duchenne's muscular dystrophy but much milder, occurring later in childhood and progressing at a much slower pace; some patients may remain ambulatory for many years; caused by mutations in the structural gene for the protein dystrophin; an X-linked recessive inheritance.

childhood muscular d. See Duchenne's muscular dystrophy.

Duchenne's muscular d. Genetic disorder occurring as an X-linked recessive inheritance and affecting males almost exclusively; characterized by progressive muscle weakness that starts in the pelvic girdle and spreads rapidly, a swaying gait, frequent falls, and difficulty arising from the floor (the child usually "climbs up his legs"); deposits of fibrofatty tissue replace muscle fibers and may occupy a greater volume than the normal muscle (pseudohypertrophy); may also involve the heart muscle; manifestations of the disorder begin between three and five years of age; death usually occurs by the end of the second decade. The defective gene is in the short arm of the X chromosome. Also called childhood muscular dystrophy.

muscular d. Any of several genetic disorders that are characterized primarily by progressive deterioration of muscle fibers.

myotonic d. Genetic disorder, occurring as an autosomal dominant inheritance (genetic defect on chromosome 19); it typically becomes evident in the second to third decades of life with varying degrees of muscular involvement and severity; symptoms include stiffness and eventual atrophy of muscles, especially of the face and neck, associated with slurred speech and cataracts.

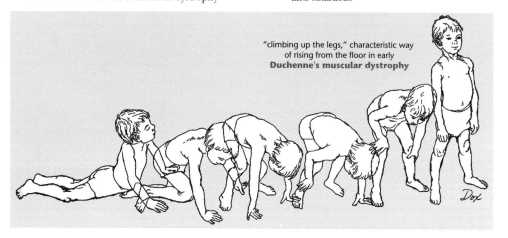

"climbing up the legs," characteristic way of rising from the floor in early **Duchenne's muscular dystrophy**

dystrophin ■ dystrophy

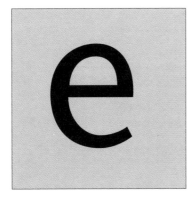

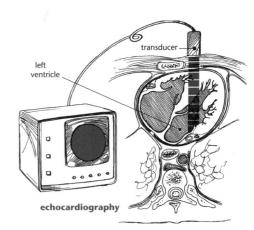

echocardiography

eardrum (ēr'drum) See tympanic membrane, under membrane.

ebonation (e-bon-na'shun) Removal of loose bone fragments from an injury.

eburnation (e-bur-na'shun) The thinning of articular cartilage followed by the transformation of bone into a shiny ivory-like substance; seen in certain degenerative joint diseases such as osteoarthritis.

echocardiogram (ek-o-kar'de-o-gram) A graphic display produced by recording the echoes returned from the heart after the application of ultrasonic impulses; the ultrasound image of the heart.

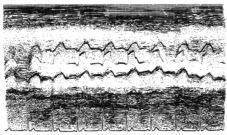

echocardiogram

echocardiography (ek-o-kar-de-og'rah-fe) The placing of an ultrasonic device on the chest wall to send sound impulses toward the walls of the heart, which in turn bounce or echo the sounds back; the patterns produced are graphically displayed for interpretation; used for determining the movement patterns of the heart and its valves, chamber size, wall thickness, and the presence of pericardial fluid.

    cross-sectional e. See two-dimensional echocardiography.

    two-dimensional e. Technique in which the ultrasound beam rapidly moves through an arc, producing a cross-sectional or fan-shaped image of heart structure. Also called cross-sectional echocardiography.

ecto- Prefix meaning on the outside; external.

ectocondyle (ek-to-kon'dīl) The outer or lateral condyle of a bone.

ectomorph (ek'to-morf) A person with a body type configuration in which the limbs predominate over the trunk, and muscles and body are thin; a body build in which the predominating tissues are derived from the ectoderm.

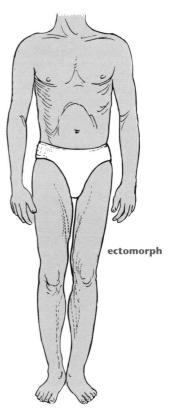

ectomorph

ectosteal (ek-tos'te-al) Relating to or situated on the outside of a bone.

ectostosis (ek-to-sto'sis) Bone formation beginning under the perichondrium and gradually replacing the cartilage model.

effector (ef-fek'tor) A tissue that reacts to a nerve impulse (e.g., a muscular contraction or a glandular secretion).

elasticity (e-las-tis'ĭ-te) The quality of being elastic.

> **physical e. of muscle** The quality of a muscle being elastic that yields to passive stretch.

> **physiologic e. of muscle** The quality of muscle that allows its length to alter in response to stimulation from the nervous system.

> **total e. of muscle** The effect of combining physical elasticity and physiologic elasticity on muscle.

elasto- Combining form meaning elasticity.

elbow (el'bo) The joint between the arm and the forearm.

> **baseball pitcher's e.** Mild cartilage degradation of the radiohumeral joint, caused by trauma, as seen in pitching a baseball repeatedly with great force.

> **bend of the e.** See cubital fossa, under fossa.

> **golfer's e.** See medial humeral epicondylitis, under epicondylitis.

> **miner's e.** See olecranon bursitis, under bursitis.

> **nursemaid's e.** Popular term for a partial dislocation (subluxation) of the head of the radius in which the radial head slips under the annular ligament at the elbow joint, with the ligament remaining intact; it is a common injury of infants and young children (under four years old) as a result of being suddenly pulled or lifted by the arm or hand. The injury is difficult, or impossible to see in x-ray pictures because the radial head may not be ossified. Also called pulled elbow.

> **point of the e.** See olecranon.

> **pulled e.** See nursemaid's elbow.

> **student's e.** See olecranon bursitis, under bursitis.

> **tennis e.** See lateral humeral epicondylitis, under epicondylitis.

electrocontractility (e-lek-tro-kon-trak-til'ĭ-te) The capacity of muscle to contract in response to an electric stimulus.

electrogastrogram (e-lek-tro-gas'tro-gram) The graphic record of the electrical activity of the stomach musculature as measured between the surface of the body and the lumen of the stomach.

electrogoniometer (e-lek-tro-go-ne-om'ĕ-ter) An instrument for measuring angular positions (extension and flexion) of an anatomic hinge joint.

electrohysterogram (e-lek-tro-his'ter-o-gram) A graphic record of electrical activity associated with contractions of the uterine musculature.

electrolaryngogram (e-lek-tro-lah-ring'go-gram) A graphic record of vocal cord activity arising from laryngeal musculature during phonation and respiration.

electromyogram (e-lek-tro-mi'o-gram) A graphic record of electric discharges generated by muscular activity.

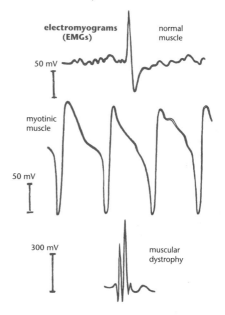

electromyography (e-lek-tro-mi-og'rah-fe) Recording of electric discharges generated by muscular activity with the use of surface or needle electrodes; useful for differentiating diseases of neuromuscular junctions from those of muscles or nerves primarily.

emedullate (e-med'u-lāt) To extract bone marrow.

eminence (em'i-nens) A rounded prominence; a raised area, especially on the surface of a bone.

> **e. of anterior semicircular canal** An arched eminence positioned transversely to the long axis of the petrous part of the temporal bone on the floor of the middle cranial fossa; it approximates the underlying anterior (superior) semicircular canal. Also called arcuate eminence.

ectosteal ■ eminence

BONES OF LEFT **ELBOW** JOINT

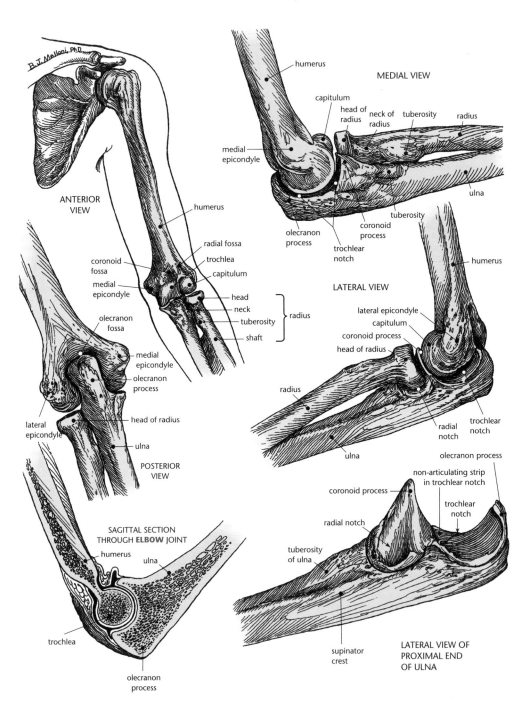

B.J. Melloni, PhD.

ANTERIOR VIEW

humerus

coronoid fossa
medial epicondyle

radial fossa
trochlea
capitulum

head
neck
tuberosity
shaft

radius

olecranon fossa

medial epicondyle
olecranon process

lateral epicondyle

head of radius

ulna

POSTERIOR VIEW

SAGITTAL SECTION THROUGH **ELBOW** JOINT

humerus
ulna

trochlea

olecranon process

MEDIAL VIEW

humerus

capitulum
head of radius
neck of radius
tuberosity
radius

medial epicondyle

ulna

olecranon process

coronoid process
trochlear notch

tuberosity

LATERAL VIEW

humerus

lateral epicondyle
capitulum
coronoid process
head of radius

radius

radial notch

trochlear notch

ulna

olecranon process

non-articulating strip in trochlear notch

coronoid process

trochlear notch

radial notch

tuberosity of ulna

supinator crest

LATERAL VIEW OF PROXIMAL END OF ULNA

arcuate e. See eminence of anterior semicircular canal.

canine e. See cuspid eminence.

coccygeal e.'s See sacral cornua, under cornu.

e. of concha An elevation on the medial surface of the auricular (ear) cartilage, formed by the depression of the concha on the lateral surface.

cruciform e. of occipital bone The cross-shaped bony ridges radiating longitudinally and transversely from the internal occipital protuberance on the inner surface of the occipital bone, creating four fossae; the upper two fossae accommodate the poles of the occipital lobes of the cerebrum; the lower two fossae accommodate the hemispheres of the cerebellum; in addition, the superior ridge contains a groove (sulcus) for the superior sagittal sinus and the horizontal ridges have grooves (sulci) for the transverse sinuses.

cuspid e. A prominent ridge on the surface of the maxilla that corresponds to the root of the cuspid tooth. Also called canine eminence; canine prominence.

deltoid e. See deltoid tuberosity of humerus, under tuberosity.

frontal e. The rounded elevation on the frontal bone of the skull on either side, a short distance above the orbit; it indicates the site where ossification of the frontal bone first occurred. Also called frontal protuberance.

hypothenar e. The fleshy eminence on the medial side of the palm, produced mostly by the three intrinsic muscles that oppose, abduct, and flex the little finger.

iliopubic e. The rounded elevation on the medial border of the hipbone that marks the union of the superior ramus of the pubic bone with the body of the ilium. Also called iliopectineal crest.

intercondylar e. of tibia A pointed elevation on the upper surface of the front of the tibia intervening between the articular surfaces of the two condyles; the lateral and medial intercondylar tubercles project upward from the eminence. Also called tibial spine; intercondylar process of tibia.

parietal e. The most prominent part of the parietal bone of the skull on either side, just above the superior temporal line; it indicates the site where ossification of the parietal bone first occurred; it can be readily felt. Also called parietal protuberance.

pyramidal e. A small, hollow, conical bony projection on the posterior wall of the middle ear chamber, immediately behind the oval window; it houses the stapedius muscle, whose tendon leaves by a small apical aperture to attach to the posterior surface of the neck of the stapes. Also called pyramid of tympanum.

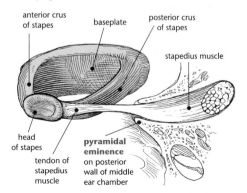

anterior crus of stapes — baseplate — posterior crus of stapes

stapedius muscle

head of stapes — tendon of stapedius muscle — **pyramidal eminence** on posterior wall of middle ear chamber

radial e. of wrist The tubercles of the scaphoid bone and trapezium bone forming an eminence on the palmar aspect of the radial (lateral) side of the wrist, and creating the lateral border of the carpal groove, which becomes the carpal tunnel when a fibrous retinaculum is attached to the bony margins.

supracondylar e. See epicondyle.

thenar e. The bulging prominence at the base of the thumb on the lateral aspect of the palm of the hand; it is created mainly by the three intrinsic muscles that flex, abduct, and oppose the thumb.

ulnar e. of wrist The pisiform bone and the hook of the hamate bone forming an

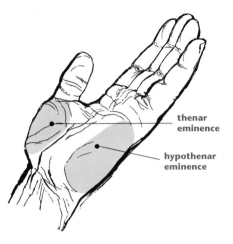

thenar eminence

hypothenar eminence

eminence ■ eminence

eminence on the palmar aspect of the ulnar (medial) side of the wrist, and creating the medial border of the carpal groove, which becomes the carpal tunnel when a fibrous retinaculum is attached to the bony margins.

enamel (en-am'el) The hard, translucent substance covering the anatomic crowns of teeth, reaching a thickness of about 2.5 mm over the cusps and diminishing markedly as it approaches the cervical margin.

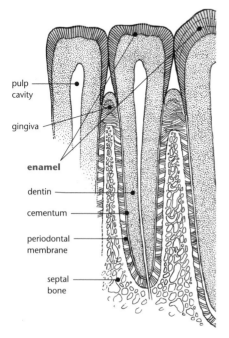

pulp
cavity

gingiva

enamel

dentin

cementum

periodontal
membrane

septal
bone

enarthrodial (en-ar-thro'de-al) Relating to a ball and socket joint (enarthrosis), as in the hip joint.

enarthrosis (en-ar-thro'sis) See ball and socket joint, under joint.

enchondroma (en-kon-dro'mah) A benign growth composed of mature cartilage developed within a bone; it is usually asymptomatic but may cause pain, bone deformity, and fracture.

enchondromatosis (en-kon-dro-mah-to'sis) A nonhereditary condition characterized by the presence of multiple enchondromas in a long bone, resulting in shortening of the limb. Also called dyschondroplasia.

enchondrosarcoma (en-kon-dro-sar-ko'mah) Malignant tumor within a bone, arising from a preexisting cartilaginous growth.

ending (end'ing) A termination, as of a nerve.

annulospiral nerve e. The principal sensory

nerve terminal in a muscle (neuromuscular) spindle, comprised of branches that coil around the intrafusal voluntary muscle fiber at its central point (nuclear region); sensitive to stretch of muscle length. Also called primary nerve ending.

flower-spray nerve e. A sensory nerve terminal in a muscle (neuromuscular) spindle, comprised of spraylike beaded configurations on the intrafusal voluntary muscle fiber at the sites away from the central point (nuclear region); sensitive to increased muscle tension. Also called secondary nerve ending.

free nerve e.'s Unmyelinated nerve endings that branch repeatedly to form networks, found in many different sites throughout the body including the skin, mucous membranes, fascia, joint capsules, ligaments, tendons, blood vessels, meninges, bones, and muscles; they are usually of small diameter and low conduction speed and respond to different stimuli including pain, light touch, tickle, and itch sensations. Also called nonencapsulated neve endings.

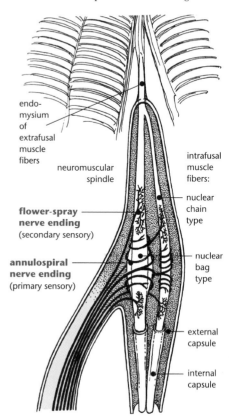

endo-
mysium
of
extrafusal
muscle
fibers

neuromuscular
spindle

intrafusal
muscle
fibers:

nuclear
chain
type

**flower-spray
nerve ending**
(secondary sensory)

**annulospiral
nerve ending**
(primary sensory)

nuclear
bag
type

external
capsule

internal
capsule

nonencapsulated nerve e.'s See free nerve endings.

primary nerve e. See annulospiral nerve ending.

secondary nerve e. See flower-spray nerve ending.

synaptic e. The knoblike terminal part of an axon where chemical transmitter substances are released from synaptic vesicles to adjoining neurons for the chemical transmission of impulses.

endo-, end- Prefixes meaning within.

endocardial (en-do-kar'de-al) 1. Relating to, or situated within, the inner lining of the heart chambers (endocardium). 2. Within the heart.

endocardium (en-do-kar'de-um) The innermost layer of the heart lining the muscular chambers, composed of endothelium and fibroelastic tissue; it is continuous with the endothelium of the great blood vessels and by folding on itself, it forms the basic structure of the heart valves.

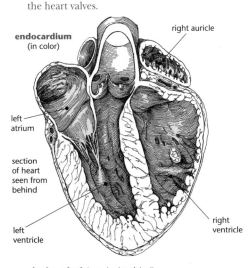

endocardium (in color)

right auricle

left atrium

section of heart seen from behind

left ventricle

right ventricle

endochondral (en-do-kon'dral) See intracartilaginous.

endocranium (en-do-kra'ne-um) The membrane lining and adhered to the inner surface of the cranium, composed of the outer zone of the dura mater; by passing through the cranial foramina, it becomes continuous with the periosteum on the outer surface of the cranium.

endolymph (en'do-limf) The fluid in the closed system of channels (membranous labyrinth) of the inner ear.

endometrium (en-do-me'tre-um) The inner mucous membrane lining the uterine musculature, divisible into three layers; the deepest

(basal) layer is not shed during menstruation and remains adhered to the muscular wall to provide a basis for regeneration after each mesntrual period.

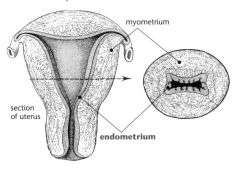

myometrium

section of uterus

endometrium

endomorph (en'do-morf) A body type in which, from a morphologic standpoint, the trunk predominates over the limbs.

endomysium (en-do-mis'e-um) The delicate connective tissue surrounding individual muscle fibers.

endoskeleton (en-do-skel'e-ton) The internal bony structures (skeleton) of vertebrates.

endosonoscopy (en-do-son-o-sko'pe) Ultrasonic scanning conducted by introducing transducers, serving as miniature probes, into hollow or tubular structures.

endosseous (en-dos'e-us) Within bone.

endosteal (en-dos'te-al) Relating to the vascular membrane lining the interior cavity of bones.

endosteitis (en-dos-te-i'tis) Inflammation of the membrane lining the inner cavities of bones.

endosteoma (en-dos-te-o'mah) Benign tumor in the internal, medullary cavity of a bone.

endosteum (en-dos'te-um) Highly vascular alveolar tissue lining the inner surface of the medullary cavity and intratrabecular spaces of bones.

endplate, end plate (end'plat) The terminal part of a motor nerve fiber that transmits nerve impulses to muscle.

motor e. See neuromuscular junction, under junction.

enostosis (en-os-to'sis) An abnormal bony growth within the medullary cavity of a bone.

ensiform (en'sĭ-form) Shaped like a sword; xiphoid.

entad (en'tad) Toward the interior; inwardly.

enthesitis (en-thĕ-si'tis) Irritation of muscular attachment to bones, usually provoked by recurring muscle stress.

enthlasis (en'thlah-sis) A comminuted depressed fracture of the skull.

epi- Prefix meaning upon.

endo-, end- ■ **epi-**

epicondyle (ep-ĭ-kon'dĭl) Any bony protuberance on or above the smooth articular eminence of a long bone (condyle). Also called supracondylar eminence.

external e. of femur See lateral epicondyle of femur.

external e. of humerus See lateral epicondyle of humerus.

internal e. of femur See medial epicondyle of femur.

internal e. of humerus See medial epicondyle of humerus.

lateral e. of femur The short, most lateral prominence of the lower femur, just above the lateral condyle; it gives attachment to the fibular (lateral) collateral ligament of the knee joint; it can be felt through the skin. Also called external epicondyle of femur.

lateral e. of humerus The blunt, most lateral prominence of the lower humerus, just above the capitulum; it gives attachment anterolaterally to the radial (lateral) collateral ligament of the elbow joint, and to the tendon common to the origin of the supinator and some of the extensor muscles of the forearm; posteriorly, it gives attachment to the anconeus muscle; it is palpable posteriorly, especially with the elbow flexed. Also called external epicondyle of humerus; lateral condyle of humerus.

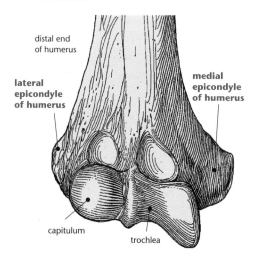

distal end of humerus

lateral epicondyle of humerus

medial epicondyle of humerus

capitulum

trochlea

medial e. of femur A large medial convex prominence of the lower femur just above the medial condyle and slightly in front of the adductor tubercle; it gives attachment to the tibial (medial) collateral ligament of the knee joint. Also called internal epicondyle of femur.

medial e. of humerus A conspicuous prominence of the lower humerus, just above and medial to the trochlea; it gives attachment to the ulnar (medial) collateral ligament of the elbow joint below, to the round pronator (pronator teres) muscle above, and to a common tendon of origin of most of the forearm's flexor muscles in the middle; it can be felt through the skin at the back of the elbow; the ulnar nerve passes directly behind it. Also called internal epicondyle of humerus; medial condyle of humerus.

epicondylitis (ep-ĭ-kon-dĭ-li'tis) Inflammation of tissues surrounding a bony prominence (epicondyle) at a joint.

lateral humeral e. Chronic pain and tenderness of tendons on the outer side of the elbow, near the lateral epicondyle of the humerus, usually due to repetitive strenuous rotatory motion of the wrist against resistance (as in manual screwdriving), or forceful extension of the wrist with the hand in a pronated position (as in playing tennis). Also called tennis elbow.

medial humeral e. Inflammation of the tissues adjoining the medial epicondyle of the humerus, especially of the flexor muscles of the forearm arising from the condyle; marked by pain and stiffness of the elbow joint accompanied by generalized tenderness of the entire forearm; seen in some golfers. Also called golfer's elbow.

epimysium (ep-ĭ-mis'e-um) Connective tissue surrounding a skeletal muscle.

epiphysiodesis (ep-ĭ-fiz-e-od'ě-sis) 1. Premature fusion of the end (epiphysis) of a long bone and its shaft (diaphysis), resulting in arrest of longitudinal bone growth. 2. Surgical destruction of the epiphyseal plate of a long bone to arrest growth of the bone shaft prematurely (e.g., to equalize the length of the legs).

epiphysiolysis (ep-ĭ-fiz-e-ol'ĭ-sis) Loosening or separation of an epiphysis from the shaft of a long bone, generally resulting in some lengthening of the bone; usually performed on the upper femoral epiphysis.

epiphysis (ě-pif'ĭ-sis), pl. epiph'yses The end of a long bone, developed and ossified separately from the shaft (diaphysis) and initially separated from the latter by a plate of cartilage.

epiphysitis (ě-pif-ĭ-si'tis) Inflammation of an epiphysis.

traumatic tibial e. A knee injury most commonly seen in adolescents active in sports; produced when the powerful vastus muscle complex, which inserts into a small area of the

epicondyle ■ epiphysitis

tibial tuberosity, exerts a sufficiently forceful contraction to separate a small portion of bone in an area of developmental bone formation; symptoms include a "knee knob" or protrusion below the patella, tenderness elicited by pressure, and pain when the knee is extended against resistance.

episternal (ep-ĭ-ster′nal) Over the sternum.

epitympanic (ep-ĭ-tim-pan′ik) Situated in the middle ear chamber above the level of the tympanic membrane; it contains most of the incus and part of the malleus ossicles.

equinocavus (e-kwi-no-kav′us) See talipes cavus, under talipes.

equinovalgus (e-kwi-no-val′gus) See talipes equinovalgus, under talipes.

equinovarus (e-kwi-no-va′rus) See talipes equinovarus, under talipes.

equinus (e-kwi′nus) See talipes equinus, under talipes.

erector (ĕ-rek′tor) A structure (e.g., a muscle) that raises and holds up a part.

eruption (e-rup′shun) The breaking out, so as to become visible, especially the appearance of a tooth piercing the gingiva.

ethmoid (eth′moid) Resembling a sieve (e.g., the ethmoid bone).

ethmoidal (eth-moi′dal) Relating to the ethmoid bone.

ethmoidectomy (eth-moi-dek′to-me) Removal of portions of the ethmoid bone.

ethmoiditis (eth-moi-di′tis) Inflammation of the mucous membrane lining the ethmoid bone.

ethmofrontal (eth-mo-fron′tal) Relating to both the ethmoid and frontal bones.

ethmolacrimal (eth-mo-lak′ri-mal) Relating to both the ethmoid and lacrimal bones.

ethmomaxillary (eth-mo-mak′sĭ-lar-e) Relating to both the ethmoid and maxillary bones.

ethmonasal (eth-mo-na′zal) Relating to both the ethmoid and nasal bones.

ethmopalatine (eth-mo-pal′ah-tin) Relating to both the ethmoid and palatine bones.

ethmosphenoid (eth-mo-sfe′noid) Relating to both the ethmoid and sphenoid bones.

ethmovomerine (eth-mo-vo′mer-in) Relating to both the ethmoid and vomer bones.

eury- Combining form meaning wide.

eurygnathic (u-rig-nath′ik) Having a wide jaw.

euryon (u′re-on) A point on the right and the left sides of the head (on each parietal bone) marking the longest transverse diameter of the head.

evertor (e-ver′tor) A muscle that turns a part, such as the hand, outward.

evulsion (e-vul′shun) Removed by force; forcible extraction.

excise (ek-sīz′) To cut away; to cut off.

excision (ek-sizh′un) Removal of a structure by cutting.

exostosis (ek-sos-to′sis) Any benign bony outgrowth from the surface of a bone, usually in response to repeated trauma or inflammation.

extension (ek-sten′shun) The straightening out of a flexed extremity.

extensor (eks-ten′sor) Any muscle that, by contracting, extends a joint, such as in the straightening of an extremity.

extortor (eks-tor′tor) An ocular muscle that causes the outward rotation of the vertical meridian of the cornea, namely, the inferior oblique muscle when the eye is abducted, and the inferior rectus muscle when it is adducted.

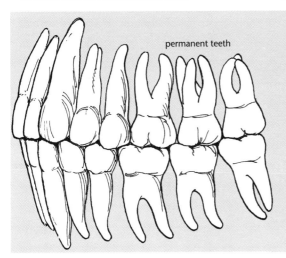

permanent teeth

eruption of permanent teeth

central incisors	6–8 years
lateral incisors	7–9 years
cuspids	9–12 years
first bicuspids	10–12 years
second bicuspids	10–12 years
first molars	6–7 years
second molars	11–13 years
third molars	17–21 years

episternal ■ extortor

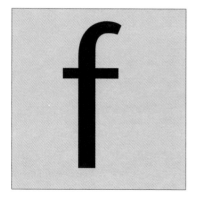

fabella (fah-bel'ah) A small sesamoid bone sometimes found in the tendon of the lateral head of the gastrocnemius muscle, behind the knee joint.

facet (fas'et) A small, highly smooth surface, such as an articulating surface on a bone.

    acromial f. The small, oval facet on the medial end of the acromion of the scapula that articulates with the lateral end of the clavicle.

    anterior articular f. of talus The small, oval, concave articular facet on the bottom of the head of the talus, often continuous with the middle articular facet, which articulates with the superior surface of the calcaneus.

    anterior calcaneal f. The small, oval articular facet on the top of the calcaneus that articulates with the overlying talus; of the three articular surfaces on the top of the calcaneus, it is the most anterior and the smallest.

    articular f. A flat or rounded facet on a bone at the site of articulation with another bone.

auricular f. of sacrum The ear-shaped articular facet on the lateral surface of the upper sacrum that, along with the ilium, forms the sacroiliac joint.

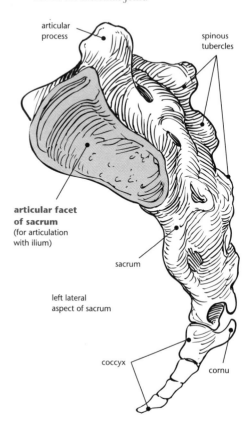

circular articular f. of atlas The small, oval, concave facet on the back of the anterior arch of the atlas (first cervical vertebra) that articulates with the dens, the toothlike process of the underlying axis (second cervical vertebra).

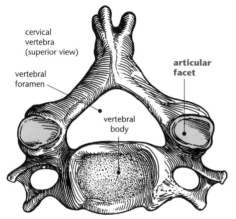

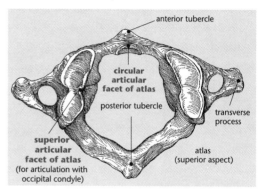

fabella ■ facet

clavicular f. The large concave facet on each side of the sternal notch of the manubrium that articulates with the medial end of the clavicle, and contains an intervening articular disk.

costal f. of sternum Any of the seven facets on each side of the lateral borders of the sternum that articulates with the first seven costal cartilages.

inferior articular f. of atlas The large, circular, slightly concave facet on the lower aspect of each side of the atlas (first cervical vertebra) that articulates with the superior facet of the axis (second cervical vertebra).

inferior costal f. of vertebra Costal facet on each side of the lower edge of the body of a vertebra; it articulates with the upper (smaller) facet of the head of a rib. Also called inferior demifacet for head of rib; inferior costal fovea.

lateral malleolar f. of talus The triangular articular facet on the lateral border of the talus (ankle bone) that articulates with the lateral malleolus of the fibula.

medial malleolar f. of talus The comma-shaped articular facet on the medial border of the talus (ankle bone) that articulates with the medial malleolus of the tibia.

middle articular f. of talus The oblong middle facet on the plantar surface of the neck of the talus, often continuous with the anterior articular facet, which articulates with the sustentaculum tali of the calcaneus.

posterior articular f. of talus The transversely-placed, concave articular facet on the bottom of the talus that articulates with the posterior articular surface of the calcaneus.

posterior calcaneal f. The large, oval, convex articular facet in the middle of the top of the calcaneus that articulates with the overlying talus; of the three articular surfaces on the top of the calcaneus, it is the most posterior.

posterior middle calcaneal f. An oval articular facet on the sustentaculum tali at the top of the calcaneus that articulates with the overlying talus; located between the anterior and posterior facets.

sternal articular f. of clavicle The quadrangular-shaped articular facet on the medial end of the clavicle that articulates with the clavicular notch of the manubrium on each side and containing an intervening articular disk.

superior articular f. of atlas The large, bean-shaped, concave articular facet on the upper aspect of each side of the atlas (first cervical vertebra) that articulates with the occipital condyle of the skull.

superior costal f. of vertebra Costal facet on each side of the upper edge of the body of a vertebra; it articulates with the lower (larger) facet of the head of a rib. Also called superior demifacet for head of rib; superior costal fovea.

f. of tubercle of rib Any of a small articular facet on the tubercle of a rib that articulates with most corresponding thoracic vertebra in forming the costotransverse joint.

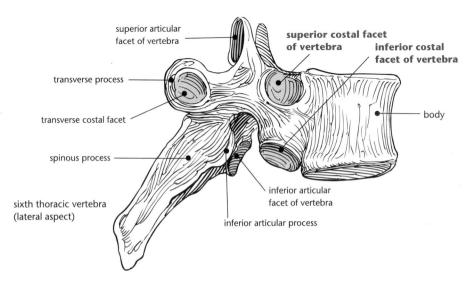

superior articular facet of vertebra

superior costal facet of vertebra

inferior costal facet of vertebra

transverse process

transverse costal facet

spinous process

body

inferior articular facet of vertebra

inferior articular process

sixth thoracic vertebra (lateral aspect)

facet ■ facet

facetectomy (fas-ĕ-tek'to-me) Surgical removal of an articular facet (e.g., of a vertebra).

fascia (fash'e-ah) An aggregation of connective tissue that lies just under the skin or forms an investment for muscles and various organs.

    f. of abdominal wall A thick subcutaneous fascia comprised of a superficial fatty layer (Camper's fascia) and a deeper membranous layer (Scarpa's fascia), between which are superficial lymph nodes, vessels, and nerves; it is continuous with the superficial fascia of the perineum and the superficial fascia of the thigh; in the male, it is continuous with the fascia in the penis and scrotum; in the female, it is continuous with the fascia in the labia majora.

    antebrachial f. See deep fascia of forearm.

    axillary f. A thick layer of fascia conforming to the concavity of the armpit; it extends from the lower border of the greater pectoral muscle (pectoralis major) in front, to the lower border of the latissimus dorsi muscle behind.

    brachial f. The deep fascia investing the muscles of the arm and epicondyles of the humerus; continuous with the axillary fascia proximally and the deep fascia of forearm distally.

    buccopharyngeal f. The thin external layer of the fibrous epimysium surrounding the constrictor muscles of the pharynx; it blends superiorly with the pharyngobasilar fascia at the base of the skull and extends forward over the buccinator muscle.

    Buck's f. See fascia of penis, deep.

    Camper's f. The thick subcutaneous fatty layer of the superficial fascia of the lower part of the anterior abdominal wall; it is continuous with the superficial fascia of the thigh and perineum, and in the male, with the penis and scrotum; in the female, with the fascia of the labia majora.

    cervical f. The superficial fascia of the neck.

    clavipectoral f. The strong fibrous fascia underlying the clavicular part of the pectoralis major muscle lying between the subclavius muscle above and the pectoralis minor muscle below; medially, it attaches to the first rib; laterally, to the coracoid process of the scapula; superiorly, to the clavicle; inferiorly, it fuses with the axillary fascia.

    f. of clitoris A dense fibrous sheath that encases the two corpora cavernosa of the clitoris; it is continuous with the suspensory ligament of the clitoris.

    Colles' f. The deep membranous layer of the superficial fascia of the perineum; it is of considerable strength and is continuous with the fascia of the penis (less demarcated with the fascia of the clitoris) and the membranous layer of the superficial fascia of the anterior abdominal wall.

    coracoclavicular f. A strong, thickened fascia situated under the clavicular portion of the greater pectoral muscle (pectoralis major); it occupies the interval between the smaller pectoral (pectoralis minor) and subclavius muscles, protecting the axillary

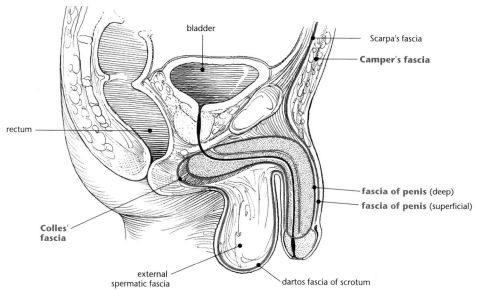

bladder

Scarpa's fascia

Camper's fascia

rectum

fascia of penis (deep)

fascia of penis (superficial)

Colles' fascia

external spermatic fascia

dartos fascia of scrotum

facetectomy ■ **fascia**

vessels and nerves. Above, it divides to enclose the subclavius muscle and the clavicle.

cremasteric f. The part of the fascia of the cremasteric muscle that invests the spermatic cord and testis; it contains discrete strands of muscle, which, when contracted elevate the testis toward the body.

crural f. See fascia of leg.

deep f. A compact fascia composed mostly of collagen fibers that lies beneath the superficial fascia and invests the trunk, neck, limbs, and parts of the head; it also covers and holds the muscles and other structures in their proper positions, separating them or joining them for independent or integrated function.

deep cervical f. The deep fascia of the neck extending between and around muscles, viscera, and vessels; it forms the pretracheal and the prevertebral fascial layers; it is continuous behind with the nuchal ligament, below it attaches to the clavicle, and above it attaches to the lower margin of the mandible and mastoid process.

deep f. of forearm The deep dense fascia of the forearm investing the muscles and sending septa between them to attach on bone. Two thickenings of the fascial sheath occur near the wrist to help retain the digital tendons in their proper position, namely the extensor retinaculum posteriorly and the flexor retinaculum anteriorly. Also called antebrachial fascia.

Denonvillier's f. Fascia located between the rectum behind and the prostate in front.

dorsal f. of foot The thin fascial layer on the dorsum of the foot, continuous above with the inferior retinaculum and extending anteriorly to ensheath the extensor tendons and to the sides of the foot where it blends with the plantar aponeurosis.

dorsal f. of hand The deep fascia on the back of the hand that blends with the deep fascia of the forearm above and fuses with the tendons on the back of the fingers.

Dupuytren's f. See palmar aponeurosis, under aponeurosis.

endothoracic f. The thin fascial sheath that lines the internal surface of the chest (thoracic) cavity, between the parietal pleura and the periosteum of the ribs and sternum.

iliac f. The fascia that covers the iliopsoas muscle; it is especially thin above, but thickens as it descends toward the inguinal ligament forming a septum that extends between the inguinal ligament and the hipbone.

inferior f. of pelvic diaphragm The layer of fascia covering the lower surface of the paired levator ani and coccygeus muscles (pelvic diaphragm). Also called inferior layer of pelvic diaphragm.

f. lata The deep, broad fascia investing the muscles of the thigh and hip; on the lateral side of the thigh, it forms the strong, thick iliotibial tract. Also called femoral aponeurosis.

f. of leg The deep fascia of the leg; above, it is continuous with the fascia lata and attaches to the patella, the condyles of the tibia and the head of the fibula; laterally, it is continuous with the anterior and posterior crural intermuscular septa and the deep transverse fascia of the leg; posteriorly, it is continuous with the thinner popliteal fascia; below, it is continuous with the extensor, flexor, and peroneal retinacula. Also called crural fascia.

lumbar f. See thoracolumbar fascia.

lumbodorsal f. See thoracolumbar fascia.

f. of nape See nuchal fascia.

nuchal f. Fascia of the back of the neck; it overlies the cervical part of the sacrospinal muscle. Also called fascia of nape.

obturator f. The parietal fascia that covers the pelvic surface of the internal obturator muscle; it is continuous with the iliac fascia and is attached to the pubic bone; it helps form the obturator canal.

palmar f. See palmar aponeurosis, under aponeurosis.

parotid f. Strong fascia that extends from the deep cervical fascia and invests the parotid gland, covers the masseter muscle and is attached to the zygomatic arch.

pectoral f. Fascia that invests the greater pectoral muscle (pectoralis major); it is attached to the sternum and clavicle and is continuous with neighboring fascia.

pelvic f. Fascia of the pelvis, composed of two layers: *Parietal pelvic f.*, fascial sheaths of the pelvic muscles, above the level of origin of the levator ani and coccygeus muscles; *Visceral pelvic f.*, fascial sheaths from around the pelvic organs and their blood vessels and nerves to the upper surface of the levator ani and coccygeus muscles.

f. of penis Connective tissue enveloping the penis, composed of two layers: *Deep f. of penis,* a deep fascial sheath of the penis, continuous with Scarpa's fascia of the abdomen and Colles' fascia of the perineum; also called Buck's fascia; *Superficial f. of penis*, the shallow, loose areolar tissue enveloping the penis, continuous with Camper's fascia, the superficial fascia of the abdominal wall.

plantar f. See plantar aponeurosis, under aponeurosis.

renal f. A sheath of fascia that surrounds the kidney and perirenal fat; formed from retroperitoneal connective tissue; connected to the fibrous capsule of the kidney by minute trabeculae.

Scarpa's f. The deep membranous or fibrous layer of the superficial fascia of the lower part of the anterior abdominal wall; it is continuous with the deep membranous layer of the superficial fascia of the perineum (Colles' fascia).

subcutaneous f. See superficial fascia.

subscapular f. The thin fascia adhered to the circumference of the subscapular fossa, and from which arise some fibers of the subscapular muscle. Also called subscapular aponeurosis.

superficial f. A loose collection or layer of connective tissue just below the skin; composed mostly of collagen fibers, it allows the skin freedom of movement and acts as a thermal insulator. Also called subcutaneous fascia; hypodermis.

superior f. of pelvic diaphragm The layer of fascia covering the upper surface of the paired levator ani and coccygeus muscles (pelvic diaphragm). Also called superior layer of pelvic diaphragm.

temporal f. A fibrous, fan-shaped investment (aponeurosis) covering the temporal muscle on the side of the head, attached above to the superior temporal line of the cranium, and below to the zygomatic arch.

thoracolumbar f. The fascia that covers the deep muscles of the back of the trunk and is continuous above with the deep fascia of the back of the neck; in the thorax the fascia is thin and attaches to the spinous processes of the thoracic vertebrae and to the angles of the ribs; in the lumbar region the fascia divides into three layers: the posterior layer is attached to the sacral and lumbar spinous processes; the middle layer to the ends of the lumbar transverse processes, as well as to the iliac crest and the lower border of the last rib; the anterior layer covers the quadrate muscle of loins (quadratus lumborum) and is attached to the lumbar transverse

processes and iliolumbar ligament; all three layers unite to form the aponeurosis of the abdominal transverse muscle. Also called the lumbar fascia; lumbodorsal fascia.

transverse f. The thin fascia between the inner surface of the transverse muscle of abdomen and the peritoneum; behind, it fuses with the thoracolumbar fascia; superiorly, with the diaphragmatic fascia; inferiorly, with the iliac fascia and is attached to the iliac crest.

triangular f. See reflex inguinal ligament, under ligament.

fasciculation (fah-sik-u-la'shun) Independent random contraction or twitching of all or most of the fibers of a motor unit of a muscle; a coarser form of muscular contraction than fibrillation.

fasciculus (fah-sik'u-lus), pl. fascic'uli A bundle of fibers all with the same orientation, especially applicable to nerve fibers or tracts, but also includes the specialized impulse-conveying muscular fibers of the heart.

fasciectomy (fas-e-ek'to-me) Surgical removal of part of a fascia (e.g., the fascia lata).

fasciitis (fas-e-i'tis) Inflammation of a fascia.

femoral (fem'or-al) Relating to the femur or to the thigh.

femur (fe'mur) The thighbone; the longest bone in the body. See also table of bones in appendix I.

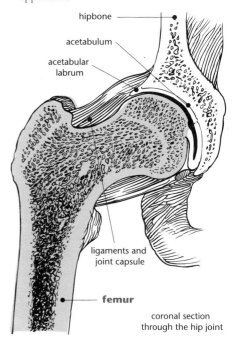

coronal section
through the hip joint

fenestra (fĕ-nes'trah), pl fenes'trae A small window-like opening in the body, especially, either of two openings in the medial wall of the middle ear chamber.

    f. of cochlea See round window, under window.

    f. ovalis See oval window, under window.

    f. rotunda See round window, under window.

    f. of vestibule See oval window, under window.

fenestrated (fen'es-trāt-ed) Having one or more small openings.

fiber (fi'ber) Any slender threadlike process, structure, or material; a filament.

    bone f.'s See Sharpey's fibers.

    bulbospiral f.'s A group of heart muscle fibers that form part of the spiral musculature of the atrial and ventricular walls of the heart.

    cardiac muscle f.'s A network of branching and anastomosing muscle fibers of the heart marked by striations similar to those of skeletal muscle fibers; their ends display conspicuous cross striations (intercalated disks).

    cardiac pressor f.'s See pressor fibers.

    collagen f.'s The white and inelastic fibers making up the principal constituent of connective tissue, the predominant component of ligaments, tendons, and fascia, as well as an essential part of bone and cartilage.

    EF f. See extrafusal muscle fiber.

    elastic f.'s Yellowish fibers that stretch easily forming a network in the substance of loose connective tissue, elastic cartilage, the dermis of the skin, and the walls of large blood vessels; composed mostly of the protein elastin along with other constituents, including traces of collagen. Also called elastin fibers.

    elastin f.'s See elastic fibers.

    extrafusal muscle f. Any skeletal muscle fiber excluding the intrafusal fibers in muscle (neuromuscular) spindles. Also called EF fiber.

    IF f. See intrafusal muscle fiber.

    intrafusal muscle f. One of six to 14 fine, small, specialized muscle fibers composing a muscle (neuromuscular) spindle; innervated by both motor and sensory nerve endings. Also called IF fiber.

    muscular f.'s Fibers composed of contractile elements of striate, cardiac, and smooth muscular tissue.

    nonstriated muscle f.'s See smooth muscle fibers.

    Purkinje's f.'s Specialized fibers formed of modified heart muscle cells, located beneath the endocardium, that are capable of transmitting excitatory impulses from the atrioventricular (A-V) node to the muscles of the ventricles.

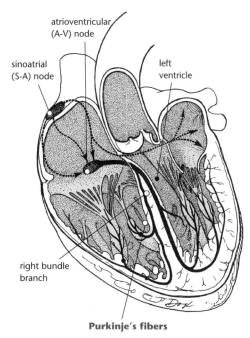

Purkinje's fibers

    red f. See type I muscle fiber.

    red muscle f. See type I muscle fiber.

    Sharpey's f.'s Thick perforating collagenous or fibroelastic bundles that attach tendons, ligaments, fascia, or periosteum to the underlying bone; they pierce the bone obliquely or at right angles to the long axis. Also called bone fibers.

    skeletal muscle f.'s Long, parallel muscle fibers with cross-sectional dimensions of about 10 to 100 μm; marked by transverse striations and nuclei positioned just under the cell membrane (sarcolemma)

    smooth muscle f.'s Narrow and tapering muscle fibers ranging in length from 20 μm in small blood vessels to 500 μm in the pregnant uterus; unlike the striated muscle fibers, the smooth muscle fibers contain no transverse striations. Also called nonstriated muscle fibers.

    type I muscle f. Small skeletal muscle fiber that is rich in large mitochondria,

fenestra ■ fiber

myoglobin, and oxidative enzymes; it is reddish in color. Also called red muscle fiber; red fiber.

type II muscle f. Large skeletal muscle fiber that is low in mitochondrial content and oxidative enzymes, but relatively rich in glycogen and phosphatase enzyme; it is whitish in color. Also called white muscle fiber; white fiber.

white f. See type II muscle fiber.

White muscle f. See type II muscle fiber.

fibril (fi'bril) A delicate thin fiber or filament.

muscle f. See myofibril.

fibrillation (fi-bri-la'shun) The rapid, uncoordinated, and ineffective contraction of single muscle fibers, not of the muscle as a whole.

atrial f. A cardiac arrhythmia in which the normal rhythmic contractions of the muscular wall of the atria are replaced by rapid uncoordinated quivers; not all of the impulses pass through the A-V node.

atrial fibrillation

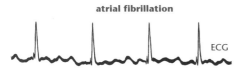

ECG

ventricular f. A cardiac arrhythmia in which rapid, irregular twitching of the muscular wall of the ventricles replaces the normal rhythmic contractions; the rhythm does not permit effective ventricular contraction.

fibrocartilage (fi-bro-kar'ti-lij) A type of cartilage containing collagen fibers; found in such structures as intervertebral disks.

intervertebral f. See intervertebral disk, under disk.

white f. Dense white fibrous tissue interspersed with scattered groups of cartilage cells (chondrocytes) between the bundles, and surrounded by relatively sparse concentrically striated areas of cartilage matrix; in bulk, it provides great tensile strength and elasticity to a structure, as in intervertebral disks, and in lesser amounts, provides considerable toughness and elasticity to a structure, as in articular disks.

yellow f. See elastic cartilage, under cartilage.

fibroid (fi'broid) 1. Commonly used term for a tumor more properly called leiomyoma, since the tumor mass is primarily composed of smooth muscle rather than fibrous tissue. See

leiomyoma. 2. Composed of or resembling fibrous tissue.

fibromuscular (fi-bro-mus'ku-lar) Denoting tissues with both fibrous and muscular components.

fibromyositis (fi-bro-mi-o-si'tis) Chronic inflammation of a muscle with overgrowth of its connective tissue.

fibrositis (fi-bro-si'tis) Inflammatory proliferation of fibrous or connective tissue in the muscles.

fibrous (fi'brus) Composed of, containing, or resembling fibers of connective tissue.

fibula (fib'u-lah) The lateral and smaller of the two bones of the leg, between the knee and the ankle; it has an insignificant role in the transmission of body weight. See also table of bones in appendix I.

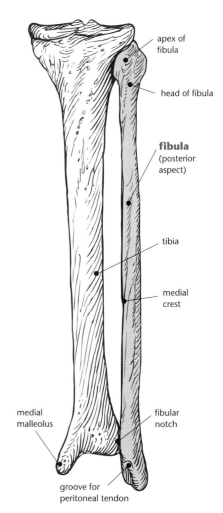

apex of fibula

head of fibula

fibula
(posterior aspect)

tibia

medial crest

medial malleolus

fibular notch

groove for peritoneal tendon

fibril ■ fibula

fibular (fib'u-lar) Relating to the fibula. Also called peroneal.

fibulocalcaneal (fib-u-lo-kal-ka'ne-al) Relating to the fibula and the calcaneus (heel bone).

filament (fil'ah-ment) A thin, threadlike structure.

    actin f. The smaller of the two contractile elements in muscle fibers, measuring about 50 Å in width; in skeletal and cardiac muscles, one end is attached to the Z line, a transverse septum that gives the muscle a characteristic striated appearance; the other free end interdigitates with the myosin filament in the contraction and relaxation of muscle.

    myosin f. The thicker of the two contractile elements in all muscle fibers; in skeletal and cardiac muscles, it measures about 100 Å in width, and traverses the central portion of each sarcomere, producing a dense A band; when interdigitating with the free ends of actin filaments, it is responsible for the contraction and relaxation of muscle.

filamentous (fil-ah-men'tus) Threadlike; filiform; consisting of filaments.

fissura (fis-su'rah) Latin for fissure; cleft; groove.

fissure (fish'ūr) A cleft, groove, depression, or slit; a sulcus or deep fold.

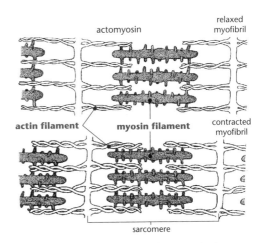

antitragohelicine f. A deep slit-like fissure in the cartilage of the ear (auricle) between the tail of the helix (cauda helicis) posteriorly and the antihelix anteriorly.

    inferior orbital f. A large fissure at the apex of the orbit separating the lateral wall from the floor, opening posteriorly into the pterygopalatine fossa and infratemporal fossa; it transmits the maxillary nerve, filaments from the pterygopalatine ganglion, and blood channels between the orbital and pterygoid venous plexuses.

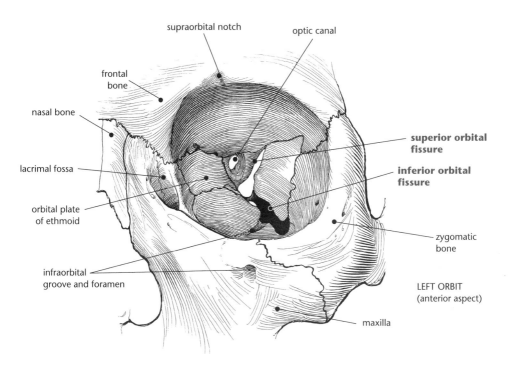

LEFT ORBIT
(anterior aspect)

petromastoid f. See tympanomastoid fissure.

petro-occipital f. A fissure extending backward from the foramen lacerum to the jugular foramen in the floor of the skull, between the petrous part of the temporal bone and the basilar part of the occipital bone; it accommodates the inferior petrosal sinus.

petrosquamous f. A superficial fissure on the floor of the middle cranial fossa designating the fusion between the petrous and squamous parts of the temporal bone.

petrotympanic f. A narrow transversal extension of the tympanosquamosal fissure, just posterior to the mandibular fossa, through which the chorda tympani and a tympanic branch of the maxillary artery pass downward and forward from the middle ear chamber (tympanic cavity) of the temporal bone.

pterygoid f. See pterygoid notch, under notch.

pterygomaxillary f. The deep cleft just behind and continuous with the inferior orbital fissure between the back of the maxilla and the lateral pterygoid plate of the sphenoid bone, through which the infratemporal fossa communicates with the pterygopalatine fossa. Also called pterygopalatine fissure.

pterygopalatine f. See pterygomaxillary fissure.

squamotympanic f. See tympanosquamous fissure.

superior orbital f. A large, irregular, narrow fissure at the apex of the orbit between the roof (lesser wing of sphenoid bone) and its lateral wall (greater wing of sphenoid bone); it connects the orbit with the middle cranial fossa and transmits the oculomotor (3rd cranial), trochlear (4th cranial), and abducent (6th cranial) nerves, as well as branches of the ophthalmic nerve, the ophthalmic veins, and some meningeal vessels.

tympanomastoid f. A fissure positioned between the tympanic part and the mastoid part of the temporal bone, on the anterior aspect of the base of the mastoid process; between the lips of the fissure is often seen the mastoid canaliculus transmitting the auricular branch of the vagus nerve. Also called petromastoid fissure.

tympanosquamous f. A transverse fissure separating the tympanic part of the temporal bone from the squamous part; easily seen in the mandibular fossa where it separates the larger medial part from the smaller tympanic part of the fossa; it is continuous medially with the petrotympanic fissure and the petrosquamous fissure. Also called squamotympanic fissure.

flank (flank) The side of the trunk bounded above by the lowest rib, and below by the iliac crest of the hipbone.

flatfoot (flat'foot) Condition marked by varying degrees of depression of the longitudinal arch of the foot, resulting in the body's weight being borne over the entire sole; it may be congenital or acquired. Also called pes planus.

flex (fleks) To approximate two parts connected by a joint.

flexion (flek'shun) 1. The act of approximating two parts connected by a joint (e.g., of a limb) or of bending forward (e.g., of the spine). 2. The condition of being bent.

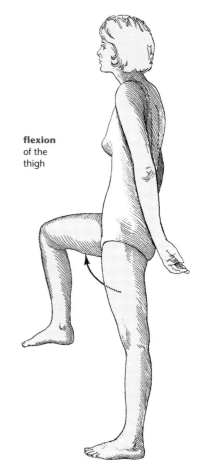

flexion of the thigh

palmar f. Flexion at the wrist, causing the hand to be bent toward the anterior surface of the forearm.

plantar f. Flexion at the ankle joint, causing the foot to be bent downward.

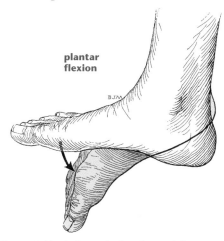

plantar
flexion

flexor (flek'sor) A muscle that flexes a joint.

f. retinaculum See under retinaculum.

flexura (flek-shoo'rah) Latin for a bend.

flexure (flek'sher) A bend, turn or curve, usually of an anatomic structure.

dorsal f. The dorsal convexity of the spine in the thoracic region.

lumbar f. The dorsal concavity of the spine in the lumbar region.

floor (flor) The lowest part or surface of a hollow structure or cavity.

f. of orbit The not quite horizontal floor of the pyramid-shaped orbit, that also serves as the roof of the underlying maxillary sinus; it is vey thin and delicate.

f. of pelvis The broad hammock of muscle sweeping down from the pelvic brim, attaching posteriorly to the sacrum and coccyx. In the female, it invests the urethra, vagina, and rectum. In the male, it invests the urethra and rectum.

f. of tympanic cavity A narrow, thin, convex bony plate that separates the tympanic cavity of the middle ear from the large superior bulb of the internal jugular vein; at its most medial aspect, it contains a small aperture for the transmission of the tympanic branch of the glossopharyngeal nerve.

fontanel, fontanelle (fon-tah-nel') Any of the normally six unossified spaces in the fetal and infant skull, covered by a fibrous tissue membrane. Commonly called soft spot.

anterior f. The largest of the six fontanels; it is diamond-shaped and located at the junction of the frontal, sagittal and coronal sutures; it normally ossifies within 18 months of birth. Also called frontal fontanel; bregmatic fontanel.

anterolateral f. See sphenoidal fontanel.

bregmatic f. See anterior fontanel.

frontal f. See anterior fontanel.

lateral f.'s The mastoid and sphenoidal fontanels.

mastoid f. An irregularly shaped, small fontanel on either side of the fetal and infant skull, between the adjacent edges of the parietal, temporal, and occipital bones; ossification generally occurs by the first year of birth. Also called posterolateral fontanel.

occipital f. See posterior fontanel.

posterior f. A triangular fontanel located at the junction of the sagittal and lambdoid sutures; it generally ossifies within two or three months of birth. Also called occipital fontanel.

posterolateral f. See mastoid fontanel.

sphenoid f. An irregularly shaped, small fontanel located on either side of the fetal and newborn skull at the junction of the frontal, parietal, temporal, and sphenoid bones; it generally ossifies within two or three months of birth. Also called anterolateral fontanel.

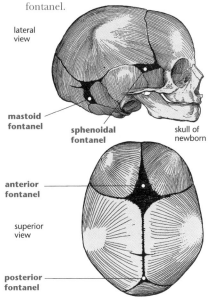

lateral
view

mastoid
fontanel

sphenoidal
fontanel

skull of
newborn

anterior
fontanel

superior
view

posterior
fontanel

footplate (foot'plāt) The base of the stapes, the smallest bone (ossicle) in the middle ear chamber.

THE **FORAMINA** AT BASE OF CRANIUM AND STRUCTURES
TRANSMITTED THROUGH THEM

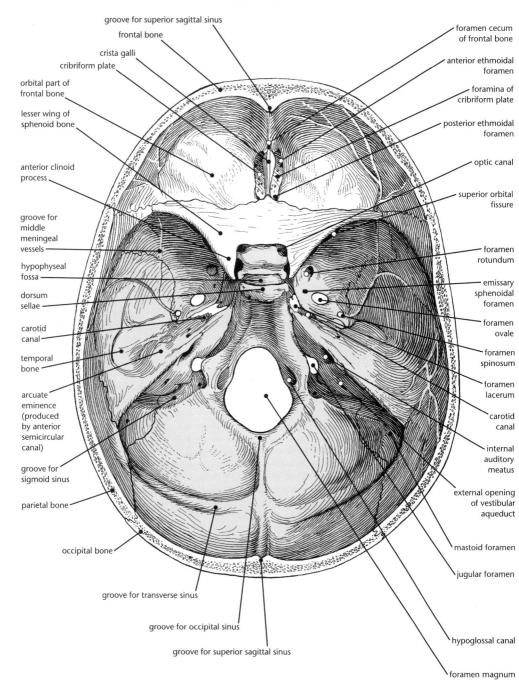

groove for superior sagittal sinus

frontal bone

crista galli

cribriform plate

orbital part of
frontal bone

lesser wing of
sphenoid bone

anterior clinoid
process

groove for
middle
meningeal
vessels

hypophyseal
fossa

dorsum
sellae

carotid
canal

temporal
bone

arcuate
eminence
(produced
by anterior
semicircular
canal)

groove for
sigmoid sinus

parietal bone

occipital bone

groove for transverse sinus

groove for occipital sinus

groove for superior sagittal sinus

foramen cecum
of frontal bone

anterior ethmoidal
foramen

foramina of
cribriform plate

posterior ethmoidal
foramen

optic canal

superior orbital
fissure

foramen
rotundum

emissary
sphenoidal
foramen

foramen
ovale

foramen
spinosum

foramen
lacerum

carotid
canal

internal
auditory
meatus

external opening
of vestibular
aqueduct

mastoid foramen

jugular foramen

hypoglossal canal

foramen magnum

foramen ■ foramen

Structures transmitted

emissary vein to superior sagittal sinus

anterior ethmoidal artery, vein and nerve

olfactory nerve

posterior ethmoidal artery, vein and nerve

optic (2nd cranial) nerve, ophthalmic artery, meninges

oculomotor (3rd cranial) nerve, trochlear (4th cranial) nerve, terminal branches of ophthalmic nerve, abducent (6th cranial) nerve, ophthalmic veins

maxillary nerve

emissary vein from cavernous sinus

mandibular nerve, accessory meningeal artery, lesser petrosal nerve (inconstant)

middle meningeal artery and vein, meningeal branch of mandibular nerve

internal carotid artery and accompanying sympathetic and venous plexus

internal carotid artery

facial (7th cranial) nerve, vestibulocochlear (8th cranial) nerve, nervus intermedius, labyrinthine vessels

endolymphatic duct

emissary vein from sigmoid sinus

glossopharyngeal (9th cranial) nerve, vagus (10th cranial) nerve, accessory (11th cranial) nerve, sigmoid sinus, inferior petrosal sinus, posterior meningeal artery

hypoglossal (12th cranial) nerve, meningeal branch of ascending pharyngeal artery

medulla oblongata, spinal roots of accessory (11th cranial) nerve, meningeal branches of vertebral arteries, meninges

foramen ■ foramen

foramen (fo-ra'men), pl. foram'ina An aperture; a natural opening through a bone or a membranous structure; a short passage.

anterior sacral foramina Four pairs of large foramina on the anterior (pelvic) surface of the sacral bone that give passage to the ventral branches of the upper four sacral nerves. Also called pelvic sacral foramina.

apical dental f. The opening at the tip of the root of a tooth through which pass the nerves and blood vessels supplying the pulp of the tooth.

f. cecum A pit or blind foramen.

f. cecum of frontal bone In the anterior cranial fossa of the skull, the depression or opening between the front of the crista galli of the ethmoid bone, and the crest of the frontal bone; occasionally an emissary vein may pass through to connect the superior sagittal sinus with veins in the nasal cavity.

dorsal sacral foramina See posterior sacral foramina.

ethmoidal foramina Two openings (anterior and posterior) in the orbit, that lead into minute bony canals passing through the orbital plate of the ethmoid bone; they transmit the ethmoidal nerves and vessels.

great f. See foramen magnum.

greater palatine f. A foramen in the vascular groove situated in the posterolateral part of the hard palate; it transmits the greater palatine nerve and vessels.

greater sciatic f. The large opening bounded by the sacrum, the greater sciatic notch of the hipbone, and the sacrotuberous and sacrospinous ligaments; the structures that pass through it when exiting the pelvis include: the piriform muscle, sciatic nerve, pudendal nerve, posterior femoral cutaneous nerves, nerves to the internal obturator muscle and quadrate muscle of thigh, superior gluteal nerve and vessels, and internal pudendal vessels.

incisive foramina Openings in the incisive fossa of the hard palate: *Lateral incisive foramina,* openings of the incisive canals leading to the lateral wall of the nasal cavity; *Median incisive foramina,* openings of the incisive canals leading to the anterior and posterior walls of the nasal cavity.

inferior dental f. See mandibular foramen.

infraorbital f. The opening of the infraorbital canal on the anterior surface of the maxilla, about one centimeter below the lower margin of the orbit and in a vertical line with the supraorbital foramen or notch; it transmits the infraorbital vessels and nerve.

intervertebral foramina Openings into the vertebral (spinal) canal between adjacent vertebrae, formed by notches on the superior and inferior borders of the vertebral pedicles; they transmit spinal vessels and nerves.

jugular f. The opening with a serrated margin at the base of the skull between the lateral part of the occipital bone and the petrous part of the temporal bone; it transmits the vagus (10th cranial), glossopharyngeal (9th cranial), and accessory (11th cranial) nerves as well as the posterior meningeal artery.

lacerated f. See foramen lacerum.

f. lacerum The irregular aperture located at the base of the skull between the apex of the petrous part of the temporal bone, the body and greater wing of the sphenoid bone, and the basilar part of the occipital bone; although normally closed by fibrocartilage, it often gives passage to the small nerve of the pterygoid canal and a small meningeal branch of the ascending pharyngeal artery. Also called lacerated foramen.

lesser palatine foramina Foramina, usually two on each side of the hard palate, situated just behind the greater palatine foramen; they transmit the lesser palatine nerves and vessels.

lesser sciatic f. The opening bounded by the lesser sciatic notch of the hipbone and the sacrotuberous and sacrospinous ligaments; it transmits the tendon of the internal obturator muscle, the nerve to the internal obturator muscle, the pudendal nerve, and the internal pudendal vessels.

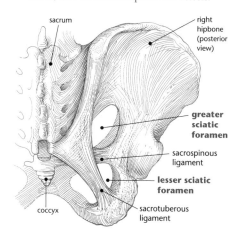

sacrum

right hipbone (posterior view)

greater sciatic foramen

sacrospinous ligament

lesser sciatic foramen

coccyx

sacrotuberous ligament

f. magnum The large median opening penetrating the occipital bone at the base of the skull, the point at which the medulla oblongata extends caudally as the spinal cord; it also transmits the vertebral arteries and the spinal roots of the accessory (11th cranial) nerves. Also called great foramen.

mandibular f. An opening located on the medial aspect of each ramus of the mandible; it transmits the inferior dental nerve and vessels, from which branches enter the roots of the teeth. Also called inferior dental foramen.

mastoid f. A foramen that pierces the mastoid process just above its base near the occipitomastoid suture; it transmits an emissary vein from the sigmoid sinus.

mental f. One of two lateral openings on the body of the lower jaw (mandible), usually beneath the second premolar tooth; it transmits the mental branch of the inferior dental nerve and vessels.

obturator f. The large opening in the hipbone bounded by the pubis and ischium (large and oval in the male, and smaller and nearly triangular in the female); it is almost completely covered by a fibrous sheath (obturator membrane) except the upper area, where a small gap (obturator canal) permits direct communication between the pelvis and the thigh; it transmits the obturator nerve and vessels.

optic f. See optic canal, under canal.

parietal f. A small opening toward the back of the parietal bone, on either side of the sagittal suture, about three to four centimeters in front of the lambdoid suture; it transmits an emissary vein from the superior sagittal sinus and an occasional small branch of the occipital artery.

pelvic sacral foramina See anterior sacral foramina.

posterior sacral foramina Four pairs of large foramina on the posterior (dorsal) surface of the sacral bone that give passage to the dorsal branches of the upper four sacral nerves. Also called dorsal sacral foramina.

f. rotundum A circular opening in the base of the skull piercing the greater wing of the sphenoid bone just behind the medial end of the superior orbital fissure; the maxillary nerve passes through it on its way to the pterygopalatine fossa.

sphenopalatine f. The foramen on the medial wall of the pterygopalatine fossa between the palatine and sphenoid bones; it permits the passage of the sphenopalatine vessels and nasal nerves from the pterygopalatine fossa to the nasal cavity posterior to the superior meatus.

f. spinosum An opening in the greater wing of the sphenoid bone, at the base of the skull, posterolateral to the foramen ovale; it transmits the middle meningeal artery and veins and the meningeal branch of the mandibular nerve.

stylomastoid f. An opening on the inferior surface of the skull between the styloid and mastoid processes; it is at the lower end of the facial canal and transmits the facial (7th cranial) nerve and the stylomastoid branch of the posterior auricular artery.

supraorbital f. A foramen in the supraorbital margin of the frontal bone on either side; it may, on occasion, be a notch; it transmits the supraorbital vessels and nerve.

vertebral f. The large enclosed space within a vertebra, between the neural arch (posterior aspect) and the body (anterior aspect); it is occupied by the spinal cord, filaments of dorsal and ventral roots, associated vessels, and adipose tissue.

zygomaticofacial f. Either of two foramina piercing the lateral surface of the zygomatic bone near its orbital border, for passage of the zygomaticofacial nerve and vessels; the canal that leads from it exits on the orbital

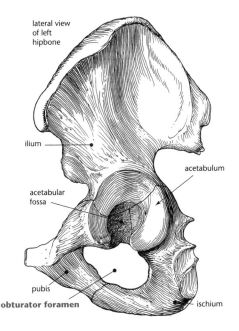

lateral view of left hipbone

ilium

acetabulum

acetabular fossa

pubis

obturator foramen

ischium

foramen ■ foramen

surface of the zygomatic bone at the zygomatico-orbital foramen.

zygomatico-orbital f. Either of two foramina piercing the lateral wall of the orbit (zygomatic bone); one canal leads to and terminates at the zygomaticofacial foramen on the lateral surface of the zygomatic bone; the other canal leads to and terminates at the zygomaticotemporal foramen on the temporal side of the zygomatic bone.

zygomaticotemporal f. The foramen that pierces the temporal surface of the zygomatic bone; it transmits the zygomaticotemporal nerve and a small branch of the lacrimal artery.

foramina (fo-ram'ĭ-nah) Plural of foramen.

forearm (for'arm) The part of the upper limb between the elbow and the wrist. Also called antebrachium.

fossa (fos'ah), pl. fos'sae A pit, hollow or depression.

acetabular f. A roughened, circular depression forming the floor of the acetabulum; it is devoid of cartilage and lodges a fibroelastic mass of fat largely covered with a synovial membrane.

f. of antihelix See triangular fossa of auricle.

articular f. A cartilage-lined depression at the end of a bone for articulation with the extremity of another bone to form a joint.

axillary f. The armpit; the axilla.

condylar f. of occipital bone The cranial depression immediately behind the occipital condyle on either side of the foramen magnum; the fossa accommodates the posterior edge of the superior facet of the atlas (first cervical vertebra) when the head is extended; it is occasionally pierced by the condylar canal for the passage of an emissary vein draining the sigmoid sinus.

coronoid f. A hollow on the front of the lower end of the humerus which accommodates the coronoid process of the ulna during flexion of the elbow joint. Also called coronoid fossa of humerus.

coronoid f. of humerus See coronoid fossa.

cranial f. Any of three depressions (anterior, middle, and posterior) of the internal surface of the base of the skull; each accommodates a different portion of the brain.

cubital f. The triangular hollow of the skin in front of the elbow joint, bounded medially by the round pronator muscle (pronator teres), laterally by the brachioradial muscle,

and above by a line joining the lateral and medial epicondyles of the humerus; it contains the median nerve and the termination and division of the brachial artery. Also called antecubital space; triangle of elbow; popularly called bend of the elbow.

cuspid f. A shallow depression on the front of the maxilla lateral to the ridge formed by the root of the cuspid tooth. Also called maxillary fossa.

digastric f. The small roughened depression on the internal surface of the lower border of the body of the mandible on each side of the mental symphysis; it affords attachment to the anterior belly of the digastric muscle.

ethmoid f. The narrow groove-shaped depression on the cribriform plate of the sphenoid bone on each side of the median triangular process (crista galli); it presents numerous foramina for the passage of the anterior olfactory nerve to the nasal cavity; the olfactory bulb lies immediately above it. Also called olfactory groove.

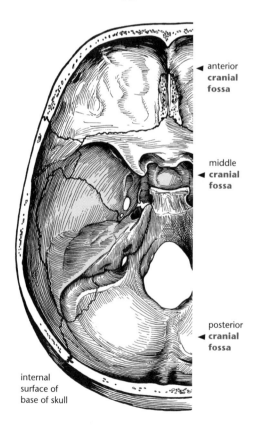

anterior ◀ **cranial fossa**

middle ◀ **cranial fossa**

posterior ◀ **cranial fossa**

internal surface of base of skull

foramina ■ fossa

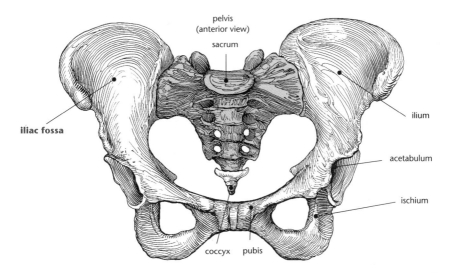

pelvis
(anterior view)

sacrum

ilium

iliac fossa

acetabulum

ischium

coccyx   pubis

glenoid f. See glenoid cavity, under cavity.

hypophyseal f. A deep depression in the sphenoid bone accommodating the pituitary (hypophysis). Sometimes written hypophysial fossa. Also called pituitary fossa.

iliac f. The smooth, concave hollow on the inner surface of the anterior and upper part of the iliac bone; it forms the posterolateral wall of the greater pelvis.

incisive f. The V-shaped depression situated in the midline of the anterior part of the bony palate immediately behind the maxillary central incisors, into which the lateral and median incisive foramina open, permitting the nasopalatine nerves and the termination of the greater palatine artery to communicate between the nasal and oral cavities.

incisive f. of maxilla The slight depression on the front of the maxilla overlying the roots of the incisor teeth; it affords attachment to the depressor muscle of the nasal septum (depressor septi nasi); it is medial to the cuspid fossa and separated from it by the cuspid eminence.

incudal f. A small depression in the lower part of the posterior wall of the epitympanic recess (above the level of the tympanic membrane in the middle ear chamber), in which the tip of the short process of the incus ossicle is attached by ligamentous fibers.

infraclavicular f. The triangular depression on the skin just below the clavicle, between the greater pectoral muscle (pectoralis major) and the deltoid muscle.

infraspinous f. The large triangular area of the dorsal surface of the scapula below the spinous crest; it is slightly concave laterally and convex medially and connects to the supraspinous fossa through the spinoglenoid notch (it is about four times larger than the supraspinous fossa); it provides attachment to the infraspinous muscle.

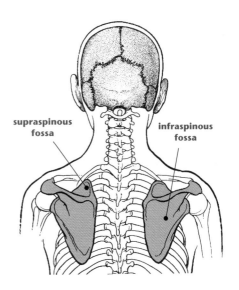

supraspinous
fossa

infraspinous
fossa

infratemporal f. A highly irregular depression on the side of the skull just below the level of the zygomatic arch, bounded medially by the lateral pterygoid plate of the sphenoid bone, laterally, by the ramus of the mandible and the zygomatic arch, anteriorly,

fossa ■ fossa

by the zygomatic process of the mandible, posteriorly, by the articular tubercle, and superiorly, by the infratemporal surface of the greater wing of the sphenoid bone; it houses the lower part of the temporal muscle as it extends to the coronoid process of the mandible. Also called zygomatic fossa.

intercondylar f. of femur The deep nonarticular posterior gap between the condyles of the femur in which the anterior and posterior cruciate ligaments are attached. Also called intercondylar notch.

jugular f. of temporal bone A deep notch on the inferior aspect of the temporal bone, just behind the carotid canal, that accommodates the superior bulb of the internal jugular vein. At its apex is seen a small canaliculus containing the perilymphatic duct.

lacrimal f. A deep fossa in the medial wall of the orbit, formed by the lacrimal bone and the frontal process of the maxilla; it communicates with the nasal cavity and houses the lacrimal sac and the upper part of the nasolacrimal duct. Also called fossa of lacrimal gland; lacrimal groove; lacrimal notch.

f. of lacrimal gland See lacrimal fossa.

f. of lateral pterygoid muscle See pterygoid fovea, under fovea.

malleolar f. A large oval depression on the medial aspect of the lower end of the fibula immediately behind its articular facet for the talus; it is pitted by numerous small vascular foramina and it affords attachment to the posterior talofibular and posterior tibiofibular ligaments.

mandibular f. One of two transversely-disposed depressions on the temporal bone at the base of the skull that accommodates the condyle of the lower jaw.

mastoid f. of temporal bone See suprameatal foveola, under foveola.

maxillary f. See cuspid fossa.

olecranon f. A deep hollow on the back of the lower end of the humerus just above the trochlea, which accommodates the tip of the olecranon of the ulna during extension of the elbow joint.

piriform f. See piriform recess, under recess.

pituitary f. See hypophyseal fossa.

popliteal f. The diamond-shaped area on the skin situated at the back of the knee joint; bounded above by the biceps muscle of thigh (biceps femoria) laterally and the semimembranous muscle medially; bounded below by the lateral and medial heads of the gastrocnemius muscle. Also called popliteal space.

pterygoid f. of sphenoid bone The large wedge-shaped interval between the lateral and medial pterygoid plates of the sphenoid bone; it affords attachment to the medial pterygoid muscle and the tensor muscle of the soft palate (tensor veli palatini).

pterygopalatine f. A small pyramidal space, bounded in front by the posterior surface of the maxilla, behind by the root of the pterygoid process of the sphenoid bone, medially by the upper part of the perpendicular plate of the palatine bone; laterally the space communicates with the infratemporal fossa, anteriorly with the orbit, and medially with the nasal cavity; it houses the pterygopalatine ganglion.

radial f. A shallow depression on the anterior aspect of the lower end of the humerus, just above the capitulum and lateral to the coronoid fossa; it accommodates the rim of the head of the radius during full extension of the forearm.

scaphoid f. The narrow longitudinal depression between the helix and the antihelix of the auricle. Also called scapha.

scaphoid f. of sphenoid bone The shallow

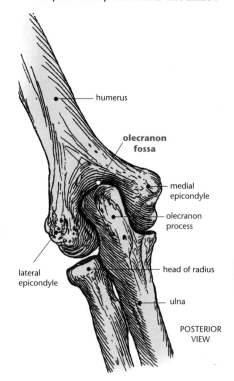

humerus

olecranon fossa

medial epicondyle

olecranon process

lateral epicondyle

head of radius

ulna

POSTERIOR VIEW

depression on the upper end of the posterior border of the medial pterygoid plate of the sphenoid bone; it affords attachment to the anterior fibers of the tensor muscle of the soft palate (tensor veli palatini).

sublingual f. A shallow, smooth triangular depression on the inner surface of the body of the mandible; it is situated on either side of the mental spine above the anterior end of the mylohyoid line; it accommodates a portion of the sublingual salivary gland. Also called sublingual fovea.

submandibular f. The slightly concave area on the inner surface of the body of the mandible, just below the middle part of the mylohyoid line; it accommodates the lateral surface of the submandibular salivary gland. Also called submandibular fovea.

supraclavicular f. Either of two depressions on the surface of the body just above the clavicle: *Major supraclavicular f.*, the depression above the clavicle and lateral to the tendon of the sternocleidomastoid muscle; *Minor supraclavicular f.*, the depression above the clavicle between the clavicular and sternal heads of the sternocleidomastoid muscle.

suprameatal f. See suprameatal foveola, under foveola.

supraspinous f. The concave depression on the dorsal surface of the scapula above the spinous process; the medial two thirds provides attachment to the supraspinous muscle.

temporal f. The region on the side of the skull below the temporal lines and bounded laterally by the zygomatic arch, anteriorly, by the frontal process of the zygomatic bone, posteriorly, by the temporal lines; inferiorly, it terminates at the level of the zygomatic arch and then becomes continuous with the infratemporal fossa; it provides attachment to the temporal muscle.

triangular f. of auricle The depression between the two ridges (crura) into which the antihelix divides superiorly. Also called fossa of antihelix.

trochanteric f. The deep, rough depression at the root of the femoral neck on the medial surface of the greater trochanter; it affords attachment to the tendon of the external obturator muscle (obturator externus).

trochlear f. A small, shallow depression on the orbital surface of the frontal bone, just behind the medial end of the supraorbital margin; it accommodates the attachment of the fibrocartilaginous pulley (trochlea) of the superior oblique tendon of the eyeball. Also

called trochlear fovea.

zygomatic f. See infratemporal fossa.

fovea (fo've-ah), pl. fo'veae A small depression.

f. of femoral head The small depression on the head of the femur below and behind its center; it affords attachment to the round ligament of the femur. Also called pit of femoral head.

inferior costal f. See inferior costal facet of vertebra, under facet.

pterygoid f. A rough depression on the inner side of the neck of the mandible, just below its articular surface; it affords insertion of the lateral pterygoid muscle; often covered by the parotid gland. Also called fossa of lateral pterygoid muscle; pterygoid pit.

f. of radial head The shallow saucer-shaped surface of the proximal head of the radius for articulation with the capitulum of the humerus.

sublingual f. See sublingual fossa, under fossa.

submandibular f. See submandibular fossa, under fossa.

superior costal f. See superior costal facet of vertebra, under facet.

trochlear f. See trochlear fossa, under fossa.

foveate, foveated (fo've-āt, fo-ve-ā'ted) Having small depressions; pitted.

foveola (fo-ve'o-lah), pl. fove'olae A minute depression, fovea, or pit.

f. of coccyx A small, shallow dimple often present in the skin at the tip of the coccyx; it represents the site of attachment of the embryonic neural tube to the skin. Also called coccygeal dimple.

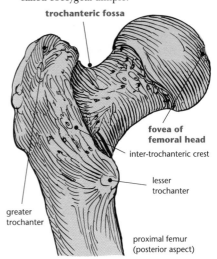

trochanteric fossa

fovea of femoral head

inter-trochanteric crest

lesser trochanter

greater trochanter

proximal femur (posterior aspect)

fossa ■ foveola

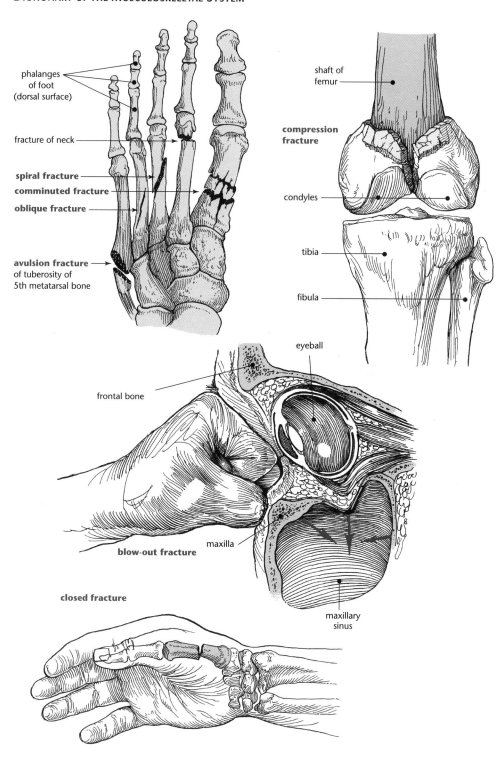

phalanges
of foot
(dorsal surface)

fracture of neck

spiral fracture

comminuted fracture

oblique fracture

avulsion fracture
of tuberosity of
5th metatarsal bone

shaft of
femur

**compression
fracture**

condyles

tibia

fibula

eyeball

frontal bone

maxilla

blow-out fracture

maxillary
sinus

closed fracture

fracture ■ fracture

granular foveolae Irregular small depressions on the internal surface of the cranial bones on each side of the sagittal sulcus; they accommodate the arachnoid granulations and become more numerous with age. Also called granular foveolae of Pacchioni.

granular foveolae of Pacchioni See granular faveolae.

suprameatal f. A small pit at the junction of the posterior and superior margins of the external auditory canal of the temporal bone, just behind the suprameatal spine. Also called suprameatal fossa; mastoid fossa of temporal bone.

fracture (frak'chur) The breaking of a bone or cartilage.

articular f. Fracture of the joint (articular) surface of a bone.

avulsion f. The tearing off of a small fragment of bone at the attachment site of a tendon or ligament, caused by a sudden forceful pull on the tendon or ligament (e.g., when the ankle is twisted or when a strong muscle contracts forcefully and suddenly). Also called sprain fracture.

Bankart f. A fracture of the shoulder blade (scapula) at the shoulder joint in which a bone fragment is detached from the anteroinferior margin of the glenoid fossa; frequently associated with anterior shoulder dislocation.

Barton's f. Intra-articular fracture of the radius at the wrist joint, involving either the front or the back of the wrist; it is usually associated with dislocation of the wrist joint but without injury to the wrist (carpal) bones.

basal f. See cervicotrochanteric fracture.

basal skull f. A fracture through the floor of the skull.

Bennett's f. An articular avulsion fracture of the base of the first metacarpal bone; a small fragment of the bone remains attached to the adjacent wrist bone (trapezium) by means of the volar oblique ligament, while the shaft fragment of the bone is displaced toward the wrist by muscle pull.

bimalleolar f. See Pott's fracture.

blowout f. A fracture through the floor of the orbit, usually caused by a blow to the eye. Also called orbital floor fracture.

boot-top f. Fracture of the tibia and fibula in the lower one third of the leg, caused by violent stress against the rim of a ski-boot.

boxer f. Fracture of the neck of the fifth metacarpal bone (on the side of the little finger), with displacement of the bone head toward the palm and protrusion of the shaft toward the back of the hand.

buckle f. See torus fracture.

bumper f. Compression fracture of the lateral articular area of the tibia at the knee, often associated with avulsion of the medial (tibial) collateral ligament of the knee joint. Also called fender fracture.

capillary f. A hairline fracture.

cervicotrochanteric f. A fracture across the base of the femoral neck, at the hip joint. Also called basal fracture.

Chance f. A horizontal splitting of the body of a lumbar vertebra and its posterior arch, frequently caused by a lap seat belt of an automobile in a traffic accident victim. Also called seat-belt fracture.

closed f. Fracture in which the overlying skin remains intact. Formerly called simple fracture.

Colles' f. Fracture of the end of the radius (at the wrist) with dorsal displacement of the distal fragment, producing the "silver fork" or "bayonet" deformity.

comminuted f. Fracture in which the bone is broken in several small pieces.

compound f. Former name for open fracture.

compression f. Fracture in which the hard shaft of a long bone (e.g., femur) is driven through the porous lower end of the bone, giving rise to a T- or V-shaped fracture.

crush f. Fracture accompanied by extensive soft tissue damage, the bone may be broken transversely or it may be extensively broken into small fragments (comminuted); when occurring in the leg or forearm, both bones (i.e., tibia and fibula or radius and ulna) are fractured at the same level.

dashboard f. Common name for a shear fracture with dislocation of the hipbone; it occurs when an automobile passenger seated in the front seat is thrown forward; the knee strikes the dashboard, transmitting axial force to the flexed and adducted thighbone (femur) and dislocating the hip either through a rent in the posterior joint capsule, or where the posterior acetabular rim is sheared by the head of the femur.

depressed skull f. Fracture of the skull with inward displacement of the fragment.

deQuervain's f. A fraction-dislocation of the wrist; specifically, fracture of the scaphoid bone with dislocation of the lunate bone.

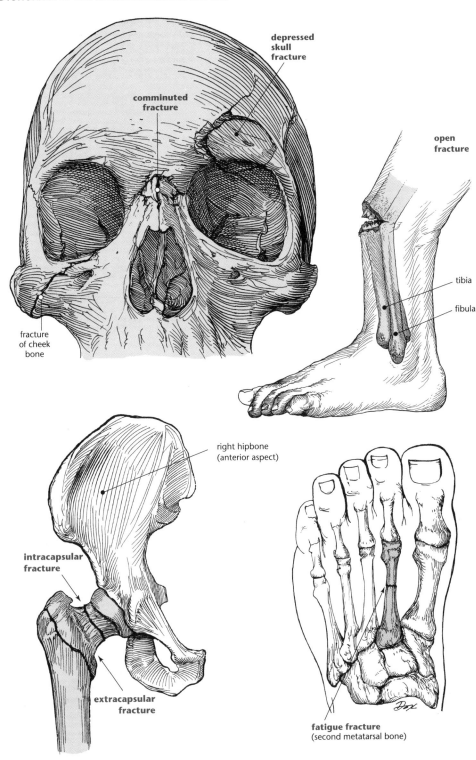

depressed
skull
fracture

comminuted
fracture

open
fracture

tibia

fibula

fracture
of cheek
bone

right hipbone
(anterior aspect)

intracapsular
fracture

extracapsular
fracture

fatigue fracture
(second metatarsal bone)

fracture ■ fracture

displaced f. Fracture in which the main bone fragments are relatively widely separated.

Dupuytren's f. Fracture of the lower end of the fibula or lateral malleolus with dislocation of the ankle joint.

epiphysial f. Traumatic separation and/or fracture of the growth (epiphysial) plate of a long bone; it may or may not involve fracture of the adjoining bone. Displacement of the bone is the only obvious indicator of a plate disruption in the x-ray image due to the radiotranslucent nature of the cartilagenous plate. Also called growth plate fracture; epiphysial separation.

extracapsular f. Fracture of a bone near but outside of the joint capsule.

fatigue f. Fracture of a metatarsal shaft, usually the second or third, associated with prolonged weightbearing activities as in walking for long periods (e.g., during basic military training), ballet dancing, and athletics; believed to be due to muscle fatigue, when the muscle action is no longer optimal and allows increased loading of the bone. Also called march fracture; stress fracture.

fender f. See bumper fracture.

fissured f. See linear fracture.

folding f. See torus fracture.

greenstick f. An incomplete fracture in which the compression side of the bone is only bent, with cortex and periosteum remaining intact; seen most frequently in children.

growth plate f. See epiphysial fracture.

hairline f. A small fracture without separation of bone fragments. Also called capillary fracture; microfracture.

hangman's f. Dislocation and fracture through the pedicles or lamina of the second cervical vertebra (C2) secondary to a traumatic forceful separation and extension of the joint surfaces.

impacted f. Fracture in which one of the bone fragments is driven into the substance of the other and is fixed in that position.

incomplete f. A fracture that involves the bone only partly, not its whole thickness or length.

intracapsular f. A fracture within a joint capsule.

linear f. A fracture running parallel with the long axis of the bone. Also called fissured fracture.

longitudinal f. One in which the direction of the fracture line is along the axis of the bone.

mandibular f. A fracture of the mandible, usually in the area of the root of the cuspid or at the angle; it is the most frequently fractured of all facial bones.

march f. See fatigue fracture.

Monteggia's f. Injury of the forearm at the elbow, characterized by fracture of the shaft of one bone (ulna) with dislocation of the head of the other bone (radius) within the elbow joint.

nightstick f. An undisplaced, or minimally displaced, fracture of the ulnar shaft alone without disruption of the interosseous membrane between ulna and radius; results most frequently from a direct blow to the forearm.

oblique f. Fracture running obliquely to the axis of the bone.

occult f. Condition in which originally there is no evidence of a fracture but after three or four weeks an x-ray image shows new bone formation, indicating a healed fracture.

open f. Fracture occurring with an open wound through which the broken bone may protrude. Formerly called compound fracture.

open book f. Fracture of the anterior portion of the pelvic ring; may range from a simple separation of the pubic symphysis to a wide separation and forward protrusion of one side of the pelvis (resembling an open book), with severe injury to the pelvic floor and genitourinary structures; caused by anteroposterior compression, either due to direct violence or to a force transmitted through the legs.

orbital floor f. See blow-out fracture.

paratrooper f. Fracture of the lower shafts of the two bones of the leg, tibia and fibula.

pathologic f. Bone fracture through an area of bone weakened by preexisting disease (e.g., malignant tumor or osteoporosis) and inflicted by relatively minor trauma, or occurring with no trauma at all.

periosteal f. Fracture occurring beneath the bone-covering membrane (periosteum), without displacement of fragments.

pertrochanteric f. Fracture of the femur at the hip joint, between the femoral neck and the greater trochanter.

Pott's f. A fracture-dislocation of the ankle joint; specifically, fracture of the lower end of the fibula (medial malleolus), associated with fracture of the lower end of the tibia (lateral malleolus) and dislocation of the ankle joint. Also called bimalleolar fracture.

fracture ■ fracture

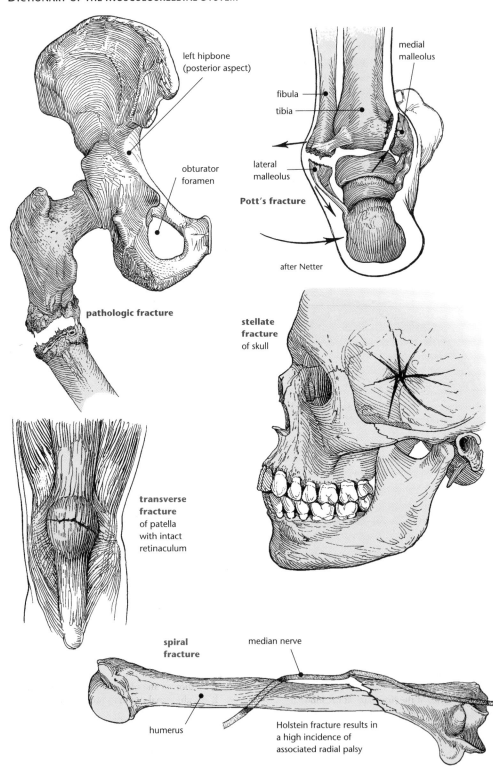

left hipbone
(posterior aspect)

obturator
foramen

pathologic fracture

medial
malleolus

fibula

tibia

lateral
malleolus

Pott's fracture

after Netter

**stellate
fracture**
of skull

**transverse
fracture**
of patella
with intact
retinaculum

**spiral
fracture**

median nerve

humerus

Holstein fracture results in
a high incidence of
associated radial palsy

fracture ■ fracture

reverse Colles' f. See Smith's fracture.

seat-belt f. See Chance fracture.

Segond f. A small avulsion-type fracture of the lateral condyle of the tibia (at the knee) associated with major ligamentous damage to the meniscus-synovial portion of the capsule on the lateral side of the knee joint.

simple f. Former name for closed fracture.

Smith f. A fracture of the distal end of the radius (at the wrist) similar to a Colles' fracture, but the end piece is displaced toward the palm, making a deformity that resembles a horizontal silver fork with its tines pointing upward. Also called reverse Colles' fracture.

spiral f. Breakage in which the fracture line is relatively spiral in direction, seen in the shaft of a long bone; caused by a twisting force.

sprain f. See avulsion fracture.

stellate f. A fracture with several break lines radiating from a central point.

stress f. See fatigue fracture.

supracondylar f. A fracture at the distal end of the humerus, near the elbow.

tapping f. Transverse fracture occurring when a force of diminishing momentum is applied to a small area; identified in the forearm or leg when only one of the two bones is broken; i.e., the radius or ulna (forearm) or the tibia or fibula (leg).

telescoping f.'s Fractures of long bones that cause an axial collapse and compaction of fragments with shortening and thickening of the bones; seen in osteogenesis imperfecta.

toddler f. A nondisplaced, usually spiral, fracture of the tibia of an infant who has just begun to walk; believed to be caused by a twisting injury to the leg.

torus f. An impact injury of childhood; it causes a longitudinal compression of the developing (metaphyseal) portion at the soft end of a long bone, near the growth plate; the compressed bone does not break completely but produces a local bulge. Also called buckle fracture; folding fracture.

transcervical f. A fracture across the midpoint of the neck of the thighbone (femur), near the hip joint.

transcondylar f. A fracture through the condyles of the humerus, at the elbow.

transepiphyseal f. A traumatic separation of a previously normal epiphysis, at the end of a long bone.

transverse f. A fracture in which the break line runs perpendicular with the axis of the bone.

unstable f. A fracture with a high likelihood of slipping after it has been reduced, producing further deformity.

fracture-dislocation (frak'chur dis-lo-ka'shun) A bone fracture accompanied by disruption of its articulating joint.

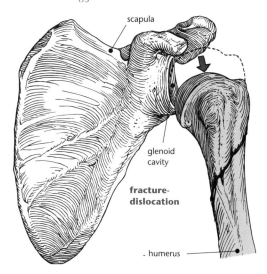

frontal (frunt'l) 1. Relating to the forehead. 2. Relating to the anterior aspect of the body.

fronto- Combining form meaning front.

frontomalar (frun-to-ma'lar) See frontozygomatic.

frontomaxillary (frun-to-mak'sĭ-lār-e) Relating to the frontal and maxillary bones.

frontonasal (frun-to-na'zal) Relating to the frontal and nasal bones.

fronto-occipital (frun-to ok-sip'ĭ-tal) Relating to the frontal and occipital bones at the front and back of the head.

frontoparietal (frun-to-pah-ri'e-tal) Relating to the frontal and parietal bones of the head. Also called parietofrontal.

frontotemporal (frun-to-tem'po-ral) Relating to the frontal and temporal bones of the head.

frontozygomatic (frun-to-zi-go-mat'ik) Relating to the frontal and zygomatic bones. Also called frontomalar.

fusion (fu'zhun) 1. A surgical joining together or formation of an ankylosis, as of two vertebrae. 2. An abnormal union of two anatomic structures.

spinal f. The permanent operative fusion of two or more vertebrae to eliminate motion between them.

fracture ■ fusion

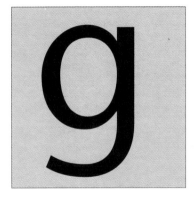

galea (ga′le-ah) A helmetlike structure.

　　g. aponeurotica See epicranial aponeurosis, under aponeurosis.

gastrocnemius (gas-trok-ne′me-us) See table of muscles in appendix II.

genial (jĕ-ni′al) Relating to the chin.

geniculum (jĕ-nik′u-lum) Latin for small knee; applied to a sharp kneelike bend of a small structure.

　　g. of facial canal The right-angled bend of the horizontal portion of the facial canal in the medial wall of the middle ear chamber; it is marked by the presence of the geniculate ganglion (sensory ganglion of the facial

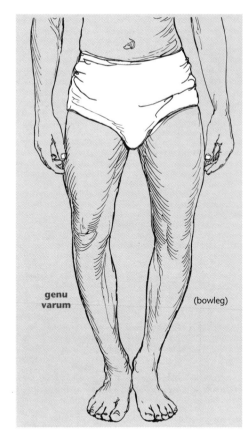

genu varum (bowleg)

nerve). Also called genu of facial canal.

genioglossus (je-ne-o-glos′us) See table of muscles in appendix II.

geniohyoglossus (je-ne-o-hi-o-glos′us) See table of muscles in appendix II.

geniohyoid (je-ne-o-hi′oid) 1. Relating to the chin and the hyoid bone. 2. See table of muscles in appendix II.

genu (je′nu) 1. Latin for knee. 2. Any structure resembling a bent knee.

　　g. of facial canal See geniculum of facial canal, under geniculum.

　　g. recurvatum Abnormal backward bending of the knee joint; back knee.

　　g. valgum A deformity of the leg, usually bilateral, in which the knees converge toward the midline while the ankles remain separated. Also called knock-knee.

　　g. varum A congenital deformity, usually bilateral, in which the leg has an outward curvature in the region of the knee, resulting in an abnormally large distance between the knees when standing with the feet close together. Also called bowleg; bandy-leg.

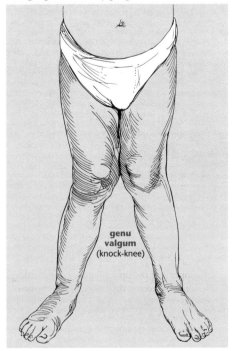

genu valgum (knock-knee)

galea ■ genu

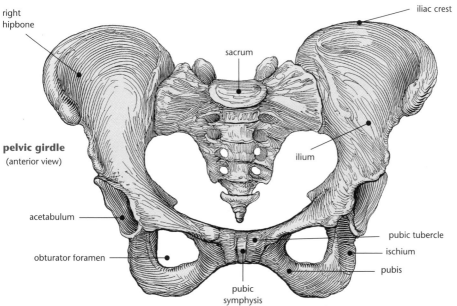

right
hipbone

iliac crest

sacrum

pelvic girdle
(anterior view)

ilium

acetabulum

pubic tubercle

ischium

obturator foramen

pubis

pubic
symphysis

shoulder girdle
(superior view)

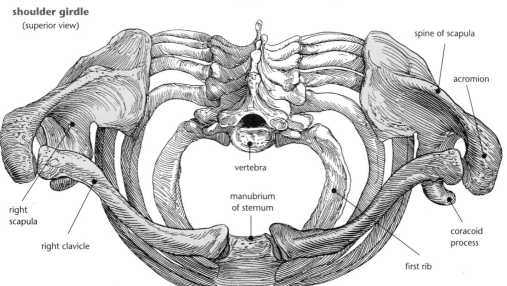

spine of scapula

acromion

right
scapula

vertebra

manubrium
of sternum

coracoid
process

right clavicle

first rib

gibbus (gib'us) A hump or kyphos.
ginglymoarthrodial (jin-gli-mo-ar-thro'de-al)
Relating to an articulation that is partly a hinge
(ginglymoid) joint and partly a plane
(arthrodial) joint.
ginglymus (jin'glĭ-mus) See hinge joint,
under joint.
girdle (ger'dl) An encircling band, structure,
region, or zone.
    pectoral g. See shoulder girdle.

    pelvic g. The bony ring supporting the
lower limbs at the hip joints, formed by the
sacrum and two hipbones.
    shoulder g. An encircling girdle
supporting the upper limbs at the shoulder
joint, formed by the two clavicles, the two
scapulas, and the upper portion of the
sternum (manubrium). Also called pectoral
girdle; thoracic girdle.
    thoracic g. See shoulder girdle.

gibbus ■ girdle

glabella (glah-bel'ah) The smooth median elevation of the frontal bone connecting the two superciliary arches just above the upper end of the nasal bones; a craniometric point.

glenohumeral (gle-no-hu'mer-al) Relating to the glenoid cavity of the scapula and the articulating humerus.

glenoid (gle'noid) Resembling a socket; applied to the articular concave depression (glenoid cavity) on the head of the scapula that articulates with the head of the humerus in the shoulder joint.

glide (glīd) An effortless movement.
  mandibular g. Lateral and protrusive movements of the lower jaw when the occluding surfaces of the teeth are in contact.

glossopharyngeal (glos-o-fah-rin'je-al) 1. Relating to the tongue and the pharynx. 2. Relating to the glossopharyngeal nerve.

glossopharyngeus (glos-o-fah-rin'je-us) The superior constrictor muscle of the pharynx. See table of muscles in appendix II.

glottis (glot'is), pl. glot'tides The vocal apparatus located in the larynx; consists of a fold of mucous membrane (vocal fold) covering the vocal ligament and muscle (vocal cord) on each side and the opening between them.

gluteal (gloo'te-al) Relating to the buttocks.

gluteofemoral (gloo-te-o-fem'or-al) Relating to the buttocks and femoral region.

gluteus (gloo'te-us) Any of the three muscles of the buttock. See table of muscles in appendix II.

gnathion (nath'e-on) The lowest point of the middle of the mandible; a craniometric point.

gnatho-, gnath- Combining forms meaning jaw.

gomphosis (gom-fo'sis) A type of fibrous articulation in which a bony process fits into a depression of another bone (e.g., a tooth and its socket). Also called socket joint of tooth.

gonio- Combining form meaning angle.

gonion (go'ne-on) The outermost point of the angle of the mandible formed by the body and the ramus; a craniometric point.

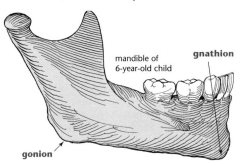

mandible of 6-year-old child

gnathion

gonion

gonycampsis (gon-ĭ-kamp'sis) Any abnormal curvature of the knee.

gout (gowt) A group of metabolic disorders that share the following features (which may occur singly or combined): an excess of uric acid in the blood, recurrent painful inflammation of joints, especially of the big toes, and deposits of sodium biurate in the cartilages of affected joints and in the kidneys.

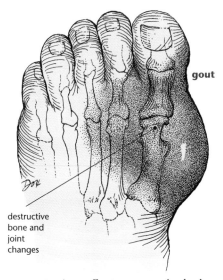

gout

destructive bone and joint changes

  saturnine g. Gout accompanying lead poisoning.

  secondary g. Gout occurring as a result of increased nucleoprotein metabolism and uric acid production.

  tophaceous g. Gout marked by the presence of deposits of sodium urate (tophi) about the joints and cartilaginous structures.

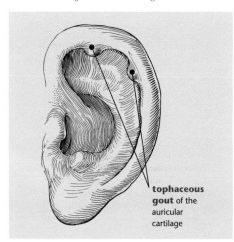

tophaceous gout of the auricular cartilage

glabella ■ gout

gracile (gras'l) Slender.

gristle (gris'l) Cartilage.

groin (groin) The inguinal region; the area around the crease formed at the junction of the anterior thigh and the anterior abdominal wall.

groove (grōōv) A narrow, elongated depression; a sulcus; a furrow; a niche.

    atrioventricular g. See coronary sulcus, under sulcus.

    g. for auditory tube See sulcus of auditory tube, under sulcus.

    bicipital g. of humerus See intertubercular sulcus of humerus, under sulcus.

    carotid g. of sphenoid bone A shallow groove on the floor of the skull that accommodates the internal carotid artery immediately upon emerging through the foramen lacerum; it also supports the cavernous sinus. Also called carotid sulcus of sphenoid bone.

    carpal g. See carpal sulcus, under sulcus.

    costal g. A groove on the lower border of the internal surface of the ribs (except the first ribs) that house the intercostal vessels and nerves. Also called costal sulcus.

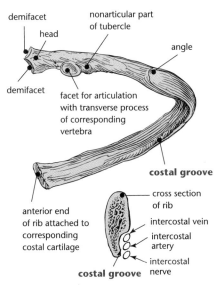

    deltopectoral g. The long groove between the deltoid muscle and the greater pectoral muscle (pectoralis major); it accommodates the cephalic vein.

    developmental g. A groove in the enamel of a tooth marking the fusion of the embryonic tooth lobes of the crown during tooth development.

    digastric g. See mastoid notch, under notch.

    ethmoidal g. A longitudinal groove on the inner surface of each nasal bone accommodating the external nasal branch of the anterior ethmoid nerve. Also called ethmoidal sulcus of nasal bone.

    greater palatine g. A groove on each side of the bony palate, medial to the posterior maxillary teeth, on both the body of the maxilla and the perpendicular plate of the palatine bone.

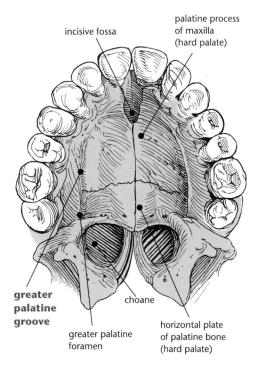

    hamular g. A smooth groove on the lateral side of the medial pterygoid plate of the sphenoid bone that accommodates the tendon of the tensor muscle of the soft palate (tensor veli palatini) that hooks around it on its way to the soft palate. Also called sulcus of pterygoid hamulus.

    infraorbital g. A groove on the floor of the orbit that passes forward and ends at the infraorbital canal; it transmits the infraorbital nerve and vessels.

    interventricular g. Any of two linear depressions on the surface of the heart separating the right from the left ventricles: *Anterior interventricular g.*, the groove on the sternocostal surface of the heart separating the ventricles; it extends from the coronary sulcus to a notch just to the right of the apex

gracile ■ groove

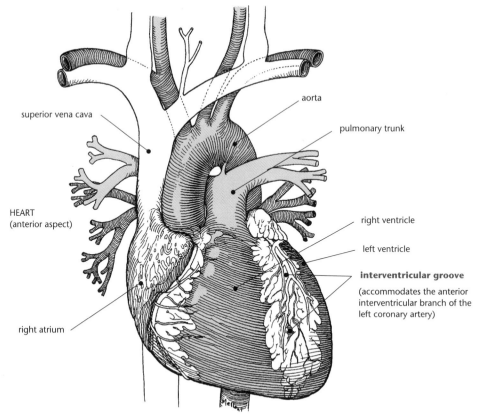

superior vena cava

aorta

pulmonary trunk

HEART
(anterior aspect)

right ventricle

left ventricle

interventricular groove

(accommodates the anterior
interventricular branch of the
left coronary artery)

right atrium

of the heart; the groove is occupied by the anterior interventricular branch of the left coronary artery. Also called anterior interventricular sulcus; *Posterior interventricular g.*, the oblique groove on the diaphragmatic surface of the heart separating the ventricles; it is continuous with the anterior interventricular groove; the groove is occupied by the posterior interventricular branch of the right coronary artery. Also called posterior interventricular sulcus.

    lacrimal g. See lacrimal fossa, under fossa.

    lateral bicipital g. A shallow longitudinal groove on the lateral side of the arm between the lateral border of the biceps muscle of the arm (biceps brachii) and the brachial muscle (brachialis); it extends from the cubital fossa at the elbow upward to about the level of the deltoid tuberosity; it accommodates the cephalic vein. Also called lateral bicipital sulcus.

    g. for long peroneal tendon An oblique groove for the long peroneal tendon on the inferior surface of the cuboid bone of the

foot, situated between the calcaneus proximally and the fourth and fifth metatarsal bones distally.

    malleolar g. See malleolar sulcus, under sulcus.

    medial bicipital g. A prominent longitudinal groove on the medial side of the arm between the medial border of the biceps muscle of the arm (biceps brachii) and the triceps muscle of the arm (triceps brachii) and continued into the cubital fossa between the biceps muscle of the arm and the round pronator muscle (pronator teres); it accommodates the median nerve, basilic vein, and brachial vessels. Also called median bicipital sulcus.

    meningeal g.'s Grooves on the inner surface of the cranial vault (calva) that transmit meningeal vessels; the deeper grooves appear in the parietal and sphenoid bones, while the smaller ones are present in the frontal, temporal and occipital bones.

    g. for middle temporal artery A somewhat vertical groove on the side of the skull, on the squama of the temporal bone, that

groove ■ groove

accommodates the middle temporal artery. Also called sulcus of middle temporal artery.

musculospiral g. See groove for radial nerve.

mylohyoid g. A groove on the inner surface of the mandibular ramus extending from the mandibular foramen, downward and forward to reach the submandibular fossa; it accommodates the mylohyoid nerve and vessels. Also called mylohyoid sulcus of mandible.

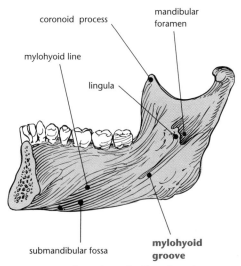

coronoid process

mandibular foramen

mylohyoid line

lingula

submandibular fossa

mylohyoid groove

nail g. See sulcus of nail, under sulcus.

nasolabial g. See nasolabial sulcus, under sulcus.

nasolacrimal g. of maxilla The groove on the nasal side of the maxilla, formed into a canal by the anterior border of the lacrimal bone and the lacrimal process of the inferior nasal concha; it accommodates the nasolacrimal duct from the lower end of the lacrimal sac downward to the anterior part of the inferior nasal meatus.

obturator g. An oblique groove that crosses the undersurface of the superior ramus of the pubic bone where it fuses with the body of the ilium; it accommodates the obturator nerve and vessels. Also called obturator canal of pubic bone; obturator sulcus of pubis.

occipital g. See groove for occipital artery.

g. for occipital artery The shallow groove medial to the mastoid notch on the undersurface of the mastoid part of the temporal bone; it accommodates the occipital artery. Also called sulcus of occipital artery.

olfactory g. See ethmoid fossa, under fossa.

optic g. See chiasmatic sulcus, under sulcus.

popliteal g. A short, deep groove at the lower end of the femur, separating the lateral epicondyle from the articular surface of the lateral condyle; it accommodates the tendon of the popliteus muscle when the knee is flexed.

preauricular g. of ilium A short, shallow groove adjacent to the front and lower borders of the auricular surface of the ilium; it affords attachment to the numerous thin bands of the anterior sacroiliac ligament. Also called preauricular sulcus.

g. for radial nerve A broad, shallow, oblique groove that spirals around the posterior surface of the mid-humeral shaft; it accommodates the radial nerve and the deep brachial artery. Also called musculospiral groove; sulcus of radial nerve.

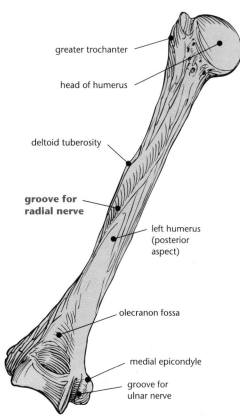

greater trochanter

head of humerus

deltoid tuberosity

groove for radial nerve

left humerus (posterior aspect)

olecranon fossa

medial epicondyle

groove for ulnar nerve

sagittal g. See groove for superior sagittal sinus.

groove ■ groove

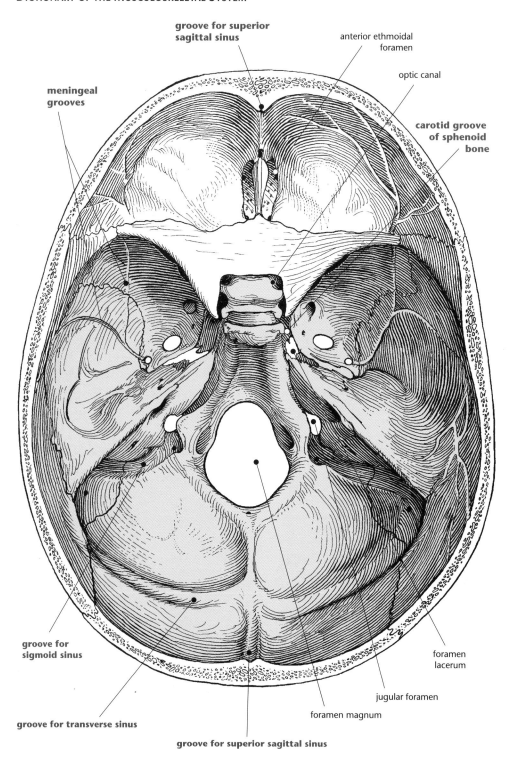

groove for superior
sagittal sinus

anterior ethmoidal
foramen

optic canal

meningeal
grooves

carotid groove
of sphenoid
bone

groove for
sigmoid sinus

foramen
lacerum

groove for transverse sinus

jugular foramen

foramen magnum

groove for superior sagittal sinus

groove ■ groove

g. for sigmoid sinus The deep, broad S-shaped groove on either side of the mastoid part of the temporal bone in the posterior cranial fossa; it is a continuation of the lateral extremity of the groove for the transverse sinus; it ends at the jugular notch of the occipital bone and accommodates the sigmoid sinus; it is usually more prominent on the right side. Also called sulcus of sigmoid sinus.

subclavian g.'s Shallow oblique grooves on the upper part of the first rib separated by the tubercle for the anterior scalene muscle. The groove in front of the tubercle accommodates the subclavian vein; the one behind the tubercle accommodates the subclavian artery. Also called subclavian sulci.

g. for superior sagittal sinus A longitudinal groove along the median plane of the cerebral surface of the skull cap from the frontal bone to the squama of the occipital bone as far as the internal occipital protuberance; it accommodates the superior sagittal sinus which widens as it progresses posteriorly. Also called sulcus for superior sagittal sinus; sagittal groove.

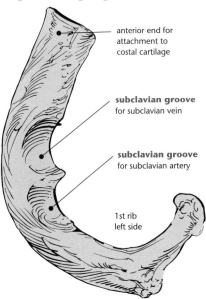

anterior end for attachment to costal cartilage

subclavian groove for subclavian vein

subclavian groove for subclavian artery

1st rib left side

g. of talus See incisure of talus, under incisure.

g. for tendon of long flexor muscle of big toe An oblique groove on the posterior surface of the talus (ankle bone) and the medial surface of the calcaneus (heel bone) that accommodates the tendon of the long flexor muscle of the big toe (flexor hallucis longus). Also called sulcus of tendon of long flexor muscle of big toe.

g. for transverse sinus A wide horizontal groove on the inner surface of the occipital bone, extending on each side of the internal occipital protuberance; it accommodates the transverse sinus and the tentorium is attached to its margins; the right groove is often larger and is a continuation of the groove for the superior sagittal sinus; it flows into the groove for the sigmoid sinus. Also called sulcus for transverse sinus.

g. for ulnar nerve A shallow vertical groove on the back surface of the medial epicondyle of the humerus; it accommodates the ulnar nerve. When the nerve is sharply pressed against the bony groove (popularly known as hitting the funny bone), a tingling sensation is generally felt. Also called sulcus of ulnar nerve.

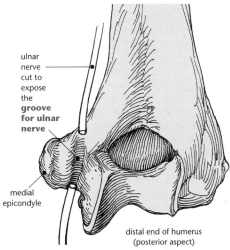

ulnar nerve cut to expose the **groove for ulnar nerve**

medial epicondyle

distal end of humerus (posterior aspect)

vertebral g. The groove on either side of the spinous processes of the vertebral column that provides attachment to the deep muscles of the back; the grooves are usually shallow in cervical and lumbar vertebrae, and deep and wide in thoracic vertebrae.

guarding (gahrd'ing) Spasm of muscles at the site of injury or disease occurring as the body's protection against further injury.

abdominal g. A sign of acute peritonitis marked by involuntary rigid contraction of the abdominal rectus muscles, occurring when the examiner gently depresses the abdomen with both hands; the muscles contract, remaining taut, rigid, and boardlike throughout deep respiration.

groove ■ guarding

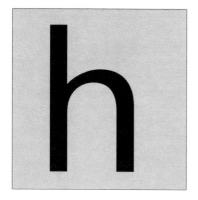

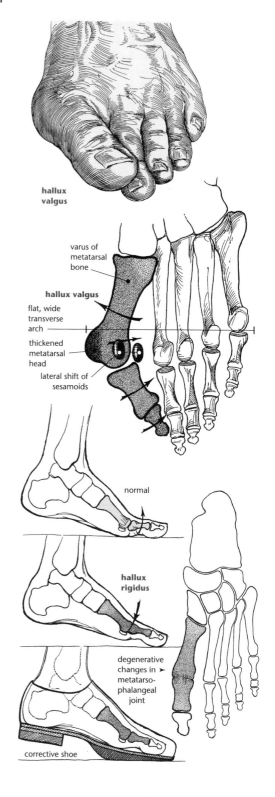

hallux valgus

varus of metatarsal bone

hallux valgus

flat, wide transverse arch

thickened metatarsal head

lateral shift of sesamoids

normal

hallux rigidus

degenerative changes in ► metatarso-phalangeal joint

corrective shoe

hallux (hal'uks), pl. hal'luces The big toe; the first or inner digit of the foot.

  h. dolorosa A painful condition, usually associated with flatfoot, in which walking causes severe discomfort in the matatarsophalangeal joint of the big toe.

  h. flexus Hammertoe of the hallux; a big toe that is congenitally bent downward. Also called hallux malleus.

  h. rigidus Stiff toe; painful flexion of the big toe due to stiffness in the metatarsophalangeal joint.

  h. valgus The most common of the painful conditions of the toes, marked by an abnormal fixed displacement (angulation) of the big toe toward the other toes of the same foot (away from the midline of the body); the big toe may ride over or under the other toes; the condition is generally attributed to the wearing of narrow or pointed shoes; predisposing congenital and familial factors may exist. COMPARE bunion.

  h. varus Abnormal fixed displacement (angulation) of the big toe away from the other toes of the same foot (toward the midline of the body).

  h. malleus See hallux flexus.
hamate (ham'āt) 1. Hooked. 2. See table of bones in appendix I.
hammertoe (ham'er-to) See hammer toe, under toe.
hamstring (ham'string) See hamstring tendon, under tendon.
hamular (ham'u-lar) Shaped like a hook.
hamulus (ham'u-lus) Any small hook-shaped process, as seen at the end of a bone; a little hook.

  h. of hamate bone A hooklike process of the hamate bone of the wrist, which projects from the distal part of the palmar surface;

hallux ■ hamulus

the flexor retinaculum attaches to its tip in the formation of the carpal tunnel.

lacrimal h. The hooklike process on the orbital surface of the lacrimal bone articulating with the maxilla and forming the upper aperture of the bony naso-lacrimal canal.

pterygoid h. The hooklike process at the bottom of the medial pterygoid plate of the sphenoid bone of the skull; the tensor muscle of the soft palate (tensor veli palatini) bends around it in passing from the sphenoid fossa to the soft palate. Also called hamular process of sphenoid bone.

h. of spiral lamina The small hooklike termination of the apex of the bony spiral lamina of the cochlea, in the inner ear.

hand (hand) The terminal part of the upper extremity below the forearm, composed of the carpus, metacarpus, and digits.

accoucheur's h. The characteristic position of the hand produced by spasm in tetany; the hand is flexed at the wrist, the fingers are flexed at the metacarpophalangeal joints, and extended at the interphalangeal joints, with the thumb tightly flexed into the palm; so called because it resembles the posture of the obstetrician's hand when examining the vagina. Also called obstetrician's hand.

obstetrician's h. See accoucheur's hand.

opera-glass h. The characteristic contracted hand of advanced rheumatoid arthritis; marked by erosion and compressive collapse of the phalanges at the base of the fingers, with consequent overriding of bones and dislocation of the metacarpophalangeal joints. May also occur in other conditions (e.g., osteoarthritis, chronic infection, and leprosy).

trident h. The characteristic hand of achondroplasia; a hand in which the fingers

are short and thick and nearly equal in length, with a deflection (at the second phalangeal joint) of the index and middle fingers toward the radial side and the ring and little fingers toward the ulnar side, and so with the thumb form the three elements of a trident.

haunch (hawnch) The region of the upper thigh, hip, and buttock regarded as a unit.

head (hed) 1. The part of the body that contains the brain, sense organs and the mouth. 2. The topmost or proximal extremity of a structure, such as a long bone. 3. The part of a muscle attached to the less movable of its two attachments. 4. The foremost part of a structure.

articular h. The cartilage-covered eminence on a bone that is able to articulate with another bone.

h. of condyloid process of mandible See head of mandible.

h. of femur The globular hemisphere at the upper end of the femur; it is mostly covered with articular cartilage and it articulates with the acetabulum of the hipbone.

h. of fibula The expanded upper extremity of the fibula that articulates with the undersurface of the lateral condyle of the tibia.

h. of humerus The expanded proximal end of the humerus, covered extensively with hyalin articular cartilage, which articulates with the glenoid cavity of the scapula at the shoulder joint.

h. of malleus The ovoid upper end of the malleus (lateral ossicle of ear) that articulates with the incus (middle ossicle of ear).

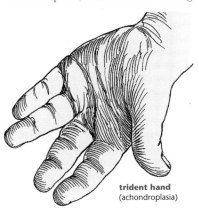

trident hand
(achondroplasia)

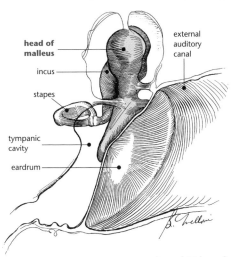

head of malleus

external auditory canal

incus

stapes

tympanic cavity

eardrum

hand ▪ head

h. of mandible The knuckle-shaped expansion at the end of the condylar process of the mandible that articulates with the mandibular fossa of the temporal bone with an articular disk intervening; it is covered with fibrocartilage. Also called head of condyloid process of mandible.

h. of metacarpus The expanded convex distal end of a metacarpal bone; it is covered by cartilage for articulation with the proximal end of the phalanx; its prominence is seen as a knuckle on the dorsal side of the hand, especially when the hand is clenched.

h. of metatarsal The expanded convex distal end of a metatarsal bone; it is covered by cartilage for articulation with the proximal end of the phalanx; the sides show a depression for the collateral ligaments of the metatarsophalangeal joint.

h. of phalanx of fingers The slightly expanded distal end of each of the proximal and middle phalanges of the fingers, which articulates with the base of the more distal phalanx.

h. of phalanx of toes The slightly expanded distal end of each of the proximal and middle phalanges of the toes, which articulate with the base of the more distal phalanx.

h. of radius The disk-shaped, expanded upper end of the radius; it possesses a shallow depression on its uppermost surface

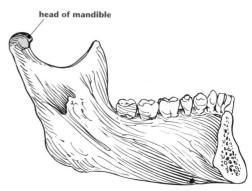

head of mandible

for articulation with the capitulum of the humerus and an articular circumference for articulation with the radial notch of the ulna.

h. of rib The expanded posterior end of a rib, usually having two articular facets that articulates with the bodies of two contiguous vertebrae; the ribs with only one facet, namely ribs number 1, 10, 11, and 12 articulate with a single vertebra.

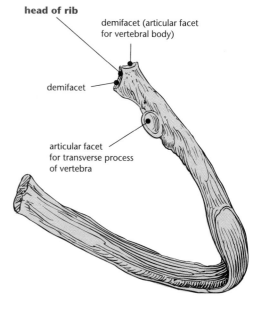

head of rib

demifacet (articular facet for vertebral body)

demifacet

articular facet for transverse process of vertebra

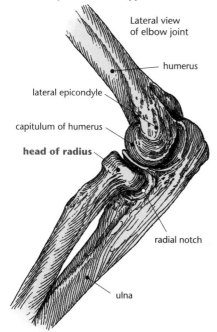

Lateral view of elbow joint

humerus

lateral epicondyle

capitulum of humerus

head of radius

radial notch

ulna

h. of stapes The knob above the neck of the stapes (medial ossicle of ear) that has a small cartilage-covered depression for articulation with the incus (middle ossicle of ear).

h. of talus The large, rounded anterior end of the talus (ankle bone), which articulates anteriorly with the proximal surface of the navicular bone of the foot.

head ■ head

h. of ulna The convex process at the distal end of the ulna; it articulates with the ulnar notch of the radius (with an intervening articular disk), to form the distal radioulnar joint.

heart (hart) The hollow, muscular, four-chambered organ covered by a membranous sac (pericardium), lying between the lungs; it receives blood from the veins and pumps it into the arteries, thus maintaining blood circulation throughout the body.

    left h. The left atrium and left ventricle considered together.

    right h. The right atrium and right ventricle considered together.

heartbeat (hart'bet) One single complete cardiac cycle; one set of contraction and dilatation of the heart muscle.

heel (hēl) The rounded posterior portion of the foot.

HEART

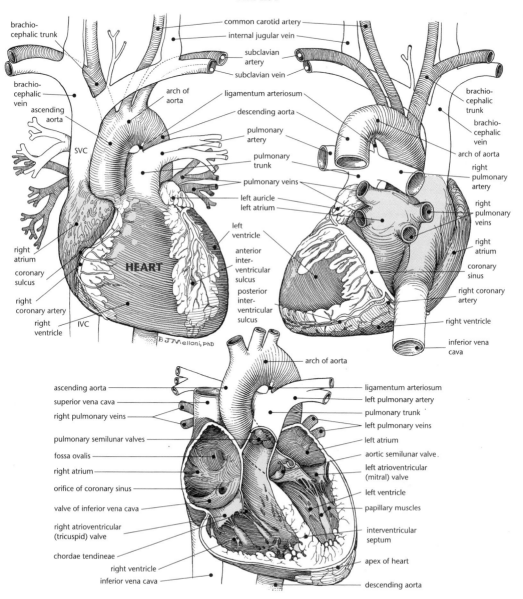

brachio-cephalic trunk · common carotid artery · internal jugular vein · subclavian artery · subclavian vein · brachio-cephalic vein · ascending aorta · arch of aorta · ligamentum arteriosum · descending aorta · pulmonary artery · pulmonary trunk · SVC · pulmonary veins · left auricle · left atrium · brachio-cephalic trunk · brachio-cephalic vein · arch of aorta · right pulmonary artery · right pulmonary veins · right atrium · coronary sulcus · left ventricle · anterior inter-ventricular sulcus · posterior inter-ventricular sulcus · HEART · right atrium · coronary sinus · right coronary artery · right coronary artery · right ventricle · IVC · right ventricle · inferior vena cava · B.J.Melloni, PhD

ascending aorta · superior vena cava · right pulmonary veins · pulmonary semilunar valves · fossa ovalis · right atrium · orifice of coronary sinus · valve of inferior vena cava · right atrioventricular (tricuspid) valve · chordae tendineae · right ventricle · inferior vena cava · arch of aorta · ligamentum arteriosum · left pulmonary artery · pulmonary trunk · left pulmonary veins · left atrium · aortic semilunar valve · left atrioventricular (mitral) valve · left ventricle · papillary muscles · interventricular septum · apex of heart · descending aorta

heart ■ heel

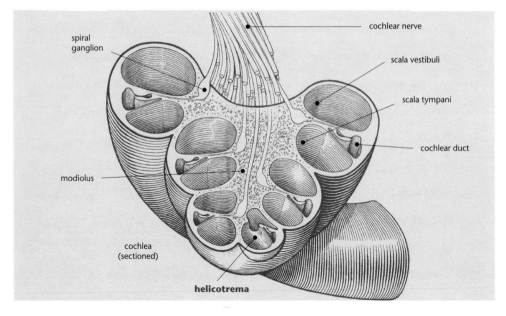

spiral ganglion

cochlear nerve

scala vestibuli

scala tympani

cochlear duct

modiolus

cochlea (sectioned)

helicotrema

helicotrema (hel-ī-ko-tre'mah) The narrow semilunar opening within the apex of the cochlea of the inner ear, connecting the scala tympani with the scala vestibuli, thereby permitting free flow of endolymph within the two passages.

hemiarthroplasty (hem-e-ar'thro-plas-te) Replacement of only part of a joint with artificial material (e.g., of the shoulder joint or hip joint).

hemarthrosis (hem-ar-thro'sis) Bleeding into a joint, or its synovial cavity.

hemi- A prefix meaning half; partial; unilateral.

hemidiaphragm (hem-e-di'ah-fram) One half of the diaphragm.

hemiparesis (hem-e-par-e'sis) Muscular weakness or mild paralysis of one side of the body.

hemiplegia (hem-e-ple'je-ah) Paralysis of one side of the body due to injury or disease.

hiatus (hi-a'tus) An opening or gap.

    adductor h. See tendinous hiatus.

    aortic h. The opening between the diaphragm and the vertebra through which pass the descending aorta, azygos vein, and thoracic duct; located at the level of the 12th thoracic vertebra.

    h. of canal for the greater petrosal nerve The opening of the narrow groove on the anterior aspect of the petrous part of the temporal bone, just lateral to the eminence of the anterior semicircular canal, it accommodates the passage of the greater petrosal nerve as it runs forward to the

foramen lacerum; the hiatus leads to the facial canal. Also called hiatus of facial canal.

    esophageal h. The opening in the diaphragm through which pass the esophagus, the right and left vagus nerves and small esophageal arteries and veins; located at the level of the 10th thoracic vertebra.

    h. of facial canal See hiatus of canal for the greater petrosal nerve.

    h. of canal for the lesser petrosal nerve The small opening in the petrous part of the temporal bone, just lateral to the hiatus for the greater petrosal nerve; it accommodates the passage of the lesser petrosal nerve from the tympanic plexus of the middle ear.

    maxillary h. A large opening between the upper medial side of the maxillary sinus and the middle meatus of the nasal cavity. Also called orifice of maxillary sinus.

    sacral h. The opening on the dorsal aspect of the lowest segment of the sacrum, leading into the vertebral canal, and through which the terminal filament (filum terminale) passes out to become attached to the coccyx; the sacral hiatus is a site for injection of epidural anesthesia.

    semilunar h. The deep, curved and narrow cleft in the lateral wall of the middle meatus of the nasal cavity, bounded below by the sharp concave ridge of the uncinate process of the ethmoid bone and above by the rounded elevation of middle ethmoid air

helicotrema ■ hiatus

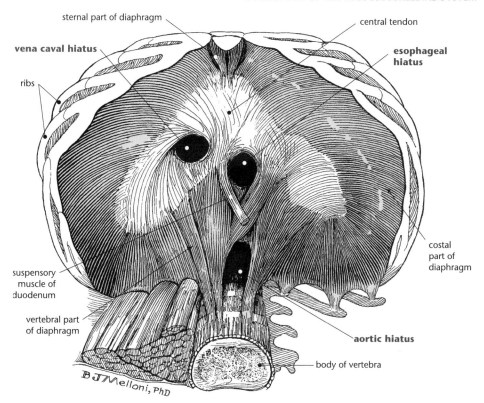

sternal part of diaphragm

central tendon

vena caval hiatus

esophageal hiatus

ribs

costal part of diaphragm

suspensory muscle of duodenum

vertebral part of diaphragm

aortic hiatus

body of vertebra

B.J.Melloni, PhD

cells (ethnoidal bulla); it is a continuation of the ethmoidal infundibulum and receives the openings of the ethmoid air cells, maxillary sinus and in 50 percent of individuals from the frontal sinus via the frontonasal duct.

tendinous h. The opening between the tendon of the great adductor muscle (adductor magnus) and the lower part of the medial surface of the femur; it transmits the femoral artery to, and the femoral vein from, the popliteal space in the back of the knee joint. Also called adductor hiatus.

vena caval h. The opening in the diaphragm through which pass the inferior vena cava and some branches of the right phrenic nerve; located at the level between the 8th and 9th thoracic vertebra.

hindfoot (hind′foot) The back part of the foot that contains the talus (ankle bone) and the calcaneus (heel bone); it is separated from the midfoot by the transverse midtarsal joint.

hip (hip) The lateral area of the body from the waist to the thigh.

hipbone (hip′bōn) The large, flattened bone enclosing the pelvic cavity; formed by the fusion of three bones (ilium, ischium, pubis).

Formerly called innominate bone; also written hip bone.

holarthritis (hol-ar-thri′tis) Inflammation of most or all joints.

homologous (ho-mol′o-gus) Corresponding in position, structure, function, origin, or development.

hook (hook) A sharply angled anatomic structure.

h. of hamate bone A hook-like process (hamulus), which projects from the distal

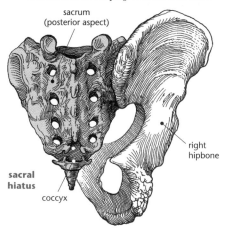

sacrum (posterior aspect)

right hipbone

sacral hiatus

coccyx

hindfoot ■ hook

part of the palmar surface of the hamate bone; it provides attachment to the flexor retinaculum.

horn (horn) Any anatomic structure projecting from a base and suggestive of a horn.

    coccygeal h.'s See coccygeal cornua, under cornu.

    greater h. of hyoid bone See greater cornu of hyoid bone, under cornu.

    inferior h. of thyroid cartilage See inferior cornu of thyroid cartilage, under cornu.

    lesser h. of hyoid bone See lesser cornu of hyoid bone, under cornu.

    pulp h. The extension of the tooth's pulp chamber toward a cusp.

    sacral h.'s See sacral cornua, under cornu.

    superior h. of thyroid cartilage See superior cornu of thyroid cartilage, under cornu.

humeral (hu'mer-al) Relating to the humerus.

humerus (hu'mer-us) The long bone of the arm, extending from the shoulder to the elbow; it has a rounded end for articulation with the scapula (shoulder blade), a shaft, and a lower end adapted for articulation with the radius and ulna at the elbow. See also table of bones in appendix I.

hyaline (hi'ah-lin) Glasslike in appearance.

hydrarthrodial (hi-drar-thro'de-al) Relating to hydrarthrosis.

hydrarthrosis (hi-drar-thro'sis) Collection of excessive synovial fluid in a joint cavity.

    intermittent h. A disorder characterized by periodic swelling of a joint due to the periodic recurrence of effusion of fluid into the cavity of the joint.

hyo- A combining form meaning hyoid or U-shaped.

hyoepiglottic (hi-o-ep-ĭ-glot'ik) Relating to the hyoid bone and the epiglottis, especially the ligament connecting them.

hyoglossal (hi-o-glos'al) 1. Relating to the hyoid bone and the tongue, especially their connecting aponeurosis. 2. Relating to the hyoglossal muscle. See also the table of muscles in appendix II.

hyoid (hi'oid) U-shaped; applied to the horseshoe-shaped bone in the throat between the thyroid cartilage and the root of the tongue. See also table of bones in appendix I.

hyolaryngeal (hi-o-lah-rin'je-al) Relating to the hyoid bone and the larynx.

hyomandibular (hi-o-man-dib'u-lar) Relating to the hyoid bone and the mandible.

hyomental (hi-o-men'tal) Relating to the hyoid bone and the chin.

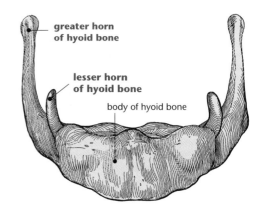

greater horn of hyoid bone

lesser horn of hyoid bone

body of hyoid bone

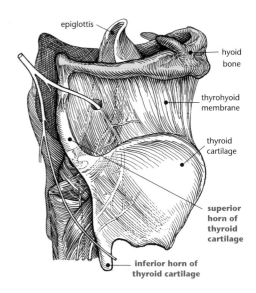

epiglottis

hyoid bone

thyrohyoid membrane

thyroid cartilage

superior horn of thyroid cartilage

inferior horn of thyroid cartilage

hyothyroid (hi-o-thi'roid) See thyrohyoid.

hyper- A prefix meaning above the normal, excessive.

hyperextension (hi-per-ek-sten'shun) Extension of a joint beyond its neutral position; it is normal in some joints (e.g., the shoulder joint) but not in others (e.g., the knee joint). Also called overextension; superextension.

hyperflexion (hi-per-flek'shun) Flexion of a body part beyond its normal limit. Also called overflexion; superflexion.

hyperostosis (hi-per-os-to'sis) Abnormal increase in the mass of bone.

    ankylosing h. See diffuse idiopathic skeletal hyperostosis.

    calvarial h. Irregular thickening of the cranial bones. Also called cranial hyperostosis.

horn ■ hyperostosis

cranial h. See calvarial hyperostosis.

diffuse idiopathic skeletal h. A variant of osteoarthritis occurring most commonly in elderly men, characterized by development of large bony outgrowth bridging the vertebrae and ossification of tendon insertions and ligaments (especially along the anterior aspect of the vertebral column). Also called ankylosing hyperostosis.

h. frontalis interna Abnormal deposition of bone in the skull, seen on the inner surface of the frontal bone.

infantile cortical h. A self-limited, benign condition of unknown cause that has its onset before the age of six months and persists for many weeks or months; characterized by bone formation on the surface of bones, typically the mandible and clavicles, but may involve any bone, especially the shafts of ribs and bones of the arm; causes irritability, fever, and tender painful swellings.

sternoclavicular h. Uncommon benign condition characterized by hyperostosis and ossification of soft tissues between the clavicles and anterior portion of ribs; often associated with eruption of vesicles on the palms and soles (bacterid); a bone infection has been suggested as a possible cause.

hypertonia (hi-per-to'ne-ah) Excessive tension of muscles.

hypo- A prefix meaning less than normal, deficient, under, beneath.

hypocalcemia (hi-po-kal-se'me-ah) Abnormally low serum calcium levels in blood or serum.

hypocalcification (hi-po-kal-sĭ-fĭ-ka'shun) A deficient calcification process; diminished calcification.

enamel h. A defect in the formation of tooth enamel, resulting in breakage of the enamel soon after tooth eruption, leaving the dentin exposed, which gives the tooth a yellow appearance.

hypodermis (hi-po-der'mis) See superficial fascia, under fascia.

hypoglossal (hi-po-glos'al) Lying below the tongue.

hypolarynx (hi-po-lar'inks) The lower part of the larynx extending from the true vocal cords to the upper part of the first tracheal ring.

hypostosis (hip-os-to'sis) An abnormal, deficient development of bone.

hypothenar (hi-poth'ĕ-nar) The fleshy part of the palm of the hand, on the side of the little finger.

hypotonia (hi-po-to'ne-ah) Lessened tone or tension, especially a reduction in the tone of skeletal muscles.

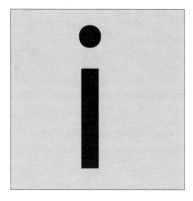

iliac (il'e-ak) Relating to the ilium, a hip bone.

ilio- Combining form meaning ilium.

iliofemoral (il-e-o-fem'or-al) Relating to the ilium (largest bone of the hip) and the femur (thighbone).

ilioinguinal (il-e-o-in'gwi-nal) Relating to the lateral area of the pelvis and the groin.

iliolumbar (il-e-o-lum'bar) Relating to the hip and the "small of the back".

iliopectineal (il-e-o-pek-tin'e-al) Relating to the ilium and the pubic bone.

iliosacral (il-e-o-sa'kral) Relating to the ilium and sacrum at the side and back of the pelvis, respectively.

ilium (il'e-um) The superior, broad bone on either side of the pelvis that supports the flank; it includes the upper part of the acetabulum and is a separate bone in early life. See also table of bones in appendix I.

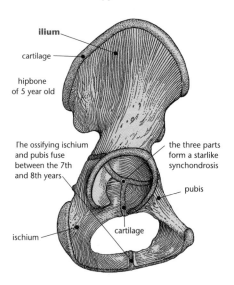

ilium

cartilage

hipbone of 5 year old

The ossifying ischium and pubis fuse between the 7th and 8th years

the three parts form a starlike synchondrosis

pubis

cartilage

ischium

impression (im-presh'un) An imprint or slight indentation on a structure that accommodates another structure with the reverse form.

    trigeminal i. A shallow depression on the internal surface of the skull, near the apex of the petrous part of the temporal bone, on which resides the trigeminal ganglion. Also called trigeminal impression of temporal bone.

    trigeminal i. of temporal bone See trigeminal impression.

incisor (in-si'zer) 1. Any of the eight front cutting teeth, four in each jaw. 2. Anything adapted for cutting.

    central i. The tooth closest to and on either side of the midline of the head, on either jaw.

    lateral i. The tooth, upper and lower, on either side of the midline of the head, situated between the central incisor and cuspid.

incisura (in-si-su'rah) See incisure.

incisure (in-si'zhur) A notch, especially on the edge of a structure.

    i. of acetabulum See acetabular notch, under notch.

    clavicular i. of sternum See clavicular notch of sternum, under notch.

    costal i. of sternum See costal notch of sternum, under notch.

    digastric i. See mastoid notch, under notch.

    ethmoidal i. of frontal bone See ethmoidal notch of frontal bone, under notch.

    fibular i. of tibia See fibular notch, under notch.

    intertragic i. of ear See intertragic notch, under notch.

    mandibular i. See mandibular notch, under notch.

    pterygoid i. See pterygoid notch, under notch.

    i. of scapula See scapular notch, under notch.

    sphenopalatine i. See sphenopalatine notch, under notch.

    i. of talus The vertical groove situated between the medial and lateral tubercles of the posterior process of the talus (ankle bone) that continues obliquely to the medial surface of the calcaneus; it accommodates the tendon of the long flexor muscle of the big toe (tendon of flexor hallucis longus). Also called groove of talus.

    terminal i. of ear See terminal notch of auricle, under notch.

iliac ■ incisure

trochlear i. of ulna See trochlear notch of ulna, under notch.

ulnar i. of radius See radial notch of ulna, under notch.

inclination (in-klĭ-na′shun) A leaning or sloping from a particular plane.

i. of pelvis The angle of the plane of the pelvic inlet to the horizontal plane, with the body in the erect position; it is usually about 55°.

inconstant (in-kon′stant) 1. Variable. 2. In anatomy, denoting a structure that may or may not be present, may have a tendency to change, or is given to change of location.

incudostapedial (ing-ku-do-sta-pe′de-al) Relating to the incus and stapes of the middle ear chamber, especially their articulation.

incudal (ing′ku-dal) Relating to the incus of the middle ear chamber.

incus (ing′kus) The middle of the three ossicles of the middle ear chamber, between the malleus and the stapes, involved in transmitting sound vibrations from the tympanic membrane (eardrum) to the inner ear; it resembles an anvil and is sometimes called by that name. See also table of bones in appendix I.

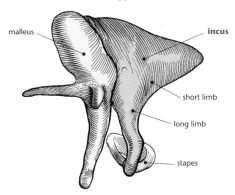

malleus · incus · short limb · long limb · stapes

indentation (in-den-ta′shun) 1. A notch, dent, or impression. 2. The act of notching or indenting.

index (in-deks), pl. in′dexes, in′dices 1. The forefinger; the second finger of the hand. 2. A value expressing the ratio of one measurement to another.

cephalic i. The ratio of the maximal breadth to the maximal length of the head of a living subject; (breadth x 100/length).

chest i. See thoracic index.

cranial i. The breadth/length ratio of a dried skull.

gnathic i. The ratio between the length from the basion (the midpoint of the anterior margin of the foramen magnum) to the prosthion (the most anterior point on the maxillary alveolar process between the central incisors), multiplied by 100 and the length from the basion to the nasion (the midpoint of the depression at the nasofrontal suture); it is an index of the degree of prominence of the upper jaw.

nasal i. A ratio of the greatest width of the nose to its length.

orbital i. The ratio of the height of the eye socket (orbit) to its width.

pelvic i. The ratio of the pelvic conjugate and transverse diameters of the maternal pelvis (conjugate diameter × 100/transverse diameter); an index to assess possible disproportion of the pelvic inlet. Also called pelvic inlet index.

pelvic inlet i. See pelvic inlet.

thoracic i. The ratio of the anteroposterior to the transverse diameter of the chest. Also called chest index.

inferior (in-fēr′e-or) 1. Directed toward the bottom; situated below in relation to another structure when the body is in the anatomic position. Also called caudal. 2. Poorer in quality; less useful.

infero- Combining form denoting inferior.

inflection (in-flek′shun) The act of inward bending. Also spelled inflexion.

inflexion (in-flek′shun) See inflection.

infra- Prefix meaning below; beneath.

infraclavicular (in-frah-klah-vik′u-lar) Below a clavicle (collarbone).

infracostal (in-frah-kos′tal) Below the ribs or a rib; subcostal.

infraglenoid (in-frah-gle′noid) Below the glenoid cavity of the scapula.

infrahyoid (in-frah-hi′oid) Below the hyoid bone, in the neck.

inframandibular (in-frah-man-dib′u-lar) Below the lower jaw; submandibular.

inframaxillary (in-frah-mak′sĭ-lār-e) Situated below the upper jaw; submaxillary.

infraorbital (in frah-or′bi-tal) Beneath or below the eye socket (orbit). Also called suborbital.

infrapatellar (in-frah-pah-tel′ar) Below the patella (kneecap).

infrascapular (in-frah-skap′u-lar) Below the scapula (shoulder blade).

infraspinous (in-frah-spi′nus) Below a spinous process.

infrasternal (in-frah-ster′nal) Situated below the sternum (breastbone).

infratemporal (in-frah-tem′po-ral) Situated beneath the temporal fossa of the skull.

inclination ■ infratemporal

infratrochlear (in-frah-trok'le-ar) Located below the pulley (trochlea) of the superior oblique muscle of the eye.

infrazygomatic (in-frah-zi-go-mat'ik) Below the zygoma (cheekbone).

inguen (ing'gwen) The groin.

inguinal (ing'gwi-nāl) Relating to the groin.

inion (in'ē-on) The most protruding point of the external occipital protuberance (at the back of the skull); used as a fixed craniometric point.

innate (in'nat) Present at birth.

innominate (ĭ-nom'ĭ-nāt) Unnamed; formerly applied to certain anatomic structures, such as the innominate bone (hipbone) and the innominate artery (brachiocephalic trunk).

inostosis (in-os-to'sis) The reformation of bony tissue to replace similar tissue that was damaged.

insertion (in-ser'shun) The site of attachment of a muscle to a bone that is most movable during the action of that muscle.

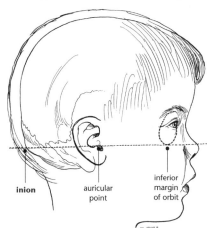

inion auricular point inferior margin of orbit

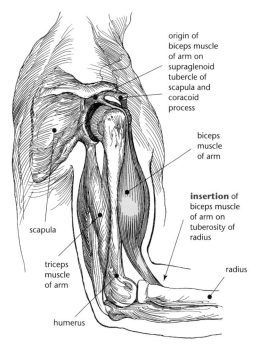

origin of biceps muscle of arm on supraglenoid tubercle of scapula and coracoid process

biceps muscle of arm

insertion of biceps muscle of arm on tuberosity of radius

scapula

triceps muscle of arm

humerus

radius

inlet (in'let) A passage leading into a cavity.

    pelvic i. The upper opening of the minor (true) pelvis; the space within the pelvis brim.

    thoracic i. The kidney-shaped inlet of the chest cavity bounded in the back by the first thoracic vertebra, at the sides by the first ribs, and in front by the upper border of the sternum. Also called superior thoracic aperture.

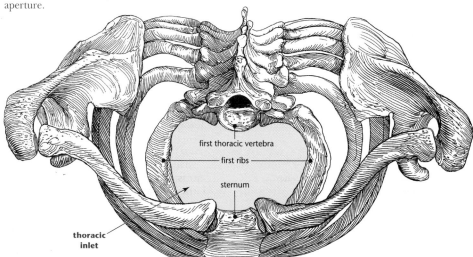

first thoracic vertebra

first ribs

sternum

thoracic inlet

infratrochlear ■ insertion

instep (in'step) The arched middle part of the dorsum of the foot.

interapophyseal (in-ter-ap-o-fiz'e-al) Situated between two bony outgrowths or projections, such as tuberosities or processes.

interarticular (in-ter-ar-tik'u-lar) Between two joints or joint surfaces.

interatrial (in-ter-a'tre-al) Between the two upper chambers (atria) of the heart.

interclavicular (in-ter-klah-vik'u-lar) Between the clavicles (collarbones).

intercondylar (in-ter-kon'di-lar) Between two condyles.

intercostal (in-ter-kos'tal) Between two successive ribs.

intercristal (in-ter-kris'tal) Between two crests of a bone.

interdental (in-ter-den'tal) Between adjacent teeth of the same dental arch.

interdigital (in-ter-dij'ĭ-tal) Between two adjacent fingers or toes.

interdigitation (in-ter-dij-i-ta'shun) 1. Interlocking of structures by means of finger-like processes. 2. The processes so interlocked.

intermalleolar (in-ter-mah-le'o-lar) Situated between the lateral and medial malleoli on either side of the ankle joint.

intermamillary (in-ter-mam'ĭ-lār-e) Between the nipples of the breasts.

intermammary (in-ter-mam'ah-re) Between the breasts.

intermetacarpal (in-ter-met-ah-kar'pal) Situated between the metacarpal bones of the hand.

intermetatarsal (in-ter-met-ah-tar'sal) Situated between the metatarsal bones of the foot.

intermuscular (in-ter-mus'ku-lar) Between the muscles or muscle groups.

interosseous (in-ter-os'e-us) Between bones; applied especially to ligaments and muscles.

interphalangeal (in-ter-fah-lan'je-al) Between two contiguous bones of fingers or toes, i.e., between two phalanges.

interpubic (in-ter-pu'bik) Situated between the two pubic bones.

interscapular (in-ter-skap'u-lar) Between the scapulas (shoulder blades).

interspinal (in-ter-spi'nal) Between the spinous processes of the vertebrae.

intertarsal (in-ter-tar'sal) Situated between adjacent tarsal bones.

intertendinous (in-ter-ten'dĭ-nus) Situated between tendons.

intertrochanteric (in-ter-tro-kan-ter'ik) Between the greater and lesser trochanters of the femur, at the hip.

intertubercular (in-ter-tu-ber'ku-lar) Situated between tubercles.

interventricular (in-ter-ven-trik'u-lar) Situated between two ventricles, e.g., interventricular septum.

intervertebral (in-ter-ver'tĕ-bral) Situated between two contiguous vertebrae; e.g., intervertebral disk.

intoe (in'to) The turning in of the feet on walking; it may be a minor self-correcting condition of toddlers, or may be a physical sign of other disorders such as metatarsus adductus, medial torsion of the tibia, bowlegs, or congenital contraction of the internal rotators of the hip. Popularly called pigeon toe.

intortor (in'tor-tor) A medial or inward rotator; applied to a muscle (e.g., an extraocular muscle) that turns a part inward.

intra- Prefix meaning within.

intra-articular (in-trah ar-tik'u-lar) Within a joint cavity.

intracapsular (in-trah-kap'su-lar) Within a capsule, especially a joint capsule.

intracarpal (in-trah-kar'pal) Situated within the wrist or among the carpal bones.

intracartilaginous (in-trah-kar-tĭ-laj'ĭ-nus) Situated or formed within cartilage or cartilaginous tissue. Also called endochondral; intrachondral.

intrachondral (in-trah-kon'dral) See intracartilaginous.

intracostal (in-trah-kos'tal) On the inner surface of a rib or ribs.

intracranial (in-trah-kra'ne-al) Within the cranium (skull).

intrafusal (in-trah-fu'zal) Within the fusiform capsule of a muscle spindle; applied to striated muscle fibers.

intramedullary (in-trah-med'u-lar-e) Situated within the bone marrow, the medulla oblongata, or the spinal cord.

intramembranous (in-trah-mem'brah-nus) Situated or formed between the layers of a membrane.

intramuscular (in-trah-mus'ku-lar) Situated or occurring within muscle tissue.

intraosseous (in-trah-os'e-us) Within bone tissue.

intrasellar (in-trah-sel'ar) Within the sella turcica, the bony cavity in the floor of the skull that houses the pituitary (hypophysis).

intraspinal (in-trah-spi'nal) See intravertebral.

intrasynovial (in-trah-si-no've-al) Within the synovial sac in a joint cavity or a synovial tendon sheath.

intratympanic (jn-trah-tim-pan'ik) Within the tympanic cavity (middle ear chamber).

instep ■ intratympanic

intravertebral (in-trah-ver'te-bral) Situated within the vertebral column or canal. Also called intraspinal.

invertor (in-ver'tor) Any muscle that turns a part inward.

ipsilateral (ip-sĭ-lat'er-al) Occurring on, or affecting the same side, as opposed to contralateral.

iridoconstriction (ir-ĭ-do-kon-strik'shun) The sphincter muscle of the iris or any agent that causes constriction of that muscle.

iridoconstrictor (ir-ĭ-do-kon-strik'tor) The dilator muscle of the iris or any agent that causes dilation of that muscle.

iris (i'ris), pl. i'rides The delicate and adjustable diaphragm of the eye that surrounds the pupil and controls the amount of light entering the eye; it is situated between the cornea and the lens; it is immersed in the aqueous humor, partially separating the anterior and posterior chambers of the eye; the concentration of pigment cells (melanocytes) is the predominant factor that determines the color of the iris.

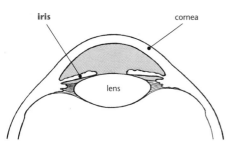

i. bombé An abnormal bulging forward of the iris; it is caused by pressure from accumulated aqueous humor in the posterior chamber of the eye, due to obstruction of the aqueous circulation by adhesion of the pupillary border of the iris to the anterior surface of the lens.

ischio- Combining form meaning ischium.

ischiococcygeal (is-ke-o-kok-sij'e-al) Relating to the ischium amd the coccyx.

ischiococcygeus (is-ke-o-kok-sij'e-us) 1. The coccygeus muscle. See also table of muscles in appendix II. 2. Part of the pelvic diaphragm; the posterior part of the levator ani.

ischiopubic (is-ke-o-pu'bik) Relating to both the ischium and the pubic bone.

ischium (is'ke-um), pl. is'chia The lower, posterior portion of the hipbone; the bone on which the body rests when sitting; it is surrounded by cartilage in early life and eventually ossifies, fusing with the ilium and pubis in the adult to form the hipbone. See also table of bones in appendix I.

isthmus (is'mus) 1. A narrow band of tissue connecting two larger parts. 2. A narrow passage between two larger cavities or tubular structures.

    i. of auditory tube The narrowest part of the auditory (eustachian) tube, at the junction of the bony and cartilaginous portions. Also called isthmus of eustachian tube.

    i. of eustachian tube See isthmus of auditory tube.

    i. of external auditory canal A narrow segment of the external auditory canal near the junction of the bony and cartilaginous portions, approximately at the outer three fourths of the canal.

    i. of fauces See isthmus of oropharynx.

    i. of oropharynx The slight constriction between the mouth and pharynx, at the palatoglossal arches. Also called isthmus of fauces.

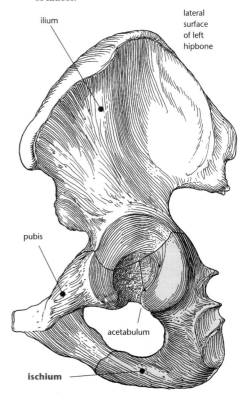

intravertebral ■ isthmus

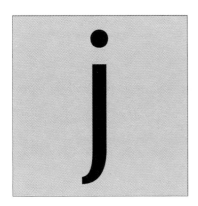

jaw (jaw) Either of two bones of the face that accommodate the teeth; the upper jaw is formed by the two maxillae and the lower jaw, the mandible.

jerk (jerk) A sudden involuntary movement, evoked when a taut tendon overlying a bone is tapped; it indicates that the local reflex nervous arc, afferent sensory and descending motor, is intact.

    Achilles j. Aee Achilles tendon reflex, under reflex.

    ankle j. See Achilles tendon reflex, under reflex.

    biceps j. See biceps reflex, under reflex.

    crossed knee j. See crossed knee reflex, under reflex.

    elbow j. See triceps reflex, under reflex.

    jaw j. See mandibular reflex, under reflex.

    knee j. See patellar reflex, under reflex.

    quadriceps j. See patellar reflex, under reflex.

    supinator j. See brachioradialis reflex, under reflex.

    tendon j. See deep reflex, under reflex.

joint (joint) The skeletal site at which two or more bones meet; an articulation.

    acromioclavicular j. The articulation between the lateral end of the clavicle and the acromion of the scapula.

    amphiarthrodal j. A joint in which the surfaces of two bones are connected by intervening cartilage, enabling slight movement, as in the articulation between two vertebrae. Also called cartilaginous joint; amphiarthrosis; slightly movable joint.

    ankle j. A hinge joint formed by the tibia and fibula and the talus (ankle bone). Also called talocrural joint; talotibiofibular joint.

    anterior talocalcanean j. See talocalcaneonavicular joint.

    arthrodial j. See plane joint.

    atlantoaxial j. Either of two articulations between the first and second cervical vertebrae (atlas and axis).

    atlantoepistrophic j. Either of two joints at the neck: *Lateral atlantoepistrophic j.*, the junction between the inferior articular processes of the atlas and the superior articular processes of the axis; *Median atlantoepistrophic j.*, the junction between the dens of the axis and the anterior arch and transverse ligament of the atlas.

    atlanto-occipital j. An ellipsoid joint between the superior articular facet of the first cervical vertebra (atlas) and the above condyle of the occipital bone on each side. Also called Cruveilhier's joint.

    ball and socket j. A synovial joint in which a rounded head (ball) of one bone fits into a cuplike cavity (socket) of another bone, permitting a wide range of movement in any direction (e.g., in the shoulder and hip joints). Also called spheroidal joint; enarthrosis; multiaxial joint.

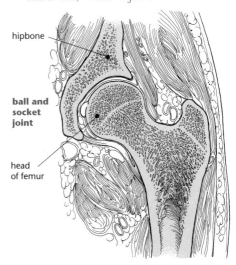

hipbone

ball and socket joint

head of femur

    biaxial j. A joint having two principal axes of movement, such as the saddle joint.

    bicondylar j. A synovial joint in which two rounded condyles of one bone fit into two shallow cavities of another bone, as in the knee or temporomandibular joints, allowing all movement except rotation. Also called condyloid joint; condylar joint.

    bilocular j. A joint in which the synovial cavity is divided into two distinct chambers by an intra-articular disk, such as the temporomandibular joint.

jaw ■ joint

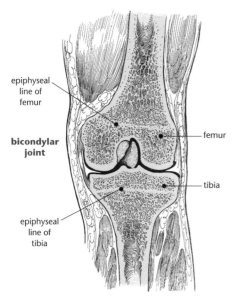

epiphyseal line of femur

bicondylar joint

— femur

— tibia

epiphyseal line of tibia

calcaneocuboid j. A saddle-shaped joint in the posterior portion of the foot between the front surface of the calcaneus (heel bone) and the back surface of the cuboid bone.

capitular j. An articulation between the head of a rib and the bodies of two adjacent thoracic vertebrae.

carpometacarpal j.'s The plane joints between the carpal bones of the wrist and the second, third, fourth, and fifth metacarpal bones of the hand.

carpometacarpal j. of thumb The joint between the trapezium of the wrist and the first metacarpal bone of the hand.

cartilaginous j. See amphiarthrodial joint.

Charcot's j. A swollen, unstable but painless joint, frequently with destruction of intra-articular ligaments and consequent abnormally increased range of motion; caused by loss of sensory innervation; the lack of sensation deprives the joint of protective reactions to undue stresses; considered a complication of a neurologic disorder (e.g., tabes dorsalis or diabetic neuropathy). Also called neuropathic joint.

Chopart's j. See transverse tarsal joint.

coccygeal j. See sacrococcygeal joint.

composite j. See compound joint.

compound j. A joint in which more than two bones articulate, as seen at the elbow joint where the humerus articulates with the ulna and radius. Also called composite joint.

condylar j. See bicondylar joint.

condyloid j. See bicondylar joint.

costochondral j. The cartilaginous articulation between the anterior end of a rib and the lateral end of a costal cartilage.

costotransverse j. The synovial articulation between the articular facet on the tubercle of a rib and the articular facet on the transverse process of the corresponding vertebra; it is a plane joint involving all ribs except the 11th and 12th.

costovertebral j.'s The joints of the ribs with the corresponding vertebrae, consisting of both the costotransverse joint and the joint of the head of the rib.

cricothyroid j. The synovial joint between the side of the cricoid cartilage and the inferior horn of the thyroid cartilage, permitting gliding and rotational movements.

Cruveilhier's j. See atlanto-occipital joint.

cubital j. See elbow joint.

cuboideonavicular j. A fibrous joint of the foot between the medial surface of the cuboid bone and the lateral surface of the navicular bone; it pemits some gliding movements.

cuneocuboid j. A plane joint between the lateral surface of the lateral cuneiform bone and the medial surface of the cuboid bone; the synovial cavity between the bones is an extension from the cuneonavicular joint; it permits some gliding movements.

cuneometatarsal j.'s See tarsometatarsal joints.

cuneonavicular j. An articulation in the posterior portion of the foot between the front surface of the navicular bone and the back surfaces of the three cuneiform bones.

diarthrodial j. See synovial joint.

dry j. A synovial joint devoid of normal synovial fluid, as one affected by chronic villous arthritis.

elbow j. The compound joint at the elbow between the distal end of the humerus and the proximal ends of the ulna and radius; it

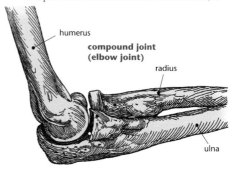

humerus

compound joint (elbow joint)

radius

ulna

joint ■ joint

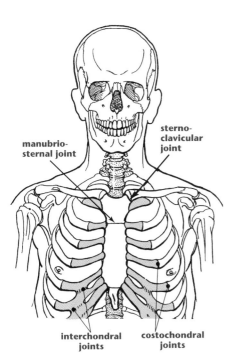

manubrio-sternal joint

sterno-clavicular joint

interchondral joints

costochondral joints

ginglymoid j. See hinge joint.
gliding j. See plane joint.
hinge j. A synovial joint that permits only a forward and backward movement similar to that of a door hinge (e.g., the bending and straightening of the fingers). Also called ginglymus; ginglymoid joint.

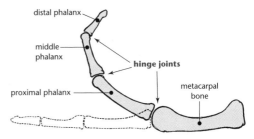

distal phalanx

middle phalanx

hinge joints

proximal phalanx

metacarpal bone

hip j. The ball and socket joint between the head of the femur and the acetabulum of the hipbone.
humeroradial j. The joint at the elbow between the humerus and the head of the radius.
humeroulnar j. The joint at the elbow between the trochlea of the humerus and the trochlear notch of the ulna.
immovable j. See fibrous joint.
incudomalleolar j. The synovial joint between the saddle-shaped facet on the body of the incus and the elliptical facet on the head of the malleus; seen in the epitympanic recess of the middle ear chamber.
incudostapedial j. The ball and socket joint between the medial surface of the cartilage-covered lenticular process of the incus and the cartilage-covered depression on the head of the stapes; it is covered by a fibroelastic capsule and is seen in the middle ear chamber close to the oval window.

consists of both the humeroulnar and humeroradial joints. Also called cubital joint.
ellipsoidal j. A joint shaped like a ball and socket, but with the articulating surfaces more closely resembling an oval; an oval-shaped part fits into an elliptic cavity permitting all types of movement except pivotal.
false j. See pseudarthrosis.
femoropatellar j. The part of the knee joint formed by the articulation between the back surface of the patella (kneecap) and corresponding anterior surface of the femur.
fibrocartilaginous j. A joint in which the bony surfaces usually covered by a thin plate of hyaline, are united by an intervening disk of fibrocartilage; it is devoid of a joint cavity and extremely limited in movement, as seen in the pubic symphysis. Also called symphysis.
fibrous j. A joint in which fibrous tissue unites two bones, permitting only slight movement, such as in the joints between the bones of the skull; the types of fibrous joints are syndesmosis, suture, and gomphosis. Also called synarthrodial joint; synarthrosis; immovable joint.
flail j. An unstabilized joint resulting from paralysis of surrounding muscles.
freely movable j. See synovial joint.
frozen j. See ankylosis.

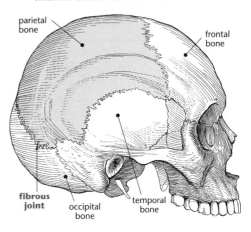

parietal bone

frontal bone

fibrous joint

occipital bone

temporal bone

joint ■ joint

inferior radioulnar j. See radioulnar joint, distal.

interarticular j. A plane synovial joint between articular processes of contiguous vertebrae. Also called zygapophyseal joint.

intercarpal j.'s The joints between the carpal bones of the wrist.

interchondral j.'s The joints between the contiguous surfaces of the 5th through 10th costal cartilages.

intercuneiform j.'s The plane synovial joints between the contiguous surfaces of the three cuneiform bones of the foot.

intermetacarpal j.'s The plane joints between the adjoining bases of the 2nd through 5th metacarpal bones of the hand.

intermetatarsal j.'s The plane joints between the adjoining bases of the five metatarsal bones of the foot.

interphalangeal j.'s The hinge joints between the phalanges of each finger and toe.

intertarsal j.'s The joints between the tarsal bones in the posterior portion of the foot. Also called tarsal joints.

jaw j. See temporomandibular joint.

knee j. A compound condylar joint formed by the two condyles and patellar surface of the femur, the posterior surface of the patella, and the superior articular surface of the tibia.

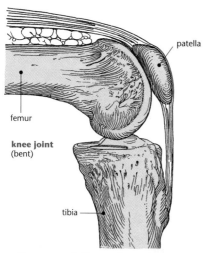

knee joint
(bent)

femur

patella

tibia

ligamentous j. See syndesmosis.

Lisfranc's j.'s See tarsometatarsal joints.

lumbosacral j. The joint between the fifth lumbar vertebra and the sacrum.

mandibular j. See temporomandibular joint.

manubriosternal j. The prominent cartilaginous joint between the manubrium and body of the sternum; it serves as an important body landmark. Also called superior sternal joint; sternal angle; angle of Louis; manubriosternal angle.

metacarpophalangeal j.'s The ellipsoidal joints between the oval, shallow concave bases of the five proximal phalanges and the convex heads of the articulating metacarpal bones.

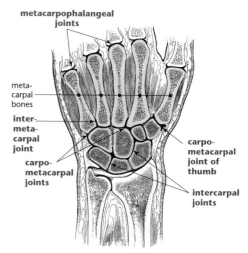

metacarpophalangeal joints

metacarpal bones

intermetacarpal joint

carpometacarpal joints

carpometacarpal joint of thumb

intercarpal joints

metatarsophalangeal j.'s The ellipsoid joints at the front of the foot between the heads of the five metatarsal bones and the concave bases of the corresponding proximal phalanges.

midcarpal j. The compound joint between the proximal and distal rows of carpal bones.

midtarsal j. See transverse tarsal joint.

movable j. See synovial joint.

multiaxial j. See ball and socket joint.

neuropathic j. See Charcot's joint.

pisiform j. See pisotriquetral joint.

pisotriquetral j. The plane synovial joint between the pisiform and triquetral bones of the wrist. Also called pisiform joint.

pivot j. See rotary joint.

plane j. A synovial joint in which the opposing articular surfaces are either flat planes or slightly curved; it allows gliding movements, as in the intermetacarpal joints. Also called gliding joint; arthrodial joint.

posterior talocalcanean j. See subtalar joint.

radiocarpal j. The ellipsoid joint at the wrist between the radius and its articular disk, and the scaphoid, lunate, and triquetral

joint ■ joint

bones. Also called wrist joint.

radioulnar j.'s The two articulations between the radius and the ulna: *Distal radioulnar j.*, the joint between the rounded head of the ulna and the ulnar notch of the radius at the distal end of the forearm, near the wrist; also called inferior radioulnar joint; *Proximal radioulnar j.*, the joint between the head of the radius and the radial notch of the ulna within the annular ligament of the radius at the proximal end of the forearm, near the elbow. Also called superior radioulnar joint.

rotary j. A joint in which a central bony projection rotates within a ring, or a ring pivots around the bony projection as in the joint between the 1st and 2nd vertebrae; movement is limited to one plane. Also called trochoid joint; pivot joint.

sacrococcygeal j. The joint between the sacrum and the coccyx (tailbone). Also called coccygeal joint.

sacroiliac j. The joint between the vertebral column and the pelvis, specifically between the two auricular surfaces on the upper part of the sacrum and each ilium on the posterior part of the pelvis.

saddle j. A synovial joint in which the opposing surfaces of two bones are reciprocally concave on one side and convex on the other as in the carpometacarpal joint of the thumb; movement is effected by the two bony surfaces opposing each other. Also called sellar joint; saddle-shaped joint.

saddle-shaped j. See saddle joint.

sellar j. See saddle joint.

shoulder j. The ball and socket joint between the rounded head of the humerus and the shallow, concave glenoid cavity of the scapula.

simple j. A synovial joint involving only two bones.

slightly movable j.
See amphiarthrodial joint.

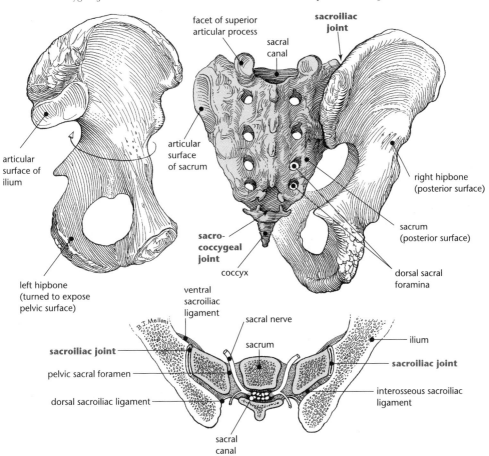

facet of superior articular process

sacral canal

sacroiliac joint

articular surface of ilium

articular surface of sacrum

right hipbone (posterior surface)

sacrum (posterior surface)

left hipbone (turned to expose pelvic surface)

sacro-coccygeal joint

coccyx

dorsal sacral foramina

ventral sacroiliac ligament

sacral nerve

sacrum

ilium

sacroiliac joint

pelvic sacral foramen

sacroiliac joint

dorsal sacroiliac ligament

interosseous sacroiliac ligament

sacral canal

joint ■ joint

socket j. of tooth See gomphosis.

spheno-occipital j. The cartilaginous joint anterior to the foramen magnum at the base of the skull, between the body of the sphenoid bone above and the basilar part of the occipital bone below; it fuses between the ages of 17 and 26 years.

spheroidal j. See ball and socket joint.

sternoclavicular j. The joint formed by the medial end of the clavicle, the manubrium of the breastbone, and the cartilage of the first rib.

sternocostal j.'s The joints between the cartilages of the first seven ribs and concavities along the lateral surface of the sternum; they are usually joined by synovial joints and through their gliding movements provide thoracic flexibility to facilitate respiration.

subtalar j. The joint between the inferior surface of the talus (ankle bone) and the superior surface of the calcaneus (heel bone). Also called talocalcanean joint; posterior talocalcanean joint.

superior radioulnar j. See radioulnar joint, proximal.

superior sternal j. See manubriosternal joint.

suture j. A fibrous joint in the skull in which apposed edges of bone are closely united by a thin layer of fibrous tissue that is continuous with the periosteum; it eventually ossifies permitting no movement to occur. Also called cranial suture.

synarthrodial j. See fibrous joint.

synovial j. A joint that usually permits free movement, characterized by a layer of hyaline cartilage or fibrocartilage and a synovial cavity between the bones, i.e., a cavity lined by a synovial membrane and containing synovial fluid; it includes most of

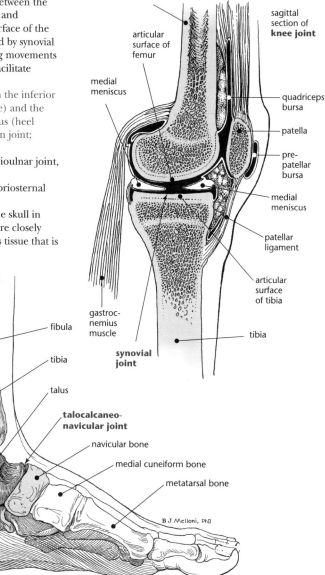

femur

sagittal section of **knee joint**

articular surface of femur

medial meniscus

quadriceps bursa

patella

pre-patellar bursa

medial meniscus

patellar ligament

articular surface of tibia

gastroc-nemius muscle

synovial joint

tibia

fibula

tibia

talus

talocrural joint (ankle joint)

talocalcaneo-navicular joint

navicular bone

subtalar joint

medial cuneiform bone

metatarsal bone

calcaneus

B J Melloni, PhD

joint ■ joint

the joints of the body. Also called diarthrosis; diarthrodial joint; movable joint; freely movable joint.

synarthrodial j. See fibrous joint.

talocalcanean j. See subtalar joint.

talocalcaneonavicular j. A joint formed by the rounded head of the talus (ankle bone), the concave surface of the navicular bone, the upper surface of the calcaneus (heel bone), and the plantar calcaneonavicular ligament. Also called anterior talocalcanean joint.

talocrural j. See ankle joint.

talonavicular j. The part of the transverse tarsal joint that is between the talus (ankle bone) and the navicular bone.

talotibiofibular j. See ankle joint.

tarsal j.'s See intertarsal joints.

tarsometatarsal j.'s The three joints between the tarsal and metatarsal bones of the foot, involving a medial joint between the 1st metatarsal bone and the medial cuneiform bone; an intermediate joint between the 2nd and 3rd metatarsal bones

and the intermediate and lateral cuneiform bones; and a lateral joint between the 4th and 5th metatarsal bones and the cuboid bone. Also called Lisfrac's joints; cuneometatarsal joints.

temporomandibular j. The synovial joint between the condyle of the mandible inferiorly and the mandibular fossa and articular tubercle of the temporal bone superiorly; separated by a thin articular disk into two cavities, each of which is lined by a synovial membrane. Also called jaw joint; mandibular joint.

tibiofibular j., inferior A fibrous joint between the medial surface of the lower end of the fibula and the triangular fibular notch on the lateral surface of the tibia; it is bound by ligaments.

tibiofibular j., superior The plane joint between the lateral condyle of the tibia and the head of the fibula, near the knee. Also called tibiofibular joint.

transverse tarsal j. The joint between the calcaneus and cuboid bone, and the talus

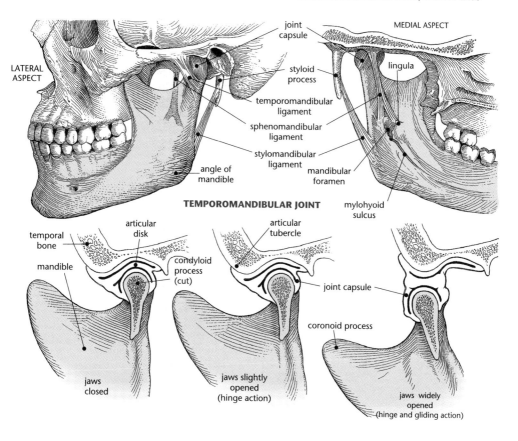

TEMPOROMANDIBULAR JOINT

LATERAL ASPECT

joint capsule

styloid process

temporomandibular ligament

sphenomandibular ligament

stylomandibular ligament

angle of mandible

mandibular foramen

MEDIAL ASPECT

lingula

mylohyoid sulcus

temporal bone

mandible

articular disk

condyloid process (cut)

jaws closed

articular tubercle

joint capsule

coronoid process

jaws slightly opened (hinge action)

jaws widely opened (hinge and gliding action)

joint ■ joint

and navicular bone of the foot. Also called Chopart's joint; midtarsal joint.

trochoid j. See rotary joint.

uniaxial j. A joint in which movement is restricted to one axis only, such as in a hinge joint.

unilocular j. A synovial joint possessing a single cavity, with or without an incomplete intra-articular disk.

wrist j. See radiocarpal joint.

xiphisternal j. The cartilaginous joint between the xiphoid process and the body of the sternum; usually by the age of 40 years, there is an osseous union of the two structures.

zygapophysial j. See interarticular joint.

joule (jool) A unit of energy equal to that consumed when a current of 1 ampere passes through a resistance of 1 ohm for 1 second.

jugal (jōō'gal) 1. Relating to the zygomatic bone. 2. Relating to the cheek. 3. Yolked together; connecting.

jugomaxillary (joo-go-mak'sĭ-lār-e) Relating to the zygomatic bone and the maxilla.

jugular (jug'u-lar) Relating to the neck.

jugum (joo'gum), pl. ju'ga A ridge or depression connecting two structures.

juga alveolaria Eminences on the front of the upper and lower jaws (maxilla and mandible) produced by the roots of incisors and cuspids within.

j. sphenoidale The raised smooth front part of the body of the sphenoid bone that connects the lesser wings of the bone; it separates the anterior cranial fossa from the sphenoid sinus.

junction (junk'shun) The point where two structures or parts unite.

cementodentinal j. The boundary between the dentin and the cementum of the root of a tooth.

cementoenamel j. The boundary between the cementum of the root of a tooth and the enamel of its crown.

costochondral j. The site of articulation between a rib and its cartilage.

dentinoenamel j. The boundary between the dentin and enamel of the crown of a tooth.

gap j. The space (about 3 nanometers wide) between certain nerve cells and cells of smooth and cardiac muscles that mediate communication by allowing passage of molecules from one cell to the next.

myoneural j. See neuromuscular junction.

myotendinal j. The junctional region between the end of the muscle fibers and the tendinous attachment.

neuromuscular j. The point of contact between the endplate of a motor nerve and a muscle fiber; specialized junctional area involved in nerve-muscle transmission. Also called myoneural junction; motor endplate.

juxta-articular (juks-tah-ar-tik'u-lar) In close proximity to a joint; in the region of a joint.

juxtaepiphyseal (juks-tah-ep-ĭ-fiz'e-al) Near or next to an end (epiphysis) of a long bone.

juxtapose (juks-tah-poz') To place in a side-by-side position.

juxtaposition (juks-tah-po-zish'un) The state of being side-by-side; apposition.

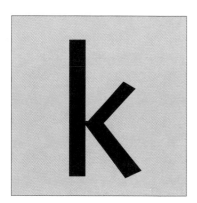

kinesio- A combining form relating to movement.

kinesiology (ki-ne-se-ol'o-je) The study of muscular movement of the human body, especially with reference to treatment.

kink (kink) 1. An unnatural sharp twist or bend. 2. A muscle spasm, often painful.

knee (ne) The articulation of the lower limb between the femur and the tibia.

> **housemaid's k.** See prepatellar bursitis, under bursitis.
>
> **jumper's k.** Inflammation of the patellar or quadriceps tendons, causing discomfort, tenderness, or pain, especially at the tendon's attachment to the patella (kneecap); may occur in athletes after jumping, kicking, climbing, or running.
>
> **knock k.** See genu valgum.
>
> **locked k.** A condition in which the flexion and extension motion of the leg is limited, due to the presence of torn cartilage in the knee joint.
>
> **runner's k.** Condition of the knee characterized by anterior knee pain or discomfort around the patella (kneecap), experienced after running or jogging a predictable distance, or when sitting with the knee flexed for long periods of time; it also occurs when walking up or down stairs; seen most commonly (not exclusively) in recreational joggers and long distance runners. The condition is considered to be caused by prolonged excessive pronation of the subtalar joint of the foot, which may occur as a compensatory mechanism for any of a variety of anatomical abnormalities of the leg.

kneecap (ne'cap) See patella.

knob (nob) A small rounded protuberance; a mass.

> **knee k.** See traumatic tibial epiphysitis, under epiphysitis.

knuckle (nuk'l) A protuberance on the dorsal surface of a clenched hand formed by a joint of the finger, especially the metacarpophalangeal joint.

kyphoscoliosis (ki-fo-sko-le-o'sis) A deformity of the spine characterized by a backward and lateral curvature, usually progressive, leading to failure of lung function and congestive heart failure, if untreated.

kyphosis (ki-fo'sis) Excessive backward curvature of the spine, affecting most frequently the upper thoracic and lower cervical vertebrae; may be caused by any of a variety of spinal disorders (e.g., fracture or tumor of the vertebrae); seen frequently in older people, especially women, affected with osteoporosis, in which case the vertebral bodies collapse upon each other. Popularly called hunchback; humpback; dowager's hump (in older women).

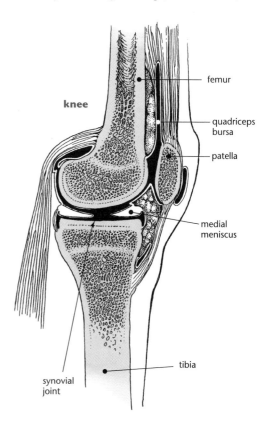

kinesio- ■ kyphosis

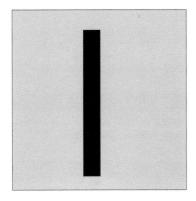

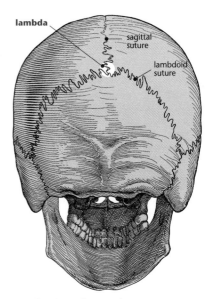

labrum (la'brum) Any liplike structure; a brim.

    acetabular l. A fibrocartilaginous rim firmly adhered to the margin of the acetabulum of the hipbone; it appreciably increases the depth of the articular cavity to accommodate the head of the femur and assists in the lubrication of the joint; it extends across the notch of the acetabulum as the transverse acetabular ligament.

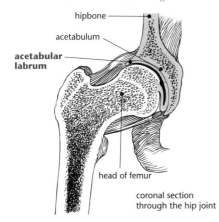

coronal section through the hip joint

    glenoid l. A fibrocartilaginous rim firmly adhered to the margin of the glenoid cavity of the scapula; it noticeably deepens the articular cavity to accommodate the head of the humerus, and assists in the lubrication of the joint.

labyrinth (lab'ĭ-rinth) A group of interconnecting channels.

    bony l. The connecting cavities and canals of the inner ear, located in the petrous portion of the temporal bone; it houses the membranous labyrinth.

    ethmoid l. The aggregation of thin-walled cavities within the ethmoid bone, near the nasal cavity and eye socket.

    membranous l. A system of communicating membranous ducts and sacs of the inner ear, situated within the bony labyrinth.

labyrinthine (lab-ĭ-rin'thĭn) Relating to a labyrinth, especially of the inner ear.

lacuna (lah-ku'nah), pl. lacu'nae 1. A small anatomic cavity or depression. 2. A defect or gap.

    cartilage l. Any of the small spaces within cartilaginous tissue, housing a chondrocyte (mature cartilage cell). Also called cartilage space.

    Howship's l. A depression in bone caused by resorption of bone tissue by residing osteoclasts. Also called resorption lacuna; osseous lacuna.

    l. of muscles The compartment between the inguinal ligament and the hipbone, lateral to the iliopectineal arch, for the passage of the iliopsoas muscle and femoral nerve into the lower extremity. Also called lacuna musculorum.

    l. musculorum See lacuna of muscles.
    osseous l. See Howship's lacuna.
    resorption l. See Howship's lacuna.
    l. vasorum See lacuna of vessels.

    l. of vessels The compartment between the inguinal ligament and the hipbone, medial to the iliopectineal arch, for the passage of femoral vessels. Also called lacuna vasorum.

lacunar (lah-ku'nar) Relating to a lacuna.

laloplegia (lal-o-ple'je-ah) Paralysis of muscles involved in production of speech.

labrum ▪ laloplegia

lambda (lam'dah) 1. The eleventh letter of the Greek alphabet. 2. A craniometric point on the back of the skull, at the junction of the sagittal and labdoid sutures.

lamella (lah-mel'ah) A thin plate, as of bone.

articular l. A compact layer of bone to which an overlying articular cartilage is attached.

basic l. See circumferential lamella.

l. of bone Any of a series of contiguous plates of bone matrix that constitutes the structural unit of mature bone; its form could be either concentric, circumferential, or interstitial.

circumferential l. One of a series of layers of bone encircling the inner and outer surfaces of compact bone; the outer layer is immediately under the periosteum while the inner layer is covered by the endosteum. Also called primary lamella; basic lamella.

concentric l. One of a series of layers of bone, arranged concentrically around the vascular (haversian) canals of compact bone; it has a predominantly longitudinal orientation. Also called secondary lamella; haversian lamella.

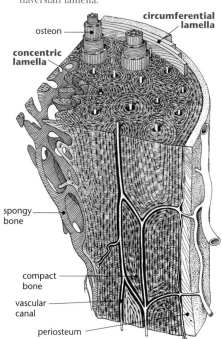

osteon

circumferential lamella

concentric lamella

spongy bone

compact bone

vascular canal

periosteum

haversian l. See concentric lamella.

interstitial l. One of the curved bony plates occupying the area between the concentric lamellae; it represents partially

resorbed concentric lamellae by the osteoclasts during bone remodeling.

primary l. See circumferential lamella.

secondary l. See concentric lamella.

lamellar (lah-mel'ar) 1. Scaly. 2. Relating to lamellae.

lamina (lam'ĭ-nah), pl.lam'inae A thin bony plate or a thin layer of cells or soft tissue.

anterior l. of rectus abdominis sheath See anterior layer of rectus abdominis sheath, under layer.

bony spiral l. A delicate flange of bone projecting from the spiral-shaped modiolus of the inner ear into the cochlear canal, and partially dividing it into an upper scala vestibuli and a lower scala tympani; the basilar membrane is attached to it and completes the separation of the two scalae; it transmits the fibers of the cochlear nerve to the spiral organ of Corti. Also called osseous spiral lamina.

laminae of cartilage of auditory tube A narrow lateral plate and a broad medial plate of the cartilaginous part of the auditory (eustachian) tube, through which the middle ear chamber communicates with the nasal part of the pharynx; on transverse section the cartilage has a hook-like appearance.

cribriform l. of ethmoid bone See cribriform plate of ethmoid bone, under plate.

l. of cricoid cartilage The wide quadrilateral lamina making up the posterior wall of the annular-shaped cricoid cartilage and the lower and back part of the larynx; its outer surface provides attachment to the posterior cricoarytenoid muscles and ligaments, and on its upper border, facets are situated to articulate with the arytenoid cartilages.

external cranial l. The outer plate of a flat cranial bone. Also called external plate of cranial bone.

horizontal l. of palatine bone See horizontal plate of palatine bone, under plate.

internal cranial l. The inner plate of a flat cranial bone. Also called internal plate of cranial bone.

interpubic fibrocartilaginous l. The fibrocartilaginous disk uniting the articular surfaces of the pubic bones at the symphysis. Also called interpubic disk.

lateral pterygoid l. See lateral pterygoid plate, under plate.

medial l. of pterygoid process A narrow,

lambda ■ lamina

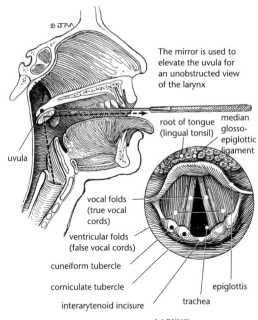

The mirror is used to elevate the uvula for an unobstructed view of the larynx

root of tongue (lingual tonsil)

median glosso-epiglottic ligament

uvula

vocal folds (true vocal cords)

ventricular folds (false vocal cords)

cuneiform tubercle

corniculate tubercle

interarytenoid incisure

epiglottis

trachea

LARYNX

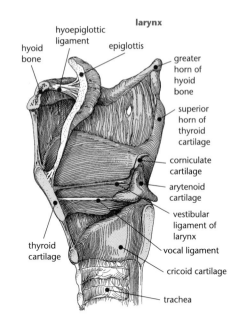

larynx

hyoepiglottic ligament

hyoid bone

epiglottis

greater horn of hyoid bone

superior horn of thyroid cartilage

corniculate cartilage

arytenoid cartilage

vestibular ligament of larynx

thyroid cartilage

vocal ligament

cricoid cartilage

trachea

long plate of the medial pterygoid process of the sphenoid bone of the skull; it curves laterally at its inferior extremity into a hooklike process, the pterygoid hamulus.

   medial pterygoid l. See medial pterygoid plate, under plate.

   orbital l. See orbital plate of ethmoid bone, under plate.

   osseous spiral l. See bony spiral lamina.

   perpendicular l. of ethmoid bone See perpendicular plate of ethmoid bone, under plate.

   perpendicular l. of palatine bone See perpendicular plate of palatine bone, under plate.

   posterior l. of rectus abdominis sheath See posterior layer of rectus abdominis sheath, under layer.

   l. of thyroid cartilage Either of the two approximately quadrilateral plates (laminae) of the thyroid cartilage, the largest of the larynx; fused in the midline anteriorly to form the laryngeal prominence (Adam's apple).

   l. of vertebral arch Two broad plates directed dorsally and medially from the right and left pedicles of a vertebra; their posterior midline fusion forms the vertebral arch and completes the vertebral foramen.

laminar (lam'ĭ-nar) 1. Arranged in layers. 2. Relating to a bony plate.

laryngopharynx (lah-ring-go-far'rinks) The lower portion of the pharynx (behind the larynx) from the level of the hyoid bone to the esophagus, with which it is continuous.

laryngospasm (lah-ring'go-spazm) An abnormal reflex contraction of the muscles of the larynx.

laryngotracheal (lah-ring-go-tra'ke-al) Relating to the larynx and trachea. Also called tracheolaryngeal.

larynx (lar'inks) The organ of voice production between the root of the tongue and the upper end of the trachea; it is composed of a cartilaginous and muscular frame, lined with mucous membrane, and contains the vocal folds. Popularly called voice box.

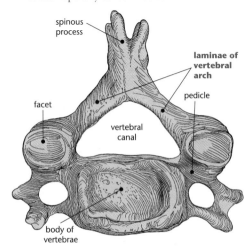

spinous process

laminae of vertebral arch

pedicle

facet

vertebral canal

body of vertebrae

laminar ■ larynx

lateral (lat'er-al) On the side; away from the midline, toward the right or left.

lateroflexion (lat-er-o-flek'shun) A bending or curving to one side of the body; lateral flexion.

latissimus (lah-tis'ĭ-mus) Latin for broadest; widest; used in naming the wide, flat muscle of the back (latissimus dorsi).

layer (la'er) A sheetlike coating; a single thickness of tissue covering a surface. Also called lamina; stratum.

　　anterior l. of rectus abdominis sheath The anterior layer of the sheath of the straight muscle of the abdomen (rectus abdominis), stretching from the margin of the lower ribs to the pubic bones. Also called anterior lamina of rectus abdominis sheath.

　　basal l. of endometrium The deepest layer of the uterine mucosa (endometrium); it accommodates the blind ends of the tubelike uterine glands, which are not shed during menstruation or at parturition and from which the endometrium regenerates.

　　circular l. of muscles of colon The strong, inner layer of circular muscle fibers of the colon.

　　circular l. of muscles of rectum The thick, inner layer of circular muscle fibers of the rectum.

　　circular l. of muscles of small intestine The relatively thick inner circular layer of the muscular coat (tunica) of the small intestine.

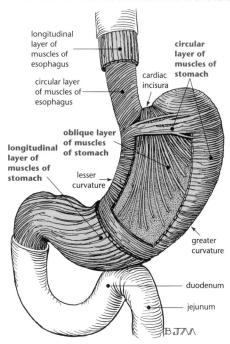

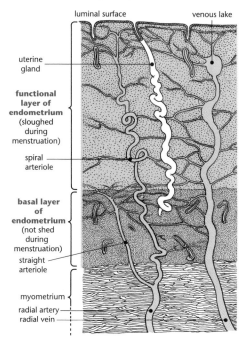

　　circular l. of muscles of stomach The strongest of three muscular layers of the stomach, comprised of a middle circular layer of smooth muscle fibers that covers the entire stomach wall (the other two layers, the superficial longitudinal and the deeper oblique layers are incomplete coats); it begins as a continuation of the circular esophageal muscle and becomes markedly thickened as it approaches the pylorus, where it forms the pyloric sphincter.

　　compact l. of endometrium The layer of the uterine endometrium nearest the surface, above the spongy layer; it contains the neck of the uterine glands and is shed during menstruation and at parturition.

　　functional l. of endometrium The compact layer of the uterine endometrium along with the spongy layer; during the secretory phase of the endometrial cycle, it becomes tremendously engorged; it is shed during menstruation.

　　inferior l. of pelvic diaphragm See inferior fascia of pelvic diaphram, under fascia.

　　longitudinal l. of muscles of colon The outer longitudinal layer of the muscular coat of the colon, being relatively thick in the areas of the teniae coli.

　　longitudinal l. of muscles of rectum The outer longitudinal layer of muscles of the rectum.

lateral ■ layer

longitudinal l. of muscles of small intestine The outer longitudinal layer of the muscular coat of the small intestine.

longitudinal l. of muscles of stomach The incomplete, outer longitudinal layer of the stomach that is continuous with the longitudinal muscle layer of the esophagus; it divides at the cardia of the stomach into two bands: the stronger band follows the lesser curvature of the stomach; the thinner band follows along the greater curvature of the stomach; both bands converge at the pyloric area to form a uniform layer.

oblique l. of muscles of stomach The incomplete, innermost oblique muscular layer of the stomach that is strongly developed in the fundus region and becomes progressively thinner as it approaches the pylorus; totally absent at the lesser curvature of the stomach and quite sparse at the greater curvature.

posterior l. of rectus abdominis sheath The posterior layer of the sheath of the straight muscle of the abdomen (rectus abdominis), stretching from the margin of the lower ribs to the arcuate line approximately halfway between the umbilicus and the pubic symphysis. Also called posterior lamina of rectus abdominis sheath.

spongy l. of endometrium The midportion of the uterine endometrium lying between the compact layer on the luminal surface and the basal layer on the myometrial side; seen especially during the late proliferative stage of the endometrial cycle, marked by growth of the stroma and engorged corkscrew convolutions of glands; it reflects heightened regenerative activity and coincides with the maturing follicle in the ovary.

superior l. of pelvic diaphragm See superior fascia of pelvic diaphragm, under fascia.

leg (leg) The lower limb, between the knee and ankle.

tennis l. Rupture of the calf muscles (gastrocnemius and soleus muscles) caused by activities in which the rapidly moving body abruptly changes directions (e.g., in tennis or soccer playing, downhill skiing); causes severe pain and accumulation of extravasated blood (hematoma); a snapping sound may be heard in the popliteal space (behind the knee).

leiomyoma (li-o-mi-o'mah) A benign grayish-white mass composed mostly of smooth muscle cells and varying degrees of collagen; although it may occur in any tissue that has an abundant smooth muscle component, the tumor is seen most frequently in the uterus; may be single or multiple and occur anywhere in the uterine wall; it tends to grow rapidly during pregnancy, often undergoing necrosis with severe abdominal pain; it usually regresses after menopause. Commonly called fibroid; also called fibroid tumor; myoma; fibromyoma; leiomyofibroma.

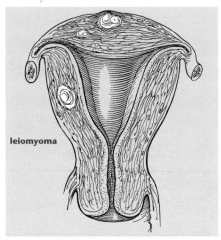

leiomyoma

levator (le-va'tor) Any muscle that raises a part.

ligament (lig'ah-ment) 1. Any band of thickened white fibrous tissue that connects bones and forms the capsule of joints. 2. A fold of peritoneum, a fascial condensation, or a cordlike fibrous band that holds an organ in position.

acromioclavicular l. A broad fibrous band extending from the acromion, a process of the scapula (shoulder blade), to the lateral end of the clavicle (collarbone); it covers the upper part of the capsule of the acromioclavicular joint at the shoulder.

alar l.'s Two short, rounded cords connecting the dens (odontoid process) of the axis (second cervical vertebra) to the occipital bone at the back of the skull. Also called odontoid ligaments.

alveolodental l. See periodontal ligament.

annular l. of base of stapes A ring of elastic fibers encircling the base of the innermost ear ossicle (stapes), attaching it to the circumference of the oval window (fenestra vestibuli); it permits movement of the ossicle during the transmission of sound vibrations from the tympanic membrane (eardrum) to the inner ear; it also serves as a hinge in response to the contraction of the stapedius muscle.

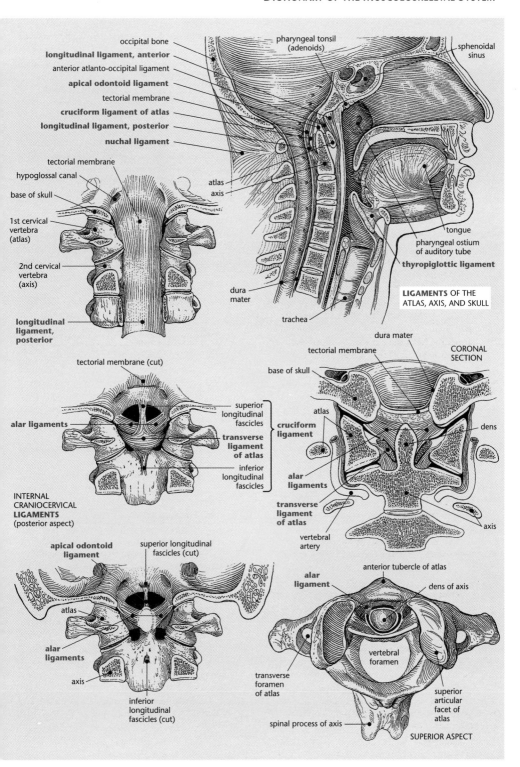

occipital bone
longitudinal ligament, anterior
anterior atlanto-occipital ligament
apical odontoid ligament
tectorial membrane
cruciform ligament of atlas
longitudinal ligament, posterior
nuchal ligament

pharyngeal tonsil
(adenoids)

sphenoidal
sinus

tectorial membrane
hypoglossal canal
base of skull
1st cervical
vertebra
(atlas)
2nd cervical
vertebra
(axis)
**longitudinal
ligament,
posterior**

atlas
axis

tongue
pharyngeal ostium
of auditory tube
thyropiglottic ligament

dura
mater

trachea

LIGAMENTS OF THE
ATLAS, AXIS, AND SKULL

tectorial membrane (cut)

alar ligaments

superior
longitudinal
fascicles
**transverse
ligament
of atlas**
inferior
longitudinal
fascicles

INTERNAL
CRANIOCERVICAL
LIGAMENTS
(posterior aspect)

dura mater

tectorial membrane

CORONAL
SECTION

base of skull

atlas

**cruciform
ligament**

dens

**alar
ligaments**

**transverse
ligament
of atlas**

vertebral
artery

axis

**apical odontoid
ligament**

superior longitudinal
fascicles (cut)

atlas

**alar
ligaments**

axis

inferior
longitudinal
fascicles (cut)

**alar
ligament**

anterior tubercle of atlas

dens of axis

vertebral
foramen

transverse
foramen
of atlas

spinal process of axis

superior
articular
facet of
atlas

SUPERIOR ASPECT

ligament ■ ligament

annular l. of radius Four-fifths of an osseofibrous band that encircles the head of the radius at the elbow and retains it in contact with the radial notch of the ulna; it blends with surrounding tissues.

anococcygeal l. A mass of fibrous and muscular tissue situated between the anal canal and the tip of the coccyx to which some of the fibers of the levator ani muscle are attached.

anterior talotibial l. See tibiotalar ligament, anterior.

apical l. of dens. See apical odontoid ligament.

apical odontoid l. A ligament that extends from the tip of the dens (odontoid process) of the axis (second cervical vertebra) to the anterior margin of the foramen magnum of the skull. Also called apical ligament of dens.

arcuate l.'s Two arched ligaments (lateral and medial) that attach the diaphragm to the first lumbar vertebra and the twelfth rib on either side, serving as the origin of the diaphragm.

arcuate l. of knee See arcuate popliteal ligament.

arcuate l. of wrist A band stretching transversely from the triangular (triquetral) bone to the scaphoid bone on the dorsal aspect of the wrist.

arcuate popliteal l. Y-shaped capsular fibers, with the stem attached to the head of the fibula, and with the posterior limb arched medially over the tendon of the popliteus muscle and the anterior limb extending to the lateral epicondyle of the femur. Also called arcuate ligament of knee.

arcuate pubic l. A thick arch of ligamentous fibers connecting the lower border of the pubic symphysis, where it intermingles with the interpubic disk of the symphysis; it forms the upper border of the pubic arch.

atlantoaxial l. The ligament extending from the anteroinferior margin of the atlas (first cervical vertebra) down to the anterosuperior margin of the axis (second cervical vertebra).

auricular l.'s Ligaments of the auricular cartilage: *Extrinsic auricular l.*, three ligaments (anterior, posterior, and superior) connecting the auricular cartilage to the side of the head; *Intrinsic auricular l.*, fibrous bands connecting various parts of the auricular cartilage (e.g., one stretching from the tragus to the helix).

bifurcate l. See bifurcated ligament.

bifurcated l. A strong band attached to the front of the upper surface of the calcaneus (heel bone) and divides (bifurcates) as it extends anteriorly to form the calcaneonavicular and calcaneocuboid ligaments, attached respectively to the navicular and cuboid bones of the foot. Also called bifurcate ligament.

broad l. of uterus One of two fibrous folds covered with peritoneum and extending from the lateral surface of the uterus to the lateral pelvic wall, on both sides, and containing the ovary, uterine (fallopian) tube, ligaments, nerves and vessels.

calcaneocuboid l. The medial part of the bifurcated ligament that connects the anterior part of the upper surface of the calcaneus (heel bone) to the dorsal part of the cuboid bone of the foot.

calcaneofibular l. A long cordlike band extending from the tip of the lateral malleolus of the fibula downward to the lateral side of the calcaneus (heel bone).

calcaneonavicular l. The lateral part of the bifurcated ligament that connects the calcaneus (heel bone) to the navicular bone of the foot: *Dorsal calcaneonavicular l.*, a band connecting the dorsal aspects of the calcaneus and navicular bones of the foot.

calcaneotibial l. See tibiocalcaneal ligament.

capsular l. Fibrous layer of ligamentous thickenings investing synovial joints.

carpometacarpal l. A series of ligaments in the hand reinforcing the joints between the distal row of carpal bones and the second to fifth metacarpal bones: *Dorsal carpometacarpal l.*, strong bands extending from the carpal to the metacarpal bones on their dorsal surfaces. *Interosseous carpometacarpal l.*, short, thick fibers connecting the capitate and hamate bones (distal row of carpus) to the adjacent surfaces of the third and fourth metacarpal bones. *Palmar carpometacarpal l.*, bands extending from the carpal to the metacarpal bones on their palmar surfaces.

collateral l.'s Collateral ligaments of the hand and foot: *Interphalangeal collateral l.*, strong, obliquely running bands along the sides of the phalangeal joints of both hand and foot. *Metacarpophalangeal collateral l.*, strong, obliquely running bands along the sides of the joint between the metacarpus and adjoining phalanx of the hand. *Metatarsophalangeal collateral l.*, strong, obliquely running bands along the sides of the joint between the metatarsus and adjoining phalanx of the foot.

conoid l. Part of the coracoclavicular ligament extending from the root of the coracoid process of the scapula (adjacent to the scapular notch) upward to the undersurface of the lateral end of the collarbone (clavicle).

Cooper's l.'s a) See suspensory ligaments of breast. b) See pectineal ligament.

coracoacromial l. A strong triangular band on the shoulder blade (scapula) extending from the tip of the acromion to the lateral edge of the coracoid process; it forms a protective arch over the shoulder joint.

coracoclavicular l. A strong band that connects the coracoid process of the shoulder blade (scapula) with the overlying undersurface of the lateral end of the clavicle; composed of two parts: the conoid and trapezoid ligaments.

coracohumeral l. A band of fibers extending from the root of the coracoid process to the front of the greater tuberosity of the humerus; it blends with the capsule of the shoulder joint.

coronary l. of knee The part of the fibrous capsule of the knee joint that extends downward to the peripheral margins of the condyle of the tibia and firmly encapsulates the periphery of each meniscus.

coronary l. of liver A ligament formed by the peritoneal reflection from the diaphragm to the superior and posterior surfaces of the right lobe of the liver; it consists of an upper and lower layer enclosing the bare area of the liver that is not covered with peritoneum.

costoclavicular l. A strong, short, flattened band extending downward from the bottom of the medial end of the collarbone (clavicle) to the upper surface of the first costal cartilage and adjoining rib.

costocoracoid l. The thickened band extending from the first rib to the coracoid process of the shoulder blade (scapula); it blends with the coracoclavicular ligament.

costotransverse l.'s Ligaments that reinforce the joints between the ribs and the vertebrae: *Lateral costotransverse l.*, the strong ligament extending from the nonarticular part of the tubercle of each rib (costal tubercle) to the tip of the thoracic transverse process of the corresponding vertebra. *Superior costotransverse l.*, the ligament extending from the neck of each rib to the

transverse process of the vertebra above.

costoxiphoid l.'s Ligaments binding the sixth and seventh costal cartilages to the front and back of the xiphoid process of the sternum (breastbone).

cricothyroid l. The median part of the cricothyroid membrane; a well defined band of elastic tissue that extends in the midline from the lower border of the thyroid cartilage down to the upper border of the cricoid cartilage. Also called cricovocal membrane; cricothyroid membrane.

cricotracheal l. A fibrous ligament that unites the lower part of the cricoid cartilage with the first ring of the trachea.

cruciate l.'s of knee Two ligaments (anterior and posterior) of considerable strength in the middle of the knee joint; they cross each other like the letter X and stabilize the tibia and femur in their anteroposterior glide upon one another; they are frequently deranged by trauma: *Anterior cruciate l. of knee,* a strong band attached below to the front of the intercondylar area of the tibia and above to the back of the medial surface of the lateral condyle of the femur; it partly blends with the anterior end of the lateral meniscus; it is tight on extension and limits excessive anterior mobility of the tibia against the femur. Rupture of the ligament is indicated if there is increased anterior mobility of the tibia when tested in flexion. *Posterior cruciate l. of knee,* a strong band (stronger, shorter and less oblique than the anterior ligament) attached below to the back of the intercondylar area of the tibia and above to the lateral surface of the medial condyle of the femur; it partly blends with the posterior end of the lateral meniscus; it limits posterior mobility and is tight on flexion. Rupture of the ligament is indicated if the tibia assumes a position of posterior displacement against the flexed femur.

cruciform l. of the atlas A cross-shaped ligament consisting of two parts: *(a)* A thick, strong transverse band which arches within the ring of the first cervical vertebra and divides the vertebral foramen into two unequal parts. The spinal cord passes through the posterior and larger part; the dens of the second cervical vertebra passes through the anterior and smaller part. Also called transverse ligament of atlas. *(b)* A vertical band (frequently called the superior longitudinal fascicles of the cruciform

ligament ■ **ligament**

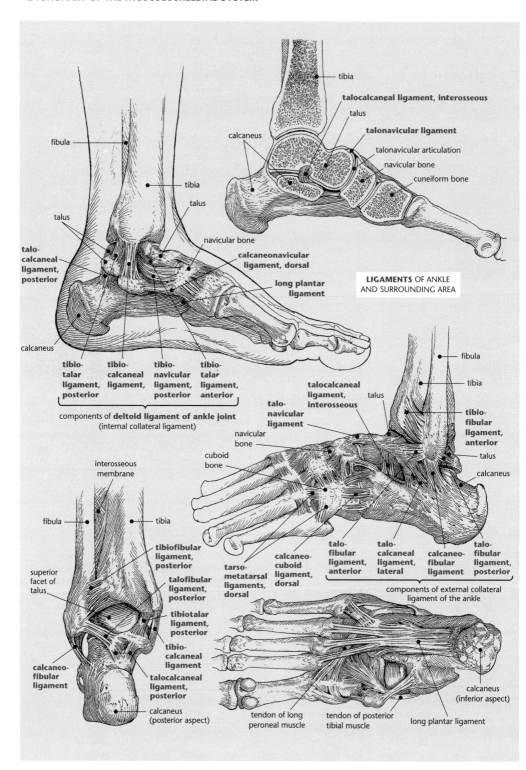

fibula

tibia

talus

talo-
calcaneal
ligament,
posterior

calcaneus

navicular bone

**calcaneonavicular
ligament, dorsal**

**long plantar
ligament**

tibia

talocalcaneal ligament, interosseous

talus

calcaneus

talonavicular ligament

talonavicular articulation

navicular bone

cuneiform bone

LIGAMENTS OF ANKLE
AND SURROUNDING AREA

**tibio-
talar
ligament,
posterior** | **tibio-
calcaneal
ligament,
posterior** | **tibio-
navicular
ligament,
posterior** | **tibio-
talar
ligament,
anterior**

components of **deltoid ligament of ankle joint**
(internal collateral ligament)

interosseous
membrane

fibula

tibia

superior
facet of
talus

**tibiofibular
ligament,
posterior**

**talofibular
ligament,
posterior**

**tibiotalar
ligament,
posterior**

**tibio-
calcaneal
ligament**

**talocalcaneal
ligament,
posterior**

calcaneus
(posterior aspect)

**calcaneo-
fibular
ligament**

**talocalcaneal
ligament,
interosseous**

talus

fibula

tibia

**tibio-
fibular
ligament,
anterior**

talus

calcaneus

**talo-
navicular
ligament**

navicular
bone

cuboid
bone

**tarso-
metatarsal
ligaments,
dorsal**

**calcaneo-
cuboid
ligament,
dorsal**

**talo-
fibular
ligament,
anterior** | **talo-
calcaneal
ligament,
lateral** | **calcaneo-
fibular
ligament** | **talo-
fibular
ligament,
posterior**

components of external collateral
ligament of the ankle

tendon of long
peroneal muscle

tendon of posterior
tibial muscle

long plantar ligament

calcaneus
(inferior aspect)

ligament ■ ligament

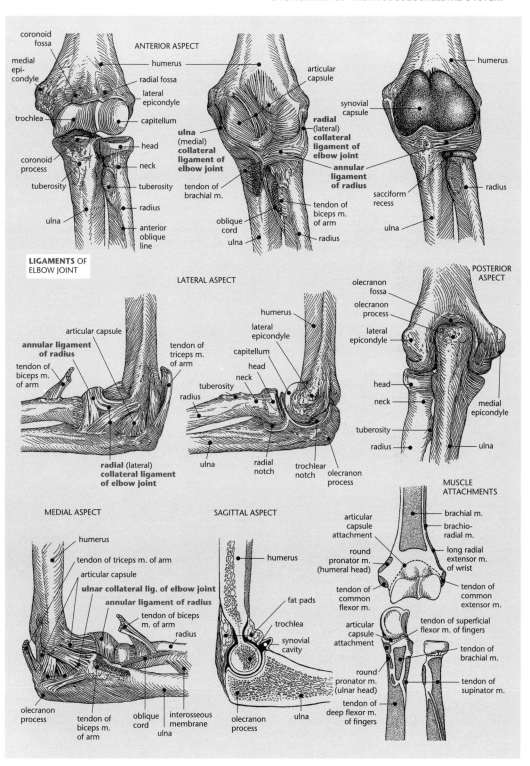

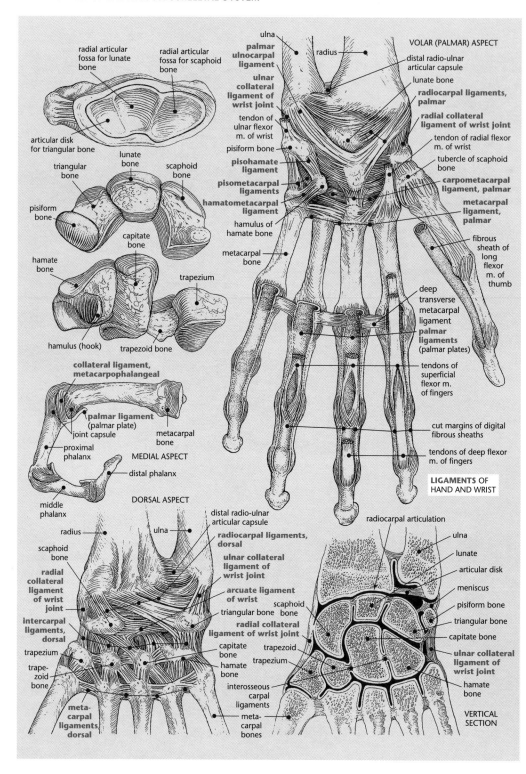

radial articular fossa for lunate bone

radial articular fossa for scaphoid bone

articular disk for triangular bone

lunate bone

triangular bone

scaphoid bone

pisiform bone

capitate bone

hamate bone

trapezium

hamulus (hook)

trapezoid bone

collateral ligament, metacarpophalangeal

palmar ligament (palmar plate)

joint capsule

metacarpal bone

proximal phalanx

MEDIAL ASPECT

distal phalanx

middle phalanx

DORSAL ASPECT

radius

ulna

scaphoid bone

radial collateral ligament of wrist joint

intercarpal ligaments, dorsal

trapezium

trapezoid bone

meta-carpal ligaments, dorsal

ulna

radius

palmar ulnocarpal ligament

ulnar collateral ligament of wrist joint

tendon of ulnar flexor m. of wrist

pisiform bone

pisohamate ligament

pisometacarpal ligaments

hamatometacarpal ligament

hamulus of hamate bone

metacarpal bone

VOLAR (PALMAR) ASPECT

distal radio-ulnar articular capsule

lunate bone

radiocarpal ligaments, palmar

radial collateral ligament of wrist joint

tendon of radial flexor m. of wrist

tubercle of scaphoid bone

carpometacarpal ligament, palmar

metacarpal ligament, palmar

fibrous sheath of long flexor m. of thumb

deep transverse metacarpal ligament

palmar ligaments (palmar plates)

tendons of superficial flexor m. of fingers

cut margins of digital fibrous sheaths

tendons of deep flexor m. of fingers

LIGAMENTS OF HAND AND WRIST

distal radio-ulnar articular capsule

radiocarpal ligaments, dorsal

ulnar collateral ligament of wrist joint

arcuate ligament of wrist

scaphoid bone

triangular bone

radial collateral ligament of wrist joint

capitate bone

hamate bone

trapezoid

trapezium

interosseous carpal ligaments

meta-carpal bones

radiocarpal articulation

ulna

lunate

articular disk

meniscus

pisiform bone

triangular bone

capitate bone

ulnar collateral ligament of wrist joint

hamate bone

VERTICAL SECTION

ligament ■ ligament

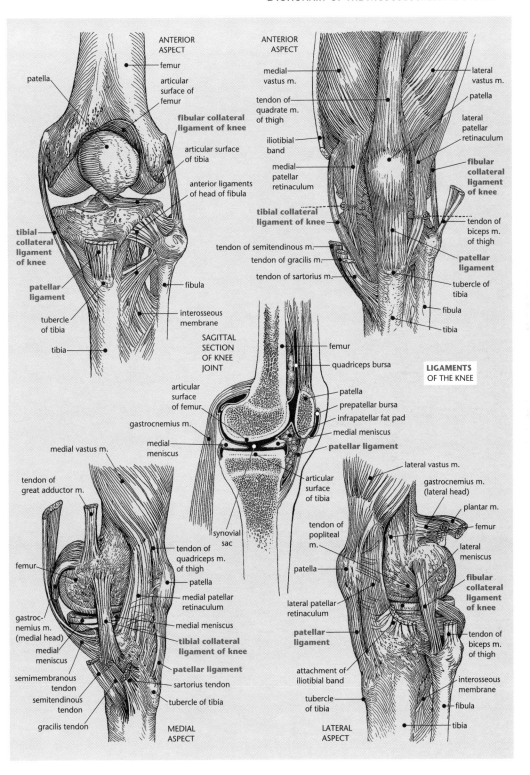

ANTERIOR ASPECT

patella
femur
articular surface of femur
fibular collateral ligament of knee
articular surface of tibia
anterior ligaments of head of fibula
tibial collateral ligament of knee
patellar ligament
tubercle of tibia
tibia
fibula
interosseous membrane

ANTERIOR ASPECT

medial vastus m.
tendon of quadrate m. of thigh
iliotibial band
medial patellar retinaculum
tibial collateral ligament of knee
tendon of semitendinous m.
tendon of gracilis m.
tendon of sartorius m.
lateral vastus m.
patella
lateral patellar retinaculum
fibular collateral ligament of knee
tendon of biceps m. of thigh
patellar ligament
tubercle of tibia
fibula
tibia

SAGITTAL SECTION OF KNEE JOINT

articular surface of femur
gastrocnemius m.
medial meniscus
femur
quadriceps bursa
patella
prepatellar bursa
infrapatellar fat pad
medial meniscus
patellar ligament
articular surface of tibia

synovial sac

tendon of popliteal m.
patella

LIGAMENTS OF THE KNEE

medial vastus m.
tendon of great adductor m.
femur
gastrocnemius m. (medial head)
medial meniscus
semimembranous tendon
semitendinous tendon
gracilis tendon
tendon of quadriceps m. of thigh
patella
medial patellar retinaculum
medial meniscus
tibial collateral ligament of knee
patellar ligament
sartorius tendon
tubercle of tibia

MEDIAL ASPECT

lateral vastus m.
gastrocnemius m. (lateral head)
plantar m.
femur
lateral meniscus
fibular collateral ligament of knee
tendon of biceps m. of thigh
lateral patellar retinaculum
patellar ligament
attachment of iliotibial band
tubercle of tibia
interosseous membrane
fibula
tibia

LATERAL ASPECT

ligament ■ ligament

137

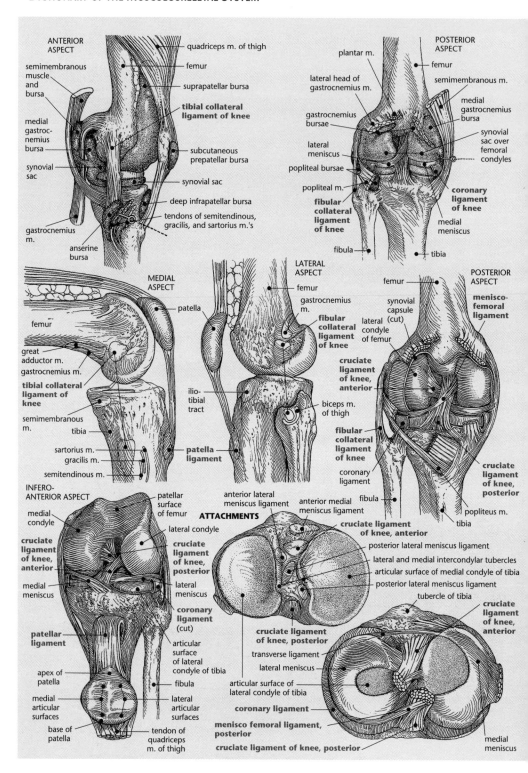

ANTERIOR ASPECT

quadriceps m. of thigh
femur
suprapatellar bursa
tibial collateral ligament of knee
subcutaneous prepatellar bursa
synovial sac
deep infrapatellar bursa
tendons of semitendinous, gracilis, and sartorius m.'s

semimembranous muscle and bursa
medial gastroc-nemius bursa
synovial sac
gastrocnemius m.
anserine bursa

POSTERIOR ASPECT

plantar m.
femur
semimembranous m.
medial gastrocnemius bursa
synovial sac over femoral condyles
coronary ligament of knee
medial meniscus
tibia

lateral head of gastrocnemius m.
gastrocnemius bursae
lateral meniscus
popliteal bursae
popliteal m.
fibular collateral ligament of knee
fibula

MEDIAL ASPECT

patella
femur
great adductor m.
gastrocnemius m.
tibial collateral ligament of knee
semimembranous m.
tibia
sartorius m.
gracilis m.
semitendinous m.

LATERAL ASPECT

femur
gastrocnemius m.
fibular collateral ligament of knee
lateral condyle of femur
cruciate ligament of knee, anterior
biceps m. of thigh
fibular collateral ligament of knee
coronary ligament
ilio-tibial tract
patella ligament

POSTERIOR ASPECT

femur
menisco-femoral ligament
synovial capsule (cut)
cruciate ligament of knee, posterior
popliteus m.
tibia
fibula

INFERO-ANTERIOR ASPECT

medial condyle
cruciate ligament of knee, anterior
medial meniscus
patellar ligament
apex of patella
medial articular surfaces
base of patella

patellar surface of femur
lateral condyle
cruciate ligament of knee, posterior
lateral meniscus
coronary ligament (cut)
articular surface of lateral condyle of tibia
fibula
lateral articular surfaces
tendon of quadriceps m. of thigh

ATTACHMENTS

anterior lateral meniscus ligament
anterior medial meniscus ligament
cruciate ligament of knee, anterior
posterior lateral meniscus ligament
lateral and medial intercondylar tubercles
articular surface of medial condyle of tibia
posterior lateral meniscus ligament
tubercle of tibia
cruciate ligament of knee, anterior

cruciate ligament of knee, posterior
transverse ligament
lateral meniscus
articular surface of lateral condyle of tibia
coronary ligament
menisco femoral ligament, posterior
cruciate ligament of knee, posterior
medial meniscus

ligament ■ ligament

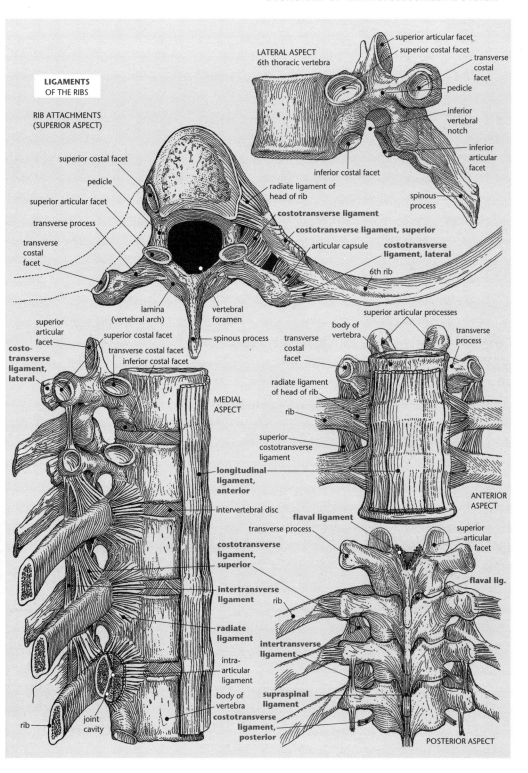

LIGAMENTS
OF THE RIBS

RIB ATTACHMENTS
(SUPERIOR ASPECT)

LATERAL ASPECT
6th thoracic vertebra

superior articular facet
superior costal facet
transverse costal facet
pedicle
inferior vertebral notch
inferior articular facet
spinous process
inferior costal facet

superior costal facet
pedicle
superior articular facet
transverse process
transverse costal facet
lamina (vertebral arch)
vertebral foramen
spinous process

radiate ligament of head of rib
costotransverse ligament
costotransverse ligament, superior
articular capsule
costotransverse ligament, lateral
6th rib

superior articular facet
costotransverse ligament, lateral
superior costal facet
transverse costal facet
inferior costal facet

MEDIAL ASPECT

transverse costal facet
radiate ligament of head of rib
rib
superior costotransverse ligament

body of vertebra
superior articular processes
transverse process

longitudinal ligament, anterior
intervertebral disc
costotransverse ligament, superior
intertransverse ligament
radiate ligament
intra-articular ligament
body of vertebra
costotransverse ligament, posterior
rib
joint cavity

rib

ANTERIOR ASPECT

flaval ligament
transverse process
costotransverse ligament, superior
rib
intertransverse ligament
supraspinal ligament

superior articular facet
flaval lig.

POSTERIOR ASPECT

ligament ■ ligament

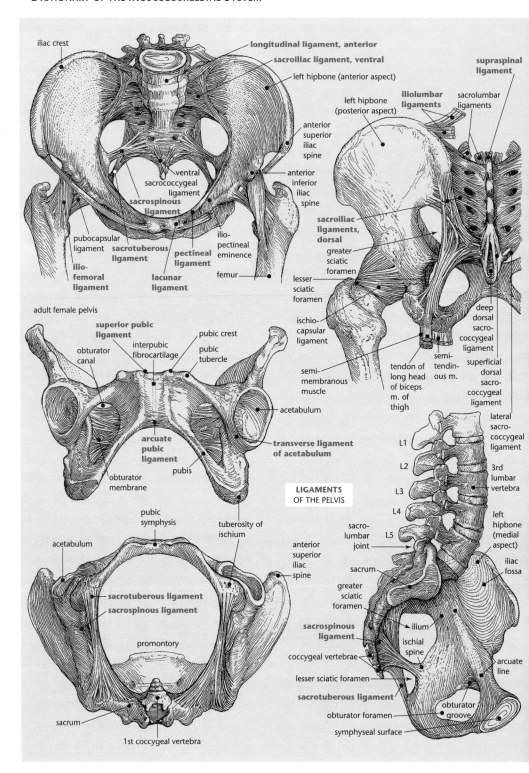

iliac crest

longitudinal ligament, anterior

sacroiliac ligament, ventral

left hipbone (anterior aspect)

supraspinal ligament

left hipbone (posterior aspect)

iliolumbar ligaments

sacrolumbar ligaments

anterior superior iliac spine

ventral sacrococcygeal ligament

sacrospinous ligament

anterior inferior iliac spine

sacroiliac ligaments, dorsal

greater sciatic foramen

pubocapsular ligament

sacrotuberous ligament

pectineal ligament

ilio-pectineal eminence

iliofemoral ligament

lacunar ligament

femur

lesser sciatic foramen

ischiocapsular ligament

deep dorsal sacro-coccygeal ligament

semi-tendinous m.

superficial dorsal sacro-coccygeal ligament

tendon of long head of biceps m. of thigh

semi-membranous muscle

adult female pelvis

superior pubic ligament

obturator canal

interpubic fibrocartilage

pubic crest

pubic tubercle

arcuate pubic ligament

pubis

obturator membrane

acetabulum

transverse ligament of acetabulum

lateral sacro-coccygeal ligament

L1

L2

3rd lumbar vertebra

L3

LIGAMENTS OF THE PELVIS

L4

pubic symphysis

acetabulum

tuberosity of ischium

sacro-lumbar joint

L5

left hipbone (medial aspect)

anterior superior iliac spine

sacrum

iliac fossa

sacrotuberous ligament

sacrospinous ligament

greater sciatic foramen

promontory

sacrospinous ligament

ilium

ischial spine

coccygeal vertebrae

arcuate line

lesser sciatic foramen

sacrotuberous ligament

sacrum

obturator foramen

obturator groove

1st coccygeal vertebra

symphyseal surface

ligament ■ ligament

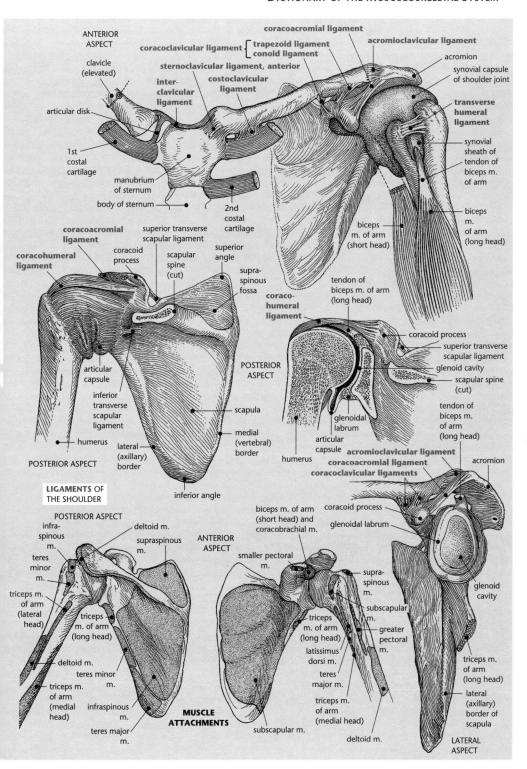

ANTERIOR
ASPECT

clavicle
(elevated)

coracoclavicular ligament

coracoacromial ligament

trapezoid ligament
conoid ligament

acromioclavicular ligament

acromion

synovial capsule
of shoulder joint

sternoclavicular ligament, anterior

inter-
clavicular
ligament

costoclavicular
ligament

transverse
humeral
ligament

articular disk

synovial
sheath of
tendon of
biceps m.
of arm

1st
costal
cartilage

manubrium
of sternum

body of sternum

2nd
costal
cartilage

biceps
m.
of arm
(long head)

biceps
m. of arm
(short head)

coracoacromial
ligament

superior transverse
scapular ligament

superior
angle

coracohumeral
ligament

coracoid
process

scapular
spine
(cut)

supra-
spinous
fossa

tendon of
biceps m. of arm
(long head)

coraco-
humeral
ligament

coracoid process

superior transverse
scapular ligament

glenoid cavity

scapular spine
(cut)

articular
capsule

inferior
transverse
scapular
ligament

POSTERIOR
ASPECT

scapula

medial
(vertebral)
border

tendon of
biceps m.
of arm
(long head)

humerus

lateral
(axillary)
border

glenoidal
labrum

articular
capsule

humerus

POSTERIOR ASPECT

acromioclavicular ligament

coracoacromial ligament

coracoclavicular ligaments

acromion

LIGAMENTS OF
THE SHOULDER

POSTERIOR ASPECT

infra-
spinous
m.

deltoid m.

supraspinous
m.

ANTERIOR
ASPECT

biceps m. of arm
(short head) and
coracobrachial m.

coracoid process

glenoidal labrum

coracoid process

teres
minor
m.

smaller pectoral
m.

glenoid
cavity

triceps m.
of arm
(lateral
head)

triceps
m. of arm
(long head)

supra-
spinous
m.

subscapular
m.

deltoid m.

teres minor
m.

triceps
m. of arm
(long head)

greater
pectoral
m.

triceps m.
of arm
(medial
head)

infraspinous
m.

teres major
m.

MUSCLE
ATTACHMENTS

latissimus
dorsi m.

teres
major m.

triceps m.
of arm
(medial head)

subscapular m.

triceps m.
of arm
(long head)

lateral
(axillary)
border of
scapula

deltoid m.

LATERAL
ASPECT

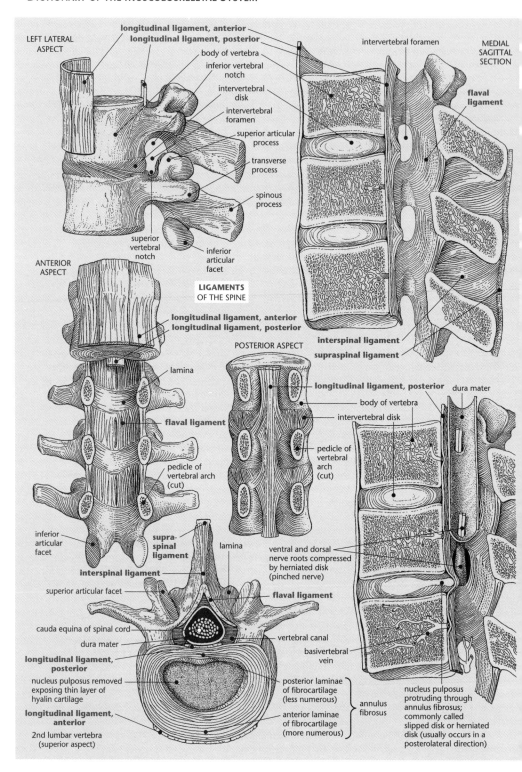

LEFT LATERAL ASPECT

longitudinal ligament, anterior
longitudinal ligament, posterior

body of vertebra
inferior vertebral notch
intervertebral disk
intervertebral foramen
superior articular process
transverse process
spinous process

superior vertebral notch
inferior articular facet

intervertebral foramen

MEDIAL SAGITTAL SECTION

flaval ligament

ANTERIOR ASPECT

LIGAMENTS OF THE SPINE

longitudinal ligament, anterior
longitudinal ligament, posterior

lamina

flaval ligament

pedicle of vertebral arch (cut)

inferior articular facet

supra-spinal ligament

interspinal ligament

superior articular facet

cauda equina of spinal cord

dura mater

longitudinal ligament, posterior

nucleus pulposus removed exposing thin layer of hyalin cartilage

longitudinal ligament, anterior

2nd lumbar vertebra (superior aspect)

POSTERIOR ASPECT

interspinal ligament
supraspinal ligament

longitudinal ligament, posterior
body of vertebra
intervertebral disk

pedicle of vertebral arch (cut)

lamina

ventral and dorsal nerve roots compressed by herniated disk (pinched nerve)

flaval ligament

vertebral canal

basivertebral vein

posterior laminae of fibrocartilage (less numerous)

anterior laminae of fibrocartilage (more numerous)

annulus fibrosus

dura mater

nucleus pulposus protruding through annulus fibrosus; commonly called slipped disk or herniated disk (usually occurs in a posterolateral direction)

ligament ■ ligament

ligament) that extends upward from the transverse band to the anterior margin of the foramen magnum and a vertical band (frequently called the inferior longitudinal fascicles of the cruciform ligament) that extends downward from the transverse band to the back of the body of the second cervical vertebra.

cuboideonavicular l.'s Ligaments that reinforce the articulation between the cuboid and navicular bones of the foot: *Dorsal cuboideonavicular l.*, ligament extending from the dorsal surface of the navicular bone, obliquely forward and laterally to the cuboid bone. *Interosseous cuboideonavicular l.*, strong transverse fibers connecting the navicular bone to the cuboid bone. *Plantar cuboideonavicular l.* , ligament extending from the plantar surface of the navicular bone, transversely to the cuboid bone.

cuneocuboid l.'s Ligaments that reinforce the articulation of the cuboid bone with the lateral cuneiform bone of the foot: *Dorsal cuneocuboid l.*, a transverse band that extends from the dorsal surface of the cuboid bone to the lateral cuneiform bone. *Interosseous cuneocuboid l.*, a strong ligament that connects the nonarticular surfaces of the cuboid bone and adjoining lateral cuneiform bone. *Plantar cuneocuboid l.*, a transverse band that extends from the plantar surface of the cuboid bone to the lateral cuneiform bone.

cuneonavicular l.'s Ligaments that bind the articulation of the navicular bone with the three adjoining cuneiform bones of the foot: *Dorsal cuneonavicular l.*, three small fasciculi extending from the dorsal surface of the navicular bone to each of the three adjoining cuneiform bones. *Plantar cuneonavicular l.*, three small fasciculi extending from the ventral surface of the navicular bone to each of the three adjoining cuneiform bones.

deep transverse metacarpal l.'s Three short, wide, flattened bands in the hand that connect transversely the palmar ligaments (plates) of the 2nd, 3rd, 4th, and 5th metacarpophalangeal joints to one another.

deep transverse metatarsal l.'s Four short, wide, flattened bands in the foot that connect the plantar ligaments (plates) of the lst, 2nd, 3rd, 4th, and 5th metatarsophalangeal joints to one another.

deltoid l. of ankle joint The medial reinforcing ligament of the ankle joint, composed of the tibiocalcaneal, anterior tibiotalar, posterior tibiotalar, and

tibionavicular ligaments; they pass downward from the medial malleolus of the tibia to the navicular bone, calcaneus and talus, respectively. Also called internal collateral ligament of ankle; medial collateral ligament of ankle.

dorsal basal metacarpal l.'s See metacarpal ligaments, dorsal.

external collateral l. of ankle See lateral collateral ligament of ankle.

falciform l. of liver A median sickle-shaped ligament composed of two layers of peritoneum connecting the liver to the diaphragm and anterior abdominal wall as low as the level of the navel (umbilicus); it contains the round ligament of the liver between its layers.

fibular collateral l. of knee A strong, round, fibrous cord, situated on the lateral side of the knee joint, extending from the lateral epicondyle of the femur to the lateral side of the head of the fibula. Also called lateral collateral ligament of knee.

flaval l. A series of yellow elastic bands that bind together the laminae of adjacent vertebrae from the first cervical vertebra to the first sacral vertebra; they serve to maintain the body in an upright position. Also called ligamentum flavum; yellow ligament.

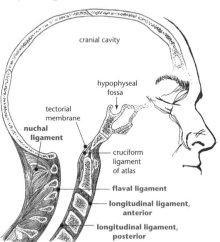

fundiform l. of penis A thickened fibroelastic tissue that is intimately adherent to the lower part of the linea alba and the top of the pubic symphysis and extends to the dorsum of the penis.

glenohumeral l.'s Three thick fibrous bands (superior, middle and inferior)

ligament ■ ligament

overlying the anterior portion of the shoulder joint capsule, extending from the anterior border of the glenoid cavity to the lesser tuberosity and neck of the humerus.

l. of head of femur A flattened intracapsular band at the hip joint originating from the head of the femur and attaching by two bands to the acetabulum, one on each side of the acetabular notch; it blends with the transverse ligament of acetabulum and relaxes when the thigh is abducted. Also called round ligament of femur.

hamatometacarpal l. A ligament that passes from the palmar aspect of the hook of the hamate bone to the base of the fifth metacarpal bone of the wrist.

hyoepiglottic l. A short triangular elastic band that unites the anterior surface of the upper epiglottic cartilage to the upper part of the hyoid bone. Also called hyoepiglottic membrane.

iliofemoral l. A strong triangular ligament overlying the hip joint and blending with its capsule; it extends from the bottom of anterior inferior iliac spine, broadening out as it descends to the trochanteric line of the femur. Also called Y-shaped ligament.

iliolumbar l.'s Strong bands extending from the transverse processes of the fourth and fifth lumbar vetebrae to the inner lip of the posterior iliac crest and the lateral side of the upper sacrum; they blend below with the ventral sacroiliac ligament.

inguinal l. The thickened upturned lower margin of the aponeurosis of the external oblique muscle, extending from the anterior superior spine of the ilium to the tubercle of the pubic bone. Also called Poupart's ligament.

intercarpal l.'s A series of dorsal, interosseous and palmar ligaments that unite the wrist (carpal) bones with one another.

interclavicular l. A strong band of curved fibers connecting the medial (sternal) ends of the two clavicles (collarbones) across the clavicular notch of the sternum (breastbone).

intercuneiform l.'s Ligamentous bands between the intermediate cuneiform bone and both the medial and lateral cuneiform bones; they are reinforced by slips from the tendon of the posterior tibial muscle.

interfoveolar l. A ligamentous band that connects the lower margin of the transverse abdominal muscle to the superior ramus of the pubic bone; it is inconstant.

intermetacarpal l.'s Ligamentous bands reinforcing the bases of the four medial metacarpal bones: *Dorsal intermetacarpal l.'s,* bands passing transversely on the dorsal surface of the bases of the second, third, fourth,and fifth metacarpal bones. *Interosseous intermetacarpal l.'s,* bands connecting the contiguous surfaces of the metacarpal bones. *Palmar intermetacarpal l.'s,* bands passing transversely on the palmar surfaces of the bases of the second, third, fourth, and fifth metacarpal bones.

internal collateral l. of ankle See deltoid ligament of ankle joint.

interspinal l.'s A series of short ligaments connecting the spinous processes of adjoining vertebrae; they abut the flaval ligament in front and the supraspinal ligament behind.

intertarsal l.'s A series of dorsal, interosseous and plantar ligaments that unite the ankle (tarsal) bones with one another.

intertransverse l.'s A series of weak ligaments connecting the tips of adjacent transverse processes of vertebrae, mainly in the lumbar region.

ischiofemoral l. A spiral ligament overlying the back of the hip joint capsule; it extends from the ischium (below and behind the acetabulum) to the back of the neck of the femur.

lacunar l. A triangular band extending from the medial end of the inguinal ligament to the iliopectineal line of the hipbone.

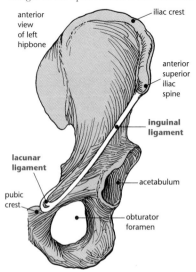

anterior view of left hipbone

iliac crest

anterior superior iliac spine

inguinal ligament

lacunar ligament

pubic crest

acetabulum

obturator foramen

ligament ■ ligament

lateral atlanto-occipital l.'s The lateral thickening of the articular capsule surrounding the joints between the occipital condyles of the skull and the superior facets of the first cervical vertebra; they limit lateral tilting of the head.

lateral collateral l. of ankle The lateral reinforcing ligament of the ankle joint, comprised of the posterior talofibular ligament, calcaneofibular ligament, and the anterior talofibular ligament. Also called external collateral ligament of ankle.

lateral collateral l. of elbow See radial collateral ligament of elbow joint.

lateral collateral l. of knee See fibular collateral ligament of knee.

lateral collateral l. of wrist See radial collateral ligament of wrist joint.

lateral temporomandibular l. See temporomandibular ligament.

longitudinal l.'s Long, broad, flat bands of fibers which reinforce the articulations of the vertebral bodies: *Anterior longitudinal l.*, a band of fibers that extends along the anterior surface of the vertebral bodies from the base of the skull to the upper part of the sacrum; it is firmly fixed to the intervertebral disks and is thickest in the thoracic area. *Posterior longitudinal l.*, a band of fibers on the posterior surface of the vertebral canal, extending from the second cervical vertebra to the upper part of the sacrum; it is attached to the intervertebral disks.

long plantar l. A strong thick band (the longest of the tarsal ligaments) extending from the plantar surface of the calcaneus and dividing into deep fibers, which attach to the plantar surface of the cuboid bone, and superficial fibers which attach to the proximal ends of the second, third, fourth and occasionally the fifth metatarsal bones; it limits the flattening of the lateral longitudinal arch of the foot.

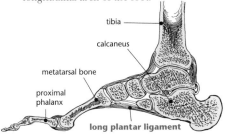

tibia

calcaneus

metatarsal bone

proximal phalanx

long plantar ligament

long posterior sacroiliac l. See sacroiliac ligament, dorsal.

medial collateral l. of ankle See deltoid ligament of ankle joint.

medial collateral l. of elbow See ulnar collateral ligament of the elbow joint.

medial collateral l. of knee See tibial collateral ligament of knee.

medial collateral l. of wrist See ulnar collateral ligament of wrist joint.

meniscofemoral l.'s Meniscus ligaments of the knee joint: *Anterior meniscofemoral l.*, an inconstant oblique band passing from the posterior end of the lateral meniscus in the knee joint to the medial condyle of the femur; it passes anterior to the posterior cruciate ligament. *Posterior meniscofemoral l.*, a strong band that passes upward and medially from the posterior end of the lateral meniscus in the knee to the medial condyle of the femur; it passes behind the posterior cruciate ligament.

meniscofibular l. An inconstant bundle of fibers extending from the posterior end of the lateral meniscus of the knee to the fibula.

metacarpal l.'s Ligaments that strengthen the proximal metacarpal articulations of the hand: *Dorsal metacarpal l.'s*, short transverse bands uniting the dorsal surface of the bases of the second, third, fourth and fifth metacarpal bones with one another. Also called dorsal basal metacarpal ligaments. *Interosseous metacarpal l.'s*, short bands connecting the contiguous surfaces of the metacarpal bones of the hand. *Palmar metacarpal l.'s*, short transverse bands uniting the palmar surface of the bases of the second to fifth metacarpal bones with one another. Also called ventral basal metacarpal ligaments.

metatarsal l.'s Ligaments that strengthen the proximal intermetatarsal articulations of the foot: *Dorsal metatarsal l.'s*, short, thin transverse bands uniting the dorsal surface of the bases of the second, third, fourth and fifth metatarsal bones of the foot. *Interosseous metatarsal l.'s*, strong, transverse bands uniting the nonarticular parts of the adjacent metatarsal bones of the foot. *Plantar metatarsal l.'s*, four transverse bands uniting the plantar surface of the bases of the metatarsal bones of the foot.

nuchal l. A broad, somewhat triangular fibroelastic septum in the back of the neck stretching from the base of the skull to the posterior tubercle of the first cervical vertebra and the spinous processes of all the other cervical vertebrae; it forms a midline septum for attachment of muscles on either

ligament ■ ligament

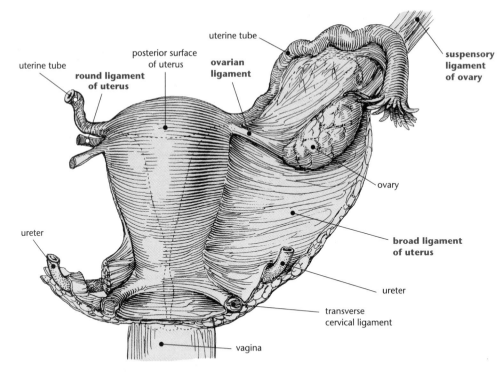

uterine tube

posterior surface
of uterus

uterine tube

round ligament
of uterus

ovarian
ligament

suspensory
ligament
of ovary

ovary

broad ligament
of uterus

ureter

ureter

transverse
cervical ligament

vagina

side of the neck. Also called ligamentum
nuchae.

oblique popliteal l. See oblique posterior
ligament of knee.

oblique posterior l. of knee A ligament
from the tendon of the semimembranous
muscle (near its insertion), extending
obliquely to the posterior part of the knee
joint capsule. Also called oblique popliteal
ligament.

odontoid l.'s See alar ligaments.

ovarian l. A cordlike bundle of fibers
between the layers of the broad ligament of
uterus, joining the uterine end of the ovary
to the lateral margin of the uterus,
immediately behind the attachment of the
uterine (fallopian) tube.

palmar l.'s Thick fibrocartilaginous plates
on the palmar surfaces of the
metacarpophalangeal plates on the palmar
surfaces of the metacarpophalangeal joints,
firmly united to the bases of the proximal
phalanges and loosely connected to the
metacarpal bones.

palmar ulnocarpal l. A rounded fibrous
band passing downward and laterally from
the base of the styloid process of the ulna
and the front of the articular disk of the

distal radioulnar joint to the palmar surface
of the lunate and triquetral bones (proximal
row of wrist bones).

palpebral l.'s Ligaments of the eyelids
(palpebrae): *Lateral palpebral l.*, a thin band
that connects the lateral ends of the tarsal
plates of the eyelids to the zygomatic bone,
just within the orbital margin. *Medial
palpebral l.*, a strong tendinous band that
connects the medial ends of the tarsal plates
of the eyelids to the frontal process of the
maxilla, in front of the nasolacrimal groove.

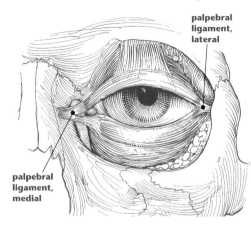

palpebral
ligament,
lateral

palpebral
ligament,
medial

ligament ■ ligament

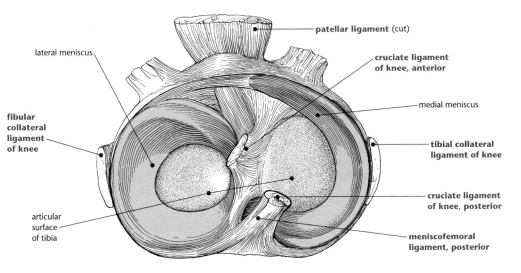

patellar ligament (cut)

lateral meniscus

cruciate ligament
of knee, anterior

medial meniscus

fibular
collateral
ligament
of knee

tibial collateral
ligament of knee

cruciate ligament
of knee, posterior

articular
surface
of tibia

meniscofemoral
ligament, posterior

patellar l. The continuation of the strong, flattened common tendon of the quadriceps muscle of thigh (quadriceps femoris) from the patella (kneecap) downward to the tuberosity of the tibia.

pectineal l. A strong fibrous band that extends from the upper border of the pectineal surface of the hipbone to the medial end of the lacunar ligament at the groin, with which it is continuous. Also called Cooper's ligament.

periodontal l. Connective tissue fibers that attach the root of a tooth to the bone of its socket. Also called periodontal membrane; alveolodental ligament.

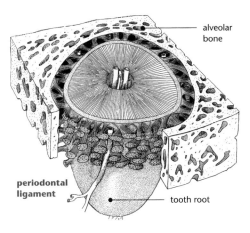

alveolar
bone

periodontal
ligament

tooth root

pisohamate l. A ligament that passes from the pisiform bone to the hook of the hamate bone at the wrist; basically it is a ligamentous

extension from the tendon of insertion of the ulnar flexor muscle of the wrist (flexor carpi ulnaris muscle).

pisometacarpal l. A ligament that passes from the pisiform bone to the base of the fifth metacarpal bone of the wrist; basically it is a ligamentous extension from the tendon of insertion of the ulnar flexor muscle of the wrist (flexor carpi ulnaris muscle).

plantar l.'s Thick, dense fibrocartilaginous plates on the plantar surfaces of the metatarsophalangeal joints, firmly united to the bases of the proximal phalanges and loosely connected to the metatarsal bones.

plantar calcaneocuboid l. The strong, short band, extending from the plantar surface of the calcaneus (heel bone) to the contiguous plantar surface of the cuboid bone. It limits flattening of the lateral longitudinal arch of the foot. Also called short plantar ligament.

plantar calcaneonavicular l. The broad, thick fibrocartilaginous band connecting the anterior margin of the calcaneus (heel bone) to the plantar surface of the navicular bone; it limits flattening of the medial longitudinal arch of the foot. Also called spring ligament.

plantar metatarsal l.'s Transverse bands over the capsules of the intermetatarsal joints and connecting the plantar surfaces of the bases of the four lateral metatarsal bones of the foot.

posterior talotibial l. See tibiotalar ligament, posterior.

Poupart's l. See inguinal ligament.

pubic l.'s See superior pubic ligament; arcuate pubic ligament.

ligament ■ ligament

pubofemoral l. A triangular ligament overlying the capsule of the hip joint on its inferior aspect; it extends from the iliopubic eminence and adjacent superior pubic ramus to blend with the hip joint capsule and iliofemoral ligament.

radial collateral l. of elbow joint A fan-shaped ligament extending from the bottom part of the lateral epicondyle of the humerus to the annular ligament of the radius and the upper end of the supinator crest of the ulna. Also called lateral collateral ligament of elbow.

radial collateral l. of wrist joint Poorly developed fibrous band extending downward from the styloid process of the radius to the scaphoid bone of the wrist. Also called lateral collateral ligament of wrist.

radiate l. A fan-shaped band that extends from the side of the bodies of two adjoining vertebrae to the head of the rib with which it articulates. Also called radiate ligament of head of rib.

radiate l. of head of rib
See radiate ligament.

radiate sternocostal l.'s
See sternocostal ligaments.

radiocarpal l.'s Ligaments of the wrist joint: *Dorsal radiocarpal l.,* a thin sheath of ligamentous tissue overlying the wrist joint extending from the distal end of the radius to the dorsal surface of the proximal row of wrist bones (triquetral, lunate, and scaphoid bones); it blends with the underlying articular disk of the inferior radioulnar articulation. *Palmar radiocarpal l.,* a broad membranous band extending from the anterior aspects of the lower end of the radius and its styloid process to the anterior surface of the proximal row of wrist bones (triquetral, lunate, and scaphoid bones), and occasionally to the capitate bone.

reflex inguinal l. The part of the inguinal ligament that extends from the lateral side of the superficial inguinal ring, passes upward and medially to interlace at the linea alba with its counterpart from the opposite side of the body. Also called triangular fascia; reflected part of inguinal ligament.

round l. of femur See ligament of head of femur.

round l. of liver A fibrous cord (the remains of the umbilical vein of the fetus) extending from the anterior abdominal wall at the level of the navel (umbilicus) to the inferior surface of the liver (in the free edge of the falciform ligament of liver). Also called ligamentum teres of liver.

round l. of uterus A fibromuscular ligamentous cord extending from the lateral margin of the uterus, on either side, passing between the two layers of the broad ligament of the uterus, it traverses the inguinal canal to become attached to the connective tissue of the labium majus. Also called ligamentum teres of uterus.

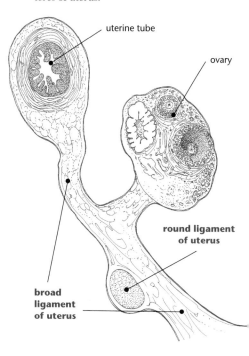

uterine tube

ovary

round ligament of uterus

broad ligament of uterus

sacroiliac l.'s Ligaments that bind the sacrum with the ilium of the hipbone: *Dorsal sacroiliac l.,* a set of thick fibrous bands overlying the interosseous sacroiliac ligament, consisting of a lower, superficial group (long posterior sacroiliac ligament) that extends from the posterior superior iliac spine of the hipbone to the transverse tubercles of the third and fourth segments of the sacrum (the bands blend with the sacrotuberous ligament); and an upper, deep group (short posterior sacroiliac ligament) that extends from the posterior inferior iliac spine and adjacent part of the ilium to the back of the sacrum. *Interosseous sacroiliac l.,* short, thick bundles of fibers interconnecting the sacral and iliac tuberosities, posterior to their articular surfaces; one of the strongest ligaments in the body, it serves as the

ligament ■ ligament

principal bond between the sacrum and ilium. *Ventral sacroiliac l.*, a thin, wide, fibrous layer reinforcing the anterior part of the articular capsule of the sacroiliac joint and stretching from the ala and pelvic surface of the sacrum to the adjoining parts of the ilium.

sacrospinous l. A strong triangular ligament attached by its apex to the spine of the ischium of the hipbone and by its base to the lateral part of the lower sacrum and coccyx.

sacrotuberous l. A long, strong triangular ligament extending from the tuberosity of the ischium of the hipbone to the lateral part of the sacrum and coccyx and to the superior and inferior posterior iliac spines.

Scarpa's l. See superior horn of falciform margin, under horn.

short plantar l.
See plantar calcaneocuboid ligament.

short posterior sacroiliac l. See sacroiliac ligament, dorsal.

sphenomandibular l. A flat, thin fibrous band that extends from the spine of the sphenoid bone, becoming broader as it descends to the lingula of the mandibular foramen.

spring l. See plantar calcaneonavicular ligament.

sternoclavicular l.'s Ligaments that reinforce the sternoclavicular joint: *Anterior sternoclavicular l.*, a short, broad band overlying the front of the sternoclavicular joint, extending from the medial end of the clavicle to the front of the upper sternum and adjoining cartilage of the first rib (costal cartilage); *Posterior sternoclavicular l.*, a short, broad band overlying the back of the sternoclavicular joint, extending from the medial end of the clavicle to the back of the upper sternum and adjoining cartilage of the first rib (costal cartilage).

sternocostal l.'s Thin, wide bands radiating from the sternal ends of the cartilages of the true ribs to the front and back surfaces of the sternum. Also called radiate sternocostal ligaments.

stylomandibular l. A condensed band of deep cervical fascia extending from the tip of the styloid process, downward to the posterior margin of the angle of the lower jaw (mandible).

superior pubic l. A transverse band that binds the two pubic bones superiorly, and extends as far as the pubic tubercles; it is firmly attached to the interpubic disk at the midline.

superior transverse l. of scapula
See suprascapular ligament.

suprascapular l. A flat ligament extending from the medial end of the scapular notch to the coracoid process, thus converting the notch into a foramen. Also called superior transverse ligament of scapula.

supraspinal l. A strong fibrous band that connects the tips of the spinous processes from the seventh cervical vetebra to the sacrum; it blends with the interspinous ligament. From the seventh cervical vertebra to the base of the skull, it expands to form the nuchal ligament.

suspensory l.'s of breast Coarse connective tissue bands distributed between the lobes of the female breast (mammary gland), extending from the overlying skin to the underlying pectoral fascia. Also called Cooper's ligaments; suspensory ligaments of mammary gland.

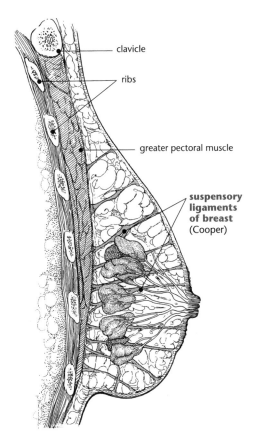

clavicle

ribs

greater pectoral muscle

suspensory ligaments of breast (Cooper)

suspensory l. of duodenum See suspensory muscle of duodenum in the table of muscles in appendix II.

suspensory l.'s of mammary gland See suspensory ligaments of breast.

suspensory l. of ovary The part of the broad ligament of the uterus arising from the tubal side of the ovary and extending upward toward the lateral wall of the pelvis; it contains the ovarian blood vessels, lymphatic vessels, and nerves.

talocalcaneal l.'s Fibrous bands that reinforce the two articulations between the talus (ankle bone) and the calcaneus (heel bone): *Anterior talocalcaneal l.*, a band extending from the upper anterior part of the neck of the talus to the upper surface of the calcaneus. *Interosseous talocalcaneal l.*, a strong, broad, flattened band extending obliquely from the deep groove of the talus to the deep groove of the calcaneus. *Lateral talocalcaneal l.*, a short, flattened band extending from the lateral process of the talus and passing downward and backward to the lateral surface of the calcaneus. *Medial talocalcaneal l.*, a band extending from the medial tubercle of the talus to the medial surface of the calcaneus; it blends with the deltoid ligament. *Posterior talocalcaneal l.*, a short, wide band extending from the posterior process of the talus, downward to the adjacent calcaneus.

talofibular l.'s Ligaments of the ankle joint: *Anterior talofibular l.*, a ligament that stretches from the anterior margin of the lateral malleolus of the fibula to the lateral aspect of the neck of the talus. *Posterior talofibular l.*, a ligament that stretches from the posterior margin of the lateral malleolus of the fibula to the posterior process of the talus.

talonavicular l. A broad, thin band, extending from the neck of the talus (ankle bone) to the dorsal surface of the adjoining navicular bone of the foot. Also called dorsal talonavicular ligament.

talotibial l.'s See tibiotalar ligaments.

tarsometatarsal l.'s Ligaments reinforcing the joints between the tarsus and the metatarsal bones of the foot: *Dorsal tarsometatarsal l.'s*, strong, flat bands connecting the dorsal surface of the proximal metatarsal bones to the distal tarsus (cuboid and three cuneiform bones). *Interosseous tarsometatarsal l.'s*, bands from the first and third cuneiform bones to the

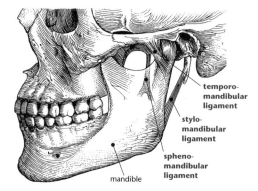

second and fourth metatarsal bones respectively. *Plantar tarsometatarsal l.'s*, oblique bands connecting the plantar surface of the proximal metatarsal bones to the distal tarsus (cuboid and three cuneiform bones).

temporomandibular l. An oblique band that reinforces the temporomandibular joint, extending downward and backward from the lower surface of the zygomatic process to the posterolateral surface margin of the neck of the lower jaw (mandible). Also called lateral temporomandibular ligament.

thyroepiglottic l. An elastic ligament that attaches the stalk (petiole) of the lower end of the epiglottic cartilage to the back of the thyroid cartilage just below the notch.

tibial collateral l. of knee A broad, flat membranous band, posteromedial to the knee joint, extending from the medial epicondyle of the femur to the medial condyle and medial surface of the tibia; consists of two parts: a short, deep, thick

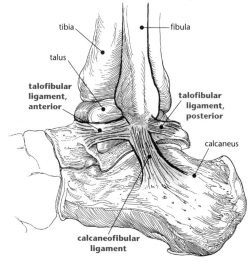

ligament ■ ligament

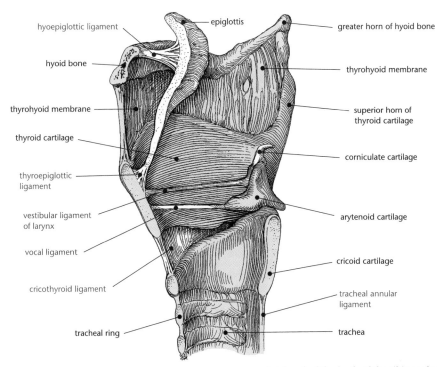

posterior band, and a longer anterior band, extending from the femoral epicondyle and fanning out into a broad expansion on the anteromedial surface of the tibia; the latter one is the most frequently injured ligament of the knee. Also called medial collateral ligament of knee.

tibiocalcaneal l. The widest part of the deltoid ligament of the ankle joint extending from the medial malleolus of the tibia to the median projection (sustentaculum tali) of the calcaneus. Also called calcaneotibial ligament.

tibiofibular l.'s Ligaments connecting the tibia and fibula at the proximal and distal ends: *Anterior (superior) tibiofibular l.*, flat bands that extend from the front of the head of the fibula to the front of the lateral condyle of the tibia. *Anterior (inferior) tibiofibular l.*, a flattened oblique band extending downward and laterally from the distal end of the front of the tibia to the adjoining fibula. *Posterior (superior) tibiofibular l.*, thick band that extends from the back of the head of the fibula to the back of the lateral condyle of the tibia. *Posterior (inferior) tibiofibular l.*, a strong oblique band extending downward and laterally from the

distal end of the back of the tibia to the adjoining fibula; its lowest part extends transversely from the fibula to the ankle bone (talus).

tibionavicular l. The part of the deltoid ligament of the ankle joint extending from the medial malleolus of the tibia to the tubercle on the dorsal side of the navicular bone.

tibiotalar l.'s Parts of the deltoid ligament of the ankle joint: *Anterior tibiotalar l.*, the deep part extending from the medial malleolus of the tibia to the medial surface of the talus. Also called anterior talotibial ligament. *Posterior tibiotalar l.*, the part that extends from the medial malleolus of the tibia, posteriorly to the medial side of the ankle bone (talus) and its tubercle. Also called posterior talotibial ligament.

tracheal annular l. The fibro-elastic membrane that posteriorly encloses and connects the ends of the incomplete tracheal rings.

transverse l. of acetabulum A strong flattened ligament that is attached to the margin of the acetabulum and crosses the acetabular notch, forming a foramen at the hip joint for the passage of nerves and vessels.

ligament ■ ligament

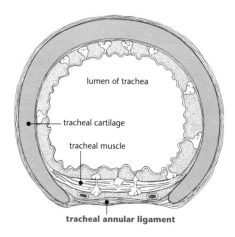

lumen of trachea

tracheal cartilage

tracheal muscle

tracheal annular ligament

transverse l. of atlas See cruciform ligament of atlas *(a)*.

transverse carpal l. A broad ligament bridging over the carpal tunnel of the wrist extending from the pisiform and hamate bones to the scaphoid and trapezium bones of the wrist.

transverse humeral l. The lowest part of the capsule of the shoulder joint, extending from the lesser to the greater tubercle of the humerus; it serves as a retinaculum for the tendon of the long head of the biceps muscle of the arm (biceps brachii) as it emerges from the capsule to enter the intertubercular sulcus of the humerus.

transverse l. of knee An inconstant bundle of fibers extending between the anterior extremities of the menisci of the knee joint by connecting the anterior convex margin of the lateral meniscus to the anterior end of the medial meniscus. Also called transverse ligament of menisci.

transverse l. of menisci See transverse ligament of knee.

trapezoid l. Part of the coracoclavicular ligament extending from the upper surface of the coracoid process upward to the undersurface of the lateral end of the clavicle.

l. of Treitz See suspensory muscle of duodenum, in table of muscles in appendix II.

ulnar collateral l. of elbow joint A strong triangular ligament on the medial side of the elbow joint, composed of anterior and posterior bands united by a thin oblique band; the anterior band extends from the front of the medial epicondyle of the humerus to the medial margin of the

coronoid process of the ulna; the posterior band extends from the lower part of the medial epicondyle to the medial surface of the olecranon; the oblique band stretches from the olecranon to the coronoid process. Also called medial collateral ligament of elbow.

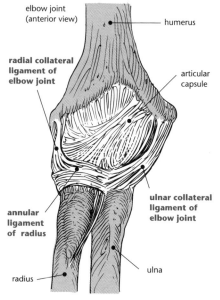

elbow joint (anterior view)

humerus

radial collateral ligament of elbow joint

articular capsule

annular ligament of radius

ulnar collateral ligament of elbow joint

radius

ulna

ulnar collateral l. of wrist joint A fibrous band extending downward from the styloid process of the ulna to the wrist; it divides into two parts, one attached to the triquetral bone and the other to the pisiform bone of the wrist. Also called medial collateral ligament of wrist.

uterosacral l. Fibromuscular band that extends backward on either side from the uterine cervix, along the lateral wall of the pelvis to the front of the sacrum. It passes by the sides of the rectum and can be palpated on rectal examination.

venous l. of liver A thin fibrous cord, the remains of the obliterated ductus venosus of the fetus, lying in a fossa on the posterior part of the diaphragmatic surface of the liver. Also called ligamentum venosum.

ventral basal metacarpal l.'s See metacarpal ligaments, palmar.

vestibular l. See vestibular ligament of larynx.

vestibular l. of larynx A thin fibrous band in the ventricular fold of the larynx that extends from the thyroid cartilage, anteriorly, to the arytenoid cartilage,

ligament ■ ligament

posteriorly. Also called vestibular ligament.

    vocal l. The elastic tissue band that extends on either side from the thyroid cartilage in front, to the vocal process of the arytenoid cartilage behind; it is situated within the vocal fold, just below the vestibular ligament.

    yellow l. See flaval ligament.

    Y-shaped l. See iliofemoral ligament.

    l. of Zinn See common annular tendon, under tendon.

ligamentous (lig-ah-men'tus) Of the nature of a ligament.

ligamentum (lig-ah-men'tum) Latin for ligament.

    l. flavum See flaval ligament, under ligament.

    l. nuchae See nuchal ligament, under ligament.

    l. teres of liver See round ligament of liver, under ligament.

    l. teres of uterus See round ligament of uterus, under ligament.

    l. venosum See venous ligament of liver, under ligament.

line (līn) 1. A thin area of demarcation designating the junction of two structures. 2. A thin, continuous strip, mark, or ridge. Also called stria. 3. An imaginary mark connecting two points or landmarks on the body or passing through them. 4. A boundary.

    arcuate l. of pelvis See iliopectineal crest of pelvis, under crest.

    arcuate l. of sheath of rectus abdominis muscle The concave lower margin of the posterior layer of the rectus abdominis sheath, located approximately halfway between the umbilicus and the pubic symphysis.

    axillary l. One of three imaginary vertical lines associated with the armpit (axilla): *Anterior axillary l.,* the line that passes through the anterior fold of the axilla. *Middle axillary l.,* the line that passes through the middle of the axilla; also called midaxillary line. *Posterior axillary l.,* the line that passes through the posterior fold of the axilla.

    basinasal l. See nasobasilar line.

    basiobregmatic l. A line joining the basion and the bregma, two craniometric points.

    bi-iliac l. A line drawn across the most prominent points between the two iliac crests.

    cervical l. The undulating line around the neck of a tooth marking the junction between the enamel of the crown and the cementum of the root.

    epiphyseal l. A line of the noncalcified cartilaginous growth plate between the

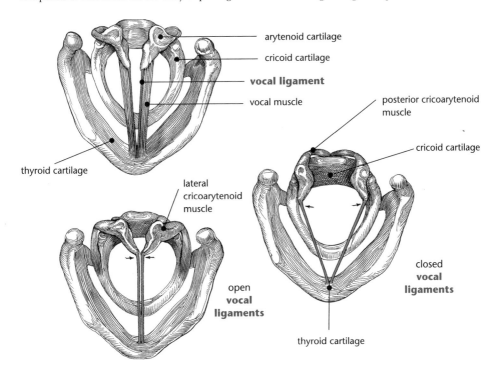

arytenoid cartilage

cricoid cartilage

vocal ligament

vocal muscle

thyroid cartilage

lateral cricoarytenoid muscle

open **vocal ligaments**

posterior cricoarytenoid muscle

cricoid cartilage

closed **vocal ligaments**

thyroid cartilage

junction of the epiphysis and the diaphysis of a long bone, where growth in length occurs.

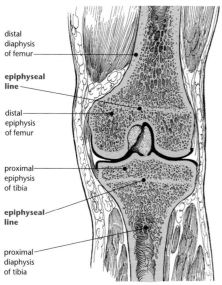

distal
diaphysis
of femur

**epiphyseal
line**

distal
epiphysis
of femur

proximal
epiphysis
of tibia

**epiphyseal
line**

proximal
diaphysis
of tibia

flexure l.'s Furrows on the external surface of the skin that correspond to habitual joint movements, seen especially on the surface of the palms, soles and digits.

gluteal l. One of the three rough curved lines on the outer surface of the iliac part of the hipbone: *Interior gluteal l.*, a rough curved line extending from the greater sciatic notch anteriorly to the notch just under the anterior superior iliac spine; it marks the lower limit of attachment of the least gluteal muscle (gluteus minimus). *Anterior gluteal l.*, the middle of the three curved lines extending from the superior margin of the great sciatic notch anteriorly to a point about five cm along the iliac crest from the anterior superior iliac spine; it marks the lower and anterior limits of attachment of the middle gluteal muscle (gluteus medius). *Posterior gluteal l.*, the posterior and shorter of the three curved lines extending from the superior margin of the greater sciatic notch to the iliac crest about five cm in front of the posterior superior iliac spine; it marks the anterior limit of attachment of the greatest gluteal muscle (gluteus maximus).

Hensen's l. See H band, under band.

Holden's l. A flexure line of the groin, below the inguinal fold, crossing the capsule of the hip joint.

iliopectineal l. See iliopectineal crest of pelvis, under crest.

infrascapular l. A horizontal line connecting the tips of the inferior angles of the two scapulas.

intercondylar l. The slight transverse ridge separating the posterior part of the intercondylar fossa from the popliteal surface of the distal femur; it provides attachment to the posterior portion of the capsule of the knee joint.

interspinal l. A horizontal line across the abdomen connecting the two anterior superior iliac spines of the hipbones.

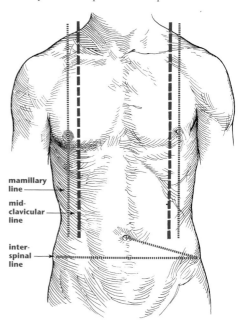

mamillary
line

mid-
clavicular
line

inter-
spinal
line

intertrochanteric l. An oblique, rough ridge on the anterior surface of the upper femur, between the neck and the shaft of the bone.

lateral sternal l. A vertical line corresponding to the lateral border of the sternum. Also called sternal line.

lateral supracondylar l. A distinct ridge on the distal third of the posterior surface of the femur that is continuous above with the linea aspera and extends down to the lateral epicondyle; the upper portion provides attachment to the biceps muscle of the thigh (biceps femoris) and the lateral intermuscular septum, while the lower portion provides attachment to the plantar muscle (plantaris). Also called lateral supracondylar ridge.

M l. A line formed by the nodular thickening of the myofilament (myosin)

line ■ line

bisecting the H central zone of striated muscle myofibrils (sarcomere).

mamillary l. An imaginary vertical line on the anterior surface of the body, passing through the nipple of either breast; it corresponds roughly to the vertical line passing through the middle of the clavicles (collarbones). Also called nipple line.

medial supracondylar l. A slight ridge (occasionally sharp) on the distal third of the posterior surface of the femur that is continuous above with the linea aspera and extends downward to the adductor tubercle; near its upper end it is interrupted to allow passage of the femoral vessels as they enter the fossa from the adductor canal; it provides attachment to the membranous expansion from the tendon of the great adductor muscle (adductor magnus).

median l. An imaginary vertical line dividing the surface of the body equally into right and left sides.

midclavicular l. An imaginary vertical line on the anterior surface of the body, passing through the midpoint of the clavicle (collarbone) on either side; it corresponds roughly to the vertical line passing through the nipple.

midsternal l. A vertical line passing through the center of the sternum (breastbone).

mylohyoid l. An oblique ridge on the inner surface of the body of the mandible, extending from the area of the third molar socket to the digastric fossa at the base of the mental symphysis; it provides attachment to the mylohyoid muscle. Above the line lies the sublingual salivary gland, and below the line lies the submandibular salivary gland. Also called mylohyoid ridge.

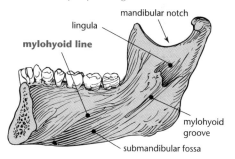

nasobasilar l. A line joining the nasion and the basion, two craniometric points. Also called basinasal line.

nasolabial l. A line extending from the ala

of the nose, obliquely downward toward the corner of the mouth.

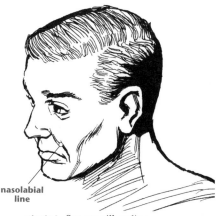

nasolabial line

nipple l. See mamillary line.

nuchal l.'s Three lines or ridges on the exterior surface of the occipital bone of the skull: *Highest nuchal l.*, the higher of the two transverse curved lines on the back of the skull, extending laterally, on both sides, from the external occipital protuberance; it provides attachment to the epicranial aponeurosis and occipital muscle. *Superior nuchal l.*, the lower of the two transverse curved lines on the back of the skull, extending laterally, on both sides, from the external occipital protuberance; it provides attachment to the trapezius muscle medially and to the sternocleidomastoid muscle and splenius muscle of head laterally. *Inferior nuchal l.*, the transverse curved line coursing on the back of the skull between the external occipital protuberance and the posterior margin of the foramen magnum.

l. of occlusion The horizontal line formed by maxillary and mandibular teeth when in normal occlusion.

pectineal l. The sharp edge on the superior ramus of the pubic bone extending from the pubic tubercle anteriorly, to the iliopubic eminence posteriorly. Also called pecten pubis.

popliteal l. of femur See pectineal crest of femur, under crest.

popliteal l. of tibia See soleal line of tibia.

rough l. See linea aspera, under linea.

scapular l. An imaginary vertical line on the posterior surface of the body, passing through the lower angle of the scapula on either side.

semilunar l. See linea semilunaris, under linea.

line ■ line

soleal l. of tibia A rough ridge that extends obliquely from the fibular facet downward and medially across the upper part of the posterior surface of the tibia; it affords attachment to the soleus muscle. Also called popliteal line of tibia.

sternal l. See lateral sternal line.

subcostal l. See subcostal plane, under plane.

temporal l.'s The two curved, transverse lines on the outer surface of the parietal bones of the skull on either side: *Inferior temporal l.*, the lower temporal line that provides attachment to the temporal muscle. *Superior temporal l.*, the upper temporal line that provides attachment to the temporal fascia. Also called temporal ridges.

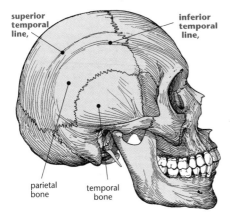

terminal l. of pelvis See iliopectineal crest of pelvis, under crest.

transverse l. of sacrum One of four transverse ridges on the pelvic surface of the sacrum; it marks the position of the intervertebral disk prior to fusion of the sacral vertebrae. Also called transverse ridge of sacrum.

Z l. See Z band, under band.

zigzag l. See Z-Z line.

Z-Z l. An irregular dentate or zigzag line between the esophagus and the stomach; it represents the transition from esophageal to gastric mucosa, easily recognized by a color change. Also called zigzag line.

linea (lin'e-ah) A line, strip, or narrow ridge, usually on the surface of a structure; a thin, continuous mark.

l. alba The narrow portion of the anterior aponeurosis extending from the midline of the xiphoid process stretching down to the pubic symphysis, formed by the interlacing aponeurotic fibers of the flat abdominal

muscles; the umbilicus (navel) is situated slightly below its midpoint.

l. aspera A broad, rough longitudinal ridge with crestlike lateral and medial lips, located on the posterior middle third surface of the shaft of the femur; it provides attachment to the short head of the biceps, long adductor, great adductor, and pectineal muscles, along with the intermuscular septa of the thigh. Also called rough line.

l. semilunaris The lateral edge of the abdominal rectus muscle, extending from the pubic tubercle to the tip of the ninth costal cartilage. Also called semilunar line.

lingula (ling'gu-lah) Any tongue-shaped process.

l. of mandible A small triangular spur of bone projecting partly over the mandibular foramen on the medial surface of the ramus of the mandible; it provides attachment to the sphenomandibular ligament. Also called spine of Spix.

l. of sphenoid A slender spur of bone that projects posteriorly between the body and greater wing of the sphenoid bone, on either side, forming the lateral margin of the carotid groove.

local (lo'kal) Confined to an area of the body; not systemic or general.

loin (loin) The region of the back between the lowest rib and the upper rim of the pelvis (iliac crest), on either side of the vertebral column.

lordoscoliosis (lor-do-sko-le-o'sis) Abnormal backward and lateral curvature of the vertebral column (spine).

lordosis (lor-do'sis) An abnormally exaggerated inward curvature of the lower vertebral column (spine). Also called swayback.

lumbar (lum'bar) Relating to the loins, i.e., the part of the back between the lowest rib and the pelvic bone on either side of the vertebral column (spine).

lumbarization (lum-ber-i-za'shun) Fusion between the transverse processes of the lowest lumbar and adjacent sacral vertebrae.

lumbo- Combining form meaning loins.

lumbocostal (lum-bo-kos'tal) Relating to the ribs and the lumbar region, especially the lumbar vertebrae.

lumbosacral (lum-bo-sa'kral) Relating to the lumbar portion of the vertebral column and the sacrum.

lumbrical (lum'bri-kal) See table of muscles in appendix II.

luxation (luk-sa'shun) Dislocation.

Malgaigne's l. Dislocation of the elbow joint with the head of the radial bone forced out of its retaining annular ligament.

linea ■ luxation

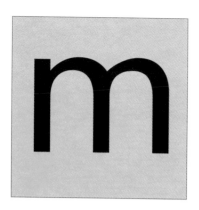

malar (ma'lar) Relating to the cheek; zygomatic bone (cheekbone).

malleolar (mal-e-o'lar) Relating to one or both bony projections on either side of the ankle.

malleolus (mal-le'o-lus), pl. malle'oli One of two bony prominences (a medial one on the lower tibia, a lateral one on the lower fibula) on either side of the ankle.

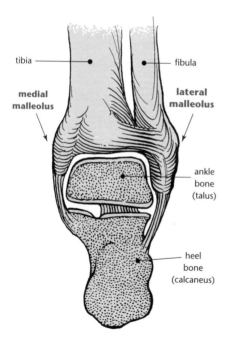

malleus (mal'e-us) The club-shaped and most lateral of the three ossicles in the middle ear chamber; it is attached to the tympanic membrane (eardrum) and articulates with the incus. See also table of bones in appendix I.

mandible (man'dĭ-bl) The horseshoe-shaped bone of the lower jaw articulating with both sides of the skull at the temporomandibular joints; it accommodates the lower teeth. Also called lower jaw; jawbone. See also table of bones in appendix I.

  prognathous m. See protruded mandible.

  protruded m. A mandible in an anterior or forward projection relative to the rest of the facial skeleton. Also called prognathous mandible.

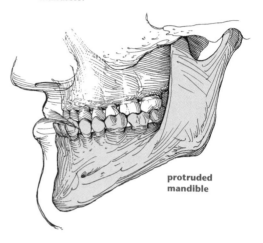

protruded
mandible

  retrognathous m. See retruded mandible.

  retruded m. A mandible in a posterior or backward position relative to the rest of the facial skeleton. Also called retrognathous mandible.

mandibular (man-dib'u-lar) Relating to the lower jaw.

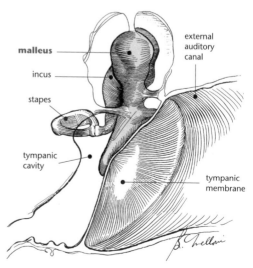

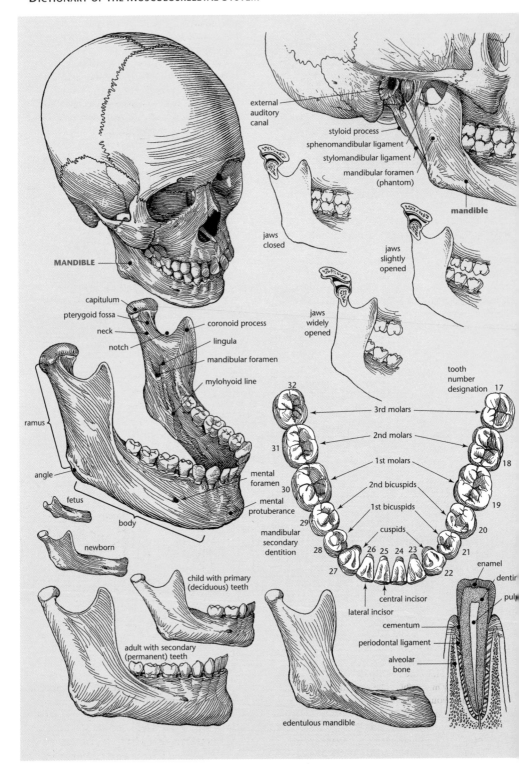

external auditory canal

styloid process
sphenomandibular ligament
stylomandibular ligament
mandibular foramen (phantom)

mandible

jaws closed

jaws slightly opened

jaws widely opened

MANDIBLE

capitulum
pterygoid fossa
neck
notch

ramus

angle

fetus

newborn

body

child with primary (deciduous) teeth

adult with secondary (permanent) teeth

coronoid process
lingula
mandibular foramen
mylohyoid line

mental foramen
mental protuberance

mandibular secondary dentition

tooth number designation

3rd molars
2nd molars
1st molars
2nd bicuspids
1st bicuspids
cuspids
central incisor
lateral incisor

32   17
31   18
30   19
29   20
28   21
27   26 25 24 23   22

enamel
dentin
pulp
cementum
periodontal ligament
alveolar bone

edentulous mandible

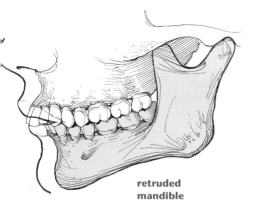

**retruded
mandible**

maniphalanx (man-ĭ-fa'lanks) One of the bones (phalanges) of the fingers.

manubriosternal (mah-nu-bre-o-ster'nal) Relating to the manubrium and the body of the sternum.

manubrium (mah-nu'bre-um) A body structure resembling a handle. When used alone, the term usually refers to the manubrium of the sternum (breastbone).

    m. of malleus The bony process of the largest of the auditory ossicles (malleus) in the middle ear chamber, attached to the inner surface of the tympanic membrane (eardrum) and articulating with the incus. Also called long process of malleus.

    m. of sternum The upper portion of the sternum, articulating with the clavicles and the cartilages of the first and second ribs on each side.

manus (ma'nus) Latin for hand.

    m. externa Backward deviation of the hand.

    m. flexa Forward deviation of the hand.

    m. valga Deviation of the hand toward the side of the little finger (ulnar side).

    m. vara Deviation of the hand toward the side of the thumb (radial side).

margin (mar'jin) The border or edge of a structure.

    anterior m. of fibula The crest on the anterior border of the fibula; the anterior intermuscular septum of the leg is secured to its upper three-fourths, and the superior retinaculum to the lower part.

    anterior m. of tibia The prominent subcutaneous ridge on the front surface of the tibia extending from the tuberosity (proximal end) to the medial malleolus (distal end); its entire length, except for the lower fourth quarter, forms a sharp crest that

is popularly known as the shin.

    anterior m. of ulna The thick, rounded anterior border of the ulna; it commences from the medial side of the ulnar tuberosity, extending downward and posteriorly to the base of the styloid process; it affords attachment to the deep flexor muscle of fingers (flexor digitorum profundus) and the quadrate pronator muscle (pronator quadratus).

    axillary m. of scapula The lateral border of the scapula, extending from the glenoid cavity to the inferior angle. Also called lateral margin of scapula.

    cervical m. An undulating line at the neck of a tooth representing the junction of enamel and cementum; it is covered by the gingiva (gum) which is attached near the cervical margin of the tooth by the epithelial attachment.

    dorsal m. of radius See posterior margin of radius.

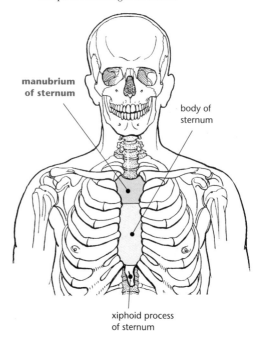

**manubrium
of sternum**

**body of
sternum**

**xiphoid process
of sternum**

    dorsal m. of ulna See posterior margin of ulna.

    falciform m. An arched fascial margin that forms the superior, lateral, and inferior boundaries of the saphenous opening (an aperture in the deep fascia at the front of the upper thigh, through which pass the great saphenous vein and other smaller vessels).

maniphalanx ■ margin

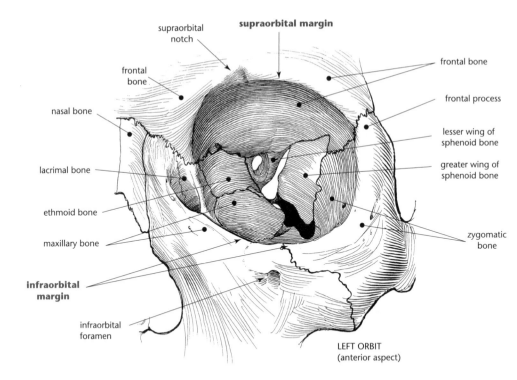

supraorbital margin

supraorbital notch

frontal bone

frontal bone

frontal process

nasal bone

lesser wing of sphenoid bone

greater wing of sphenoid bone

lacrimal bone

ethmoid bone

maxillary bone

zygomatic bone

infraorbital margin

infraorbital foramen

LEFT ORBIT
(anterior aspect)

infraorbital m. The lower border of the orbit formed by the maxillary and zygomatic bones.

lateral m. of humerus The outer ridge of the humerus that extends from the posterior surface of the greater tubercle downward to the lateral epicondyle; near the middle of the ridge, it is interrupted by the sulcus for the radial nerve.

lateral orbital m. The lateral edge of the orbit formed by the frontal process of the zygomatic bone (almost entirely) and the zygomatic process of the frontal bone.

lateral m. of scapula See axillary margin of scapula.

medial orbital m. The medial edge of the orbit formed above by the frontal bone and below by the frontal process of the maxilla.

medial m. of scapula See vertebral margin of scapula.

medial m. of tibia The inner margin of the tibia; it commences at the medial condyle and extends downward to the posterior border of the medial malleolus; its middle section is distinctly sharp in contrast to the rounded upper and lower parts of the margin.

posterior m. of fibula The ridge on the posterior surface of the fibula, extending from the head of the fibula downward to the medial margin of the groove for the peroneal tendons on the distal extremity.

posterior m. of radius The ridge most evident in the middle third of the posterior border of the shaft of the radius, extending obliquely upward and medially toward the radial tuberosity. Also called dorsal margin of radius.

posterior m. of ulna The rounded posterior border of the ulna, extending from the back of the olecranon to the styloid process; it separates the posterior from the medial surface of the ulna. Also called dorsal margin of ulna.

right m. of heart The indefinite curved border of the right side of the heart between the sternocostal and diaphragmatic surfaces.

superior m. of scapula The thin, sharp upper edge of the scapula, extending from the coracoid process to the superior angle; it affords attachment to the omohyoid muscle at its lateral end near the suprascapular notch.

supraorbital m. The superior edge of the orbit formed entirely by the frontal bone; it contains the supraorbital notch (or foramen)

margin ■ margin

which transmits the supraorbital vessels and nerves.

vertebral m. of scapula The medial border of the scapula, extending from the superior angle to the inferior angle. Also called medial margin of scapula.

marrow (mar'o) A medulla, especially of bone.

bone m. The soft tissue occupying the cavities of bones; it produces most of the cells that circulate in the blood (erythrocytes, leukocytes, and megakaryocytes). Also called marrow; medulla of bone.

red m. The marrow found mainly within the spongy tissues of ribs, sternum, and the ends of the long bones; it is the site of production of red blood cells and granular white blood cells.

yellow m. The material located mainly within the large cavities of large bones; consists mainly of fat cells and a few immature blood cells.

mass (mas) A body of coherent material.

lateral m. of atlas The solid parts of the first cervical vertebra on either side, articulating above with the occipital condyles of the skull and below with the second cervical vertebra.

lateral m. of ethmoid bone Either of the paired lateral masses of thin-walled air cells of the ethmoid bone, forming part of the lateral wall of the nasal cavity and part of the medial wall of the orbit.

lateral m. of occipital bone An expansion of bone situated on both sides of the foramen magnum of the skull; the inferior surface possesses a convex, reniform process (occipital condyle) for articulation with the superior facet of the first cervical vertebra (atlas). Also called condylar part of occipital bone.

lateral m. of sacrum See sacral crest, lateral, under crest.

masseter (mas-se'ter) See table of muscles in appendix II.

masseteric (mas-e-ter'ik) Relating to the masseter muscle.

mastoid (mas'toid) 1. Shaped like a nipple or breast. 2. The mastoid portion of the temporal bone.

matrix (ma'triks) The ground substance of a tissue or the tissue from which a structure is formed.

bone m. The intercellular substance of bone tissue, consisting of collagen fibers embedded in amorphous ground substance

and inorganic bone salts; the content of the fibers and salt increases with the maturation of the bone. Also called medulla of bone.

cartilaginous m. The intercellular substance of cartilage, consisting of extracellular fibers, cells and an amorphous ground substance.

mature (mah-chur') Completely developed; fully grown.

maxilla (mak-sil'ah), pl. maxil'lae One of a pair of bones forming the upper jaw; it accommodates the upper teeth and contains a central sinus. See also table of bones in appendix I.

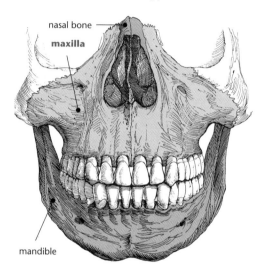

maxillary (mak's ĭ-ler-e) Relating to the maxilla (upper jaw).

maxillofacial (mak-sil-o-fa'shal) Relating to the maxilla (upper jaw) and the face.

meatus (me-a'tus), pl. mea'tuses, mea'tus A passageway in the body, or its external opening.

external auditory m. See external auditory canal, under canal.

inferior nasal m. The part of the nasal cavity below and lateral to the inferior nasal concha; it allows the nasolacrimal duct to communicate with the nasal cavity. Also called inferior meatus of nose.

inferior m. of nose See inferior nasal meatus.

internal auditory m. See internal auditory canal, under canal.

middle nasal m. The part of the nasal cavity below and lateral to the middle nasal concha; it serves as the passageway from which the anterior ethmoidal cells and the frontal and maxillary sinuses communicate

marrow ■ meatus

with the nasal cavity. Also called middle meatus of nose.

middle m. of nose
See middle nasal meatus.

nasopharyngeal m. The passage in the posterior part of the nasal cavity from the back part of the turbinates to the choanae.

superior nasal m. The part of the nasal cavity below and lateral to the superior nasal concha; it serves as the passageway from which the posterior ethmoidal cells communicate with the nasal cavity. Also called superior meatus of nose.

superior m. of nose
See superior nasal meatus.

mediad (me'de-ad) Toward the midline.

medial (me'de-al) 1. Relating to the middle. 2. Situated near the median plane of the body or an organ.

median (me'de-an) 1. Situated in the middle or midline; central. 2. In statistics, denoting the middle value, i.e., the point at which half of the plotted values are on one side and half on the other.

mediastinal (me-de-as-ti'nal) Relating to the mediastinum.

mediastinum (me-de-as-ti'num), pl. mediasti'na The central space in the chest bounded anteriorly by the sternum, posteriorly by the vertebral column, and laterally by the pleural sacs.

anterior m. The portion of the lower mediastinum bounded behind by the pericardium, in front by the body of the sternum, and on each side by the pleura; it contains, among other structures, part of the thymus gland, a few lymph nodes, and loose areolar tissue.

inferior m. See lower mediastinum.

lower m. The three lower portions of the mediastinum (below the plane that extends from the manubriosternal joint to the lower border of the fourth vertebra); it is subdivided into anterior, middle, and posterior mediastina. Also called inferior mediastinum.

middle m. The broadest portion of the lower mediastinum; it contains, among other structures, the bifurcation of the trachea into two bronchi, a large part of the roots of the lungs, some tracheobronchial lymph nodes, the heart enclosed in the pericardium, and adjacent parts of the great vessels.

posterior m. The portion of the lower mediastinum behind the heart, in front of the vertebral column, and between the

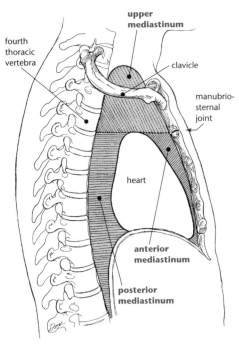

pleurae of the lungs; it contains, among other structures, the esophagus, descending thoracic aorta, thoracic duct, vagus nerves, and many lymph nodes.

superior m. See upper mediastinum.

upper m. The portion of the mediastinum from the level of the manubriosternal joint to the root of the neck (plane of thoracic inlet); it contains among other structures, the aortic arch (with its branches), brachiocephalic veins, upper half of the superior vena cava, vagus nerves, trachea, esophagus, thoracic duct, thymus gland, and some lymph nodes. Also called superior mediastinum.

mediocarpal (me-de-o-kar'pal) See midcarpal.

medulla (me-dul'ah), pl. medul'lae 1. Any centrally located soft tissue. 2. The marrow of bone or any similar structure. 3. Any part of an organ situated more centrally than the cortex.

m. of bone See bone marrow, under marrow.

medullary (med'u-lār-e) 1. Relating to a medulla. 2. Resembling bone marrow.

medullated (med'u-lāt-ed) Containing, or covered with, a soft marrow-like substance.

medullation (med-u-la'shun) The formation of marrow or a medulla.

medullization (med-u-li-za'shun) Abnormal enlargement of bone marrow spaces (e.g., in rarefying osteosis).

mediad ■ medullization

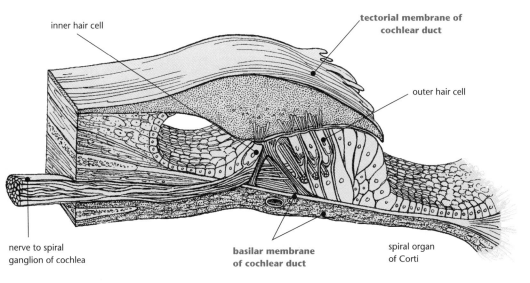

inner hair cell

tectorial membrane of cochlear duct

outer hair cell

nerve to spiral ganglion of cochlea

basilar membrane of cochlear duct

spiral organ of Corti

membrane (mem'brăn) A thin, pliable layer of tissue that covers a surface, lines a cavity, connects two structures, or divides a space or organ.

atlanto-occipital m. Any of two membranes (anterior and posterior) extending from the margin of the foramen magnum of the skull to the upper margin of the arch of the first cervical vertebra (atlas); the anterior fibers corresponds below with the anterior longitudinal ligament and the posterior fibers correspond below with the flaval ligament.

basement m. A thin transparent noncellular layer of the basal surface of epithelium; a composite structure consisting of a basal lamina (a thin amorphous collagen-containing sheath) and a reticular lamina (which varies in composition and appearance according to location); generally, the basement membrane serves to stabilize tissue shapes, but may have specialized functions in select areas, such as in the glomerulus of the kidney, where it serves as a selective permeability barrier for ultrafiltration of plasma in forming urine; it also invests muscle, fat, and Schwann cells.

basilar m. of cochlear duct The fibrous membrane that forms the greater part of the floor of the cochlear duct and the roof of the scala tympani, extending from the tip of the bony spiral lamina to the spiral ligament on the lateral wall; it is about 35 mm in length and accommodates the spiral organ of Corti within the cochlear duct.

cell m. A delicate structure about 90 Å in thickness that envelopes the cell, separating the contents of the cell from the surrounding environment; it is comprised of lipids and proteins with associated glycoproteins on the outer surface; it regulates the passage of substances into and out of the cell. Also called plasma membrane; plasmalemma.

cricothyroid m. See cricothyroid ligament, under ligament.

cricovocal m. See cricothyroid ligament, under ligament.

crural interosseous m. See interosseous membrane of leg.

fibrous m. of articular capsule The outer of the two layers of the articular capsule of a synovial joint; it fuses with the periosteum of the bones of the joint.

hyoepiglottic m. See hyoepiglottic ligament, under ligament.

hyoglossal m. A fibrous membrane that connects the undersurface of the root of the tongue with the hyoid bone.

interosseous m. of forearm A broad, thin sheet of fibers connecting the shafts of the radius and ulna of the forearm, running downward and medially from the interosseous border of the radius to that of the ulna. Also called radioulnar interosseous membrane.

interosseous m. of leg A dense membrane connecting the shafts of the tibia and fibula, running downward and laterally for the most part, from the interosseous borders of the

membrane ■ membrane

tibia and fibula; it divides the front muscles from those on the back of the leg. Also called crural interosseous membrane.

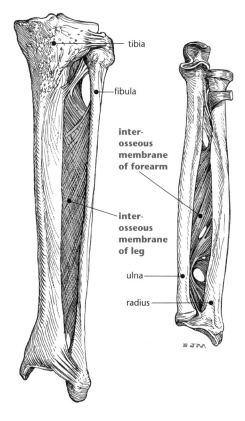

Nasmyth's m. The primary enamel cuticle; an extremely thin membrane covering the entire enamel of recently erupted teeth; it is quickly abraded by mastication.

obturator m. The thin interlacing membrane of white fibers that almost completely closes the obturator foramen of the hipbone; it leaves a small canal for the passage of the obturator nerve and vessels.

perineal m. The lower layer of fascia of the urogenital diaphragm stretched across the anterior half of the pelvic outlet, filling the gap of the pubic arch; it is situated between the ischiopubic rami and covers the under surface of the urethral sphincter and deep transverse perineal muscles; in the male, it is penetrated by the urethra and the ducts of the bulbourethral glands; in the female, by the urethra and the vagina.

periodontal m. See periodontal ligament, under ligament.

periorbital m. See periorbita.
plasma m. See cell membrane.
radioulnar interosseous m. See interosseous membrane of forearm.
Reissner's m. See vestibular membrane of cochlear duct.
secondary tympanic m. The membrane that closes the round window between the blind end of the scala tympani of the inner ear and the medial wall of the middle ear chamber; the membrane normally bulges slightly into the scala tympani.

spiral m. of cochlear duct See vestibular membrane of cochlear duct.

synovial m. The smooth connective tissue membrane that lines the cavity of a synovial joint, except the articular cartilages of bones; it produces a pale yellow viscous (synovial) fluid as a lubricant which increases joint efficiency and reduces erosion of surfaces.

tectorial m. of cochlear duct A delicate gelatinous membrane in the cochlear duct of the inner ear; it is attached to the limbus of the bony spiral lamina and its free end extends over the sensory part of the spiral organ of Corti where it embeds some of the underlying stereocilia from the outer hair cells.

thyrohyoid m. A broad fibroelastic membrane that fills the interval between the hyoid bone and the thyroid cartilage.

tympanic m. The thin, oblique, semitransparent membrane separating the external auditory canal from the middle ear chamber; it is kept taut for better reception of sound vibrations by the tensor muscle of the tympanum (tensor tympani); an ear ossicle (the malleus) is attached to its depressed center on its inner surface. Also called eardrum.

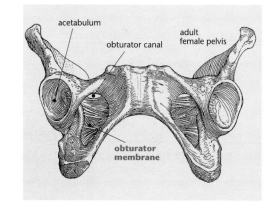

membrane ■ membrane

vestibular m. See vestibular membrane of cochlear duct.

vestibular m. of cochlear duct The delicate membrane of the inner ear separating the endolymph-filled cochlear duct from the perilymph-filled scala vestibuli; it consists of a basal lamina with flattened epithelial cells on both sides. Also called Reissner's membrane; vestibular membrane; spiral membrane of cochlear duct.

epiglottis

hyoid bone

thyrohyoid membrane

thyroid cartilage

cricothyroid ligament

trachea

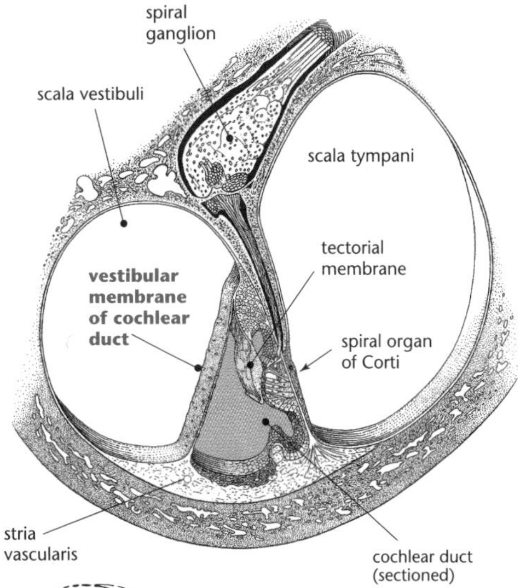

spiral ganglion

scala vestibuli

scala tympani

vestibular membrane of cochlear duct

tectorial membrane

spiral organ of Corti

stria vascularis

cochlear duct (sectioned)

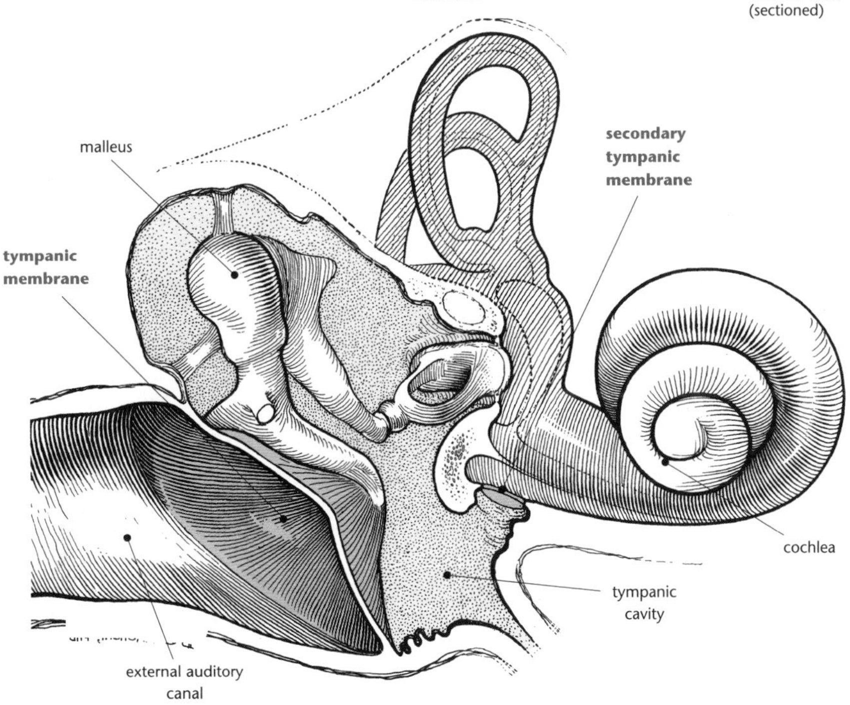

malleus

secondary tympanic membrane

tympanic membrane

cochlea

tympanic cavity

external auditory canal

membrane ■ membrane

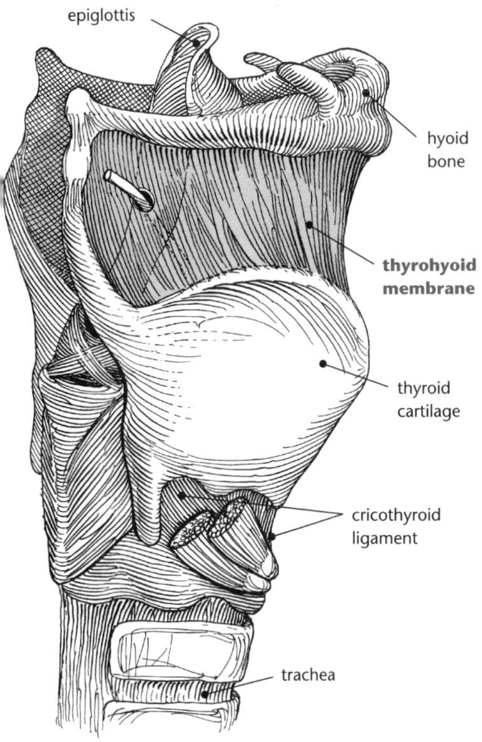

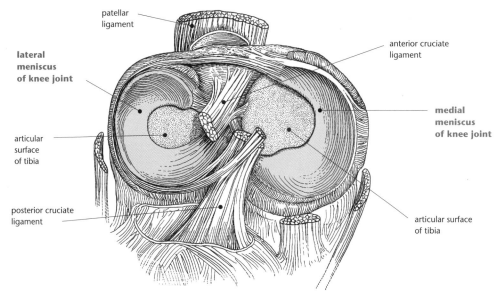

patellar ligament

lateral meniscus of knee joint

anterior cruciate ligament

medial meniscus of knee joint

articular surface of tibia

posterior cruciate ligament

articular surface of tibia

membranocartilaginous (mem-brah-no-kar-tĭ-laj'ĭ-nus) Composed of or derived from both membrane and cartilage.

membranous (mem'brah-nus) Relating to a membrane.

menisci (men-is'ki) Plural of meniscus.

meniscus (mĕ-nis'kus), pl. menis'ci A crescent-shaped structure, such as a fibrocartilage serving as a cushion between two bones meeting at a joint.

    lateral m. of knee joint A nearly circular, crescent-shaped fibrocartilage attached to the lateral articular surface of the upper end of the tibia. Also called lateral semilunar cartilage of knee; external semilunar cartilage of knee joint.

    medial m. of knee joint A crescent-shaped fibrocartilage attached to the medial articular surface of the upper end of the tibia. Also called medial semilunar cartilage of knee; internal semilunar cartilage of knee joint.

    temporomandibular m. See temporomandibular articular disk, under disk.

mesial (me'ze-al) Toward the median plane (e.g., of the dental arch).

metacarpal (met-ah-kar'pal) Relating to the metacarpus.

metacarpophalangeal (met-ah-kar-po-fah-lan'je-al) Relating to the bones in the broad part of the hand (metacarpus) and those of the fingers (phalanges); applied to their articulations.

metacarpus (met-ah-kar'pus) The five bones of the hand between those of the wrist (carpus) and of the fingers (phalanges).

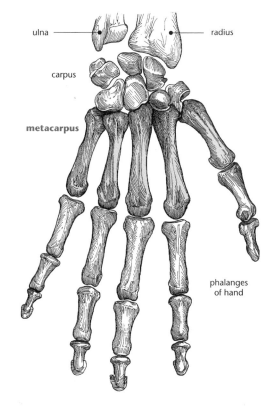

ulna

radius

carpus

metacarpus

phalanges of hand

membranocartilaginous ■ metacarpus

metaphysis (mĕ-taf´ĭ-sis), pl. metaph´yses
The active growth area of a long bone at the junction of the epiphysis with the shaft (diaphysis); it becomes fused with the epiphysis and the diaphysis upon cessation of growth.

metatarsal (met-ah-tar´sal) Relating to the metatarsus.

metatarsophalangeal (met-ah-tar-so-fah-lan´je-al) Relating to the metatarsus and the bones of the toes.

metatarsus (met-ah-tar´sus) The five bones in the anterior part of the foot between the tarsus, at the back of the foot, and the bones of the toes (phalanges).

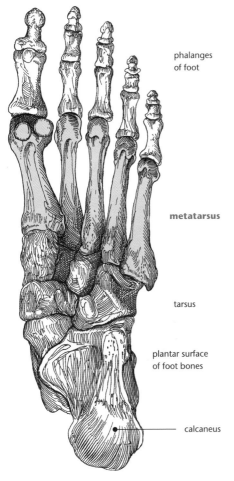

phalanges of foot

metatarsus

tarsus

plantar surface of foot bones

calcaneus

m. adductus Foot deformity in which only the front part of the foot (at the tarsometatarsal joints) is drawn toward the midline. Also called metatarsus varus.

m. varus See metatarsus adductus.

metopion (me-to´pe-on) Craniometric point on the sagittal plane between the two frontal eminences; glabella.

microfracture (mi-kro-frak´chur) See hairline fracture, under fracture.

midcarpal (mid-kar´pal) Between the two rows of bones forming the wrist. Also called mediocarpal.

midclavicular (mid-klah-vik´u-lar) Relating to the middle of the clavicle.

midoccipital (mid-ok-sip´ĭ-tal) Relating to the central portion of the back of the head.

midsection (mid-sek´shun) A cut through the middle of an organ.

midphalangeal (mid-fah-lan´je-al) 1. Pertaining to the middle phalanx of a finger or toe. 2. Pertaining to the middle of a phalanx of a finger or toe.

midsternum (mid-ster´num) The middle, largest portion of the sternum; the body of the sternum.

modiolus (mo-di´o-lus) The spongy bone around which the spiral canals of the cochlea turn; situated lateral to the internal auditory canal.

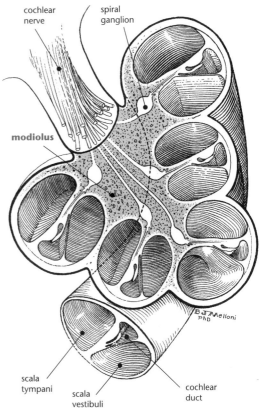

cochlear nerve

spiral ganglion

modiolus

scala tympani

scala vestibuli

cochlear duct

B.J.Melloni PhD

metaphysis ■ modiolus

molar (mo'lar) One of the eight back teeth in the deciduous dentition, or one of the 12 back teeth in the permanent dentition.

deciduous m. One of the eight back teeth in the deciduous (primary) dentition.

first permanent m. The largest permanent tooth in the mouth; first permanent tooth to erupt, usually at the age of six years. Also called six-year molar.

impacted m. A molar that fails to erupt or erupt fully because of an obstruction.

permanent m. One of the 12 back teeth in the permanent (secondary) dentition.

second permanent m. A permanent molar immediately distal to the first molar; it usually erupts at the age of 12 years. Also called twelve-year molar.

six-year m. See first permanent molar.

third permanent m. Last permanent back tooth in the mouth; it generally erupts between the ages of 17 and 21 years. Also called wisdom tooth.

twelve-year m.
See second permanent molar.

monarticular (mon-ar-tik'u-lar) Relating to one joint; monarthric.

multifid (mul'ti-fid) Divided into many parts.

multifidus (mul-tif'i-dus) See table of muscles in appendix II.

muscle (mus'el) Tissue that serves to produce movement by its contraction; composed primarily of contractile cells. See table of muscles for individual muscles in appendix II.

abductor m. A muscle that draws a part away from the median plane, or in the fingers and toes, away from the axial line of the limb.

adductor m. A muscle that draws a part toward the median plane, or in the fingers and toes, toward the axial line of the limb.

agonistic m. A muscle that is constantly active in both the initiation and maintenance of a particular movement of an anatomic part, such as the brachial muscle in flexion of the forearm at the elbow joint; the action of the agonistic muscle can be opposed by that of another muscle called antagonistic. Also called prime mover.

antagonistic m. A muscle with opposing force that counteracts the action of another muscle, called the agonistic muscle, or that initiates and maintains a movement opposite to that of the agonist.

antigravity m.'s Muscles maintaining the normal posture of the body characteristic of a given species by resisting the constant pull of gravity.

bipennate m. Muscle with a central tendon in which the muscle fibers converge in barb-like fashion (e.g., the rectus muscle of the thigh).

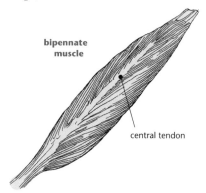

bipennate muscle

central tendon

cardiac m. Muscle of the heart (myocardium), composed of striated fibers identical in organization with those of skeletal muscle but with conspicuous cross striations (intercalated disks) marking the junctions between the ends of the cells.

congenerous m.'s Muscles that perform the same action or function.

constrictor m. A muscle that makes a passage smaller or narrower by contracting (e.g., the constrictor muscles of the pharynx).

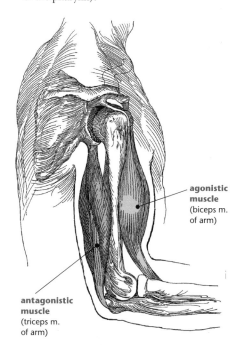

agonistic muscle (biceps m. of arm)

antagonistic muscle (triceps m. of arm)

molar ■ muscle

depressor m. A muscle that serves to depress the structure into which it is inserted.

dilator m. A muscle that dilates an opening, such as the pupil of the eye.

emergency m.'s Muscles that assist agonistic muscles when considerable force is required.

extensor m. A muscle that straightens out (extends) a joint to full length.

extrinsic m. A muscle that does not originate in the same part or limb to which it is inserted (e.g., superior rectus muscle of eyeball).

facial m.'s Muscles of facial expression that affect movements of the skin, eyelids, eyebrows, nose, lips, and scalp.

fast twitch m. See white muscle.

fixator m.'s Agonistic and antagonistic muscles collaborating in stabilizing the position of a joint or part; they contract together to hold the joint in position when powerful external forces are encountered.

flexor m. A muscle that bends (flexes) a joint.

fusiform m. A muscle with a fleshy belly tapering upon a tendon at either end. Also called spindle-shaped muscle.

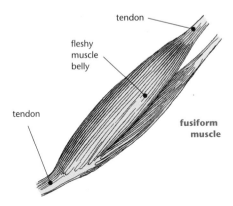

fusiform muscle

hamstring m.'s The three muscles at the back of the thigh: the biceps muscle of the thigh (biceps femoris), the semitendinous muscle, and the semimembranous muscle; they flex the leg and rotate it medially and laterally at the knee joint, and extend the thigh at the hip joint. Also called posterior femoral muscles.

intrinsic m. A muscle in which both origin and insertion are lying wholly within the same part or limb (e.g., ciliary muscle of eyeball).

involuntary m. See smooth muscle.

levator m. A muscle that elevates a structure into which it is inserted.

longitudinal m. A muscle in which the fiber bundles are lengthwise, i.e., parallel to the long axis of the body or part.

multipennate m. A muscle in which the fiber bundles converge to several tendons, e.g., deltoid muscle.

nonstriated m. See smooth muscle.

papillary m.'s The fleshy columns of muscles arising from the inner walls of the cardiac ventricles, attached to the triangular cusps of the atrioventricular valves by the chordae tendinae; there are two major papillary muscles in each ventricle.

posterior femoral m.'s See hamstring muscles.

red m. Skeletal muscle of dark reddish color, due to the presence of large amounts

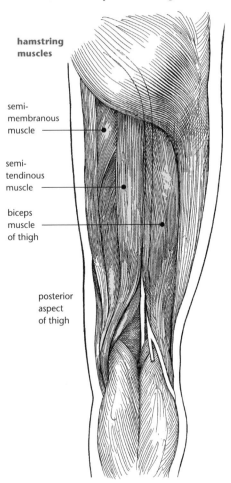

hamstring muscles

semi-membranous muscle

semi-tendinous muscle

biceps muscle of thigh

posterior aspect of thigh

muscle ■ muscle

of the protein pigment myoglobin; characterized by slow contractability (with a twitch duration of 70 msec) and resistance to fatigue; well suited to a repetitive type of contraction (e.g., muscles that sustain posture). Also called type I muscle; slow twitch muscle. COMPARE white muscle.

skeletal m. A striated voluntary muscle that is attached to bones, usually crossing at least one joint on which it acts; when viewed microscopically, the muscle fibers exhibit regularly spaced transverse bands. Also called voluntary muscle.

slow twitch m. See red muscle.

smooth m. Nonstriated muscle that is not under voluntary control, but responds to the autonomic nervous system; mainly concerned with movements and contractions of blood vessels, alimentary canal, respiratory, urogenital systems and of glands. Also called nonstriated muscle; unstriated muscle; involuntary muscle.

sphincter m. A circular band of muscle arranged around an orifice or tube (e.g., sphincter muscle of the anus; the sphincter muscle of the bile duct).

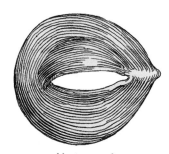

sphincter muscle
(orbicular muscle of eye)

spindle-shaped m. See fusiform muscle.

strap m. Any flat muscle, especially those of the neck associated with the hyoid bone and thyroid cartilage.

striated m. Skeletal and cardiac muscle in which cross striations occur in the fibers; with the exception of the cardiac muscle, striated muscles are voluntary, as opposed to the smooth muscles under the control of the autonomic nervous system.

synergistic m. A muscle that acts in conjunction with the agonist muscle (prime mover) to maximize a mutually helpful action.

type I m. See red muscle.
type II m. See white muscle.

unipennate m. Muscle with a tendon attached to one side only (e.g., extensor muscle of the little finger).

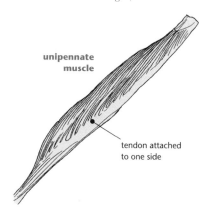

unipennate
muscle

tendon attached
to one side

unstriated m. See smooth muscle.
voluntary m. See skeletal muscle.
white m. Skeletal muscle of pale color, due to the presence of relatively small amounts of the protein pigment myoglobin; characterized by fast contractability (with a twitch duration of 25 msec) and rapid onset of fatigue; generally involved in large scale movements of body segments. Also called type II muscle; fast twitch muscle. COMPARE red muscle.

muscular (mus'ku-lar) 1. Relating to muscles. 2. Having well-developed muscles.

musculature (mus'ku-lah-chur) The system of muscles in the body or a body part.

musculoaponeurotic (mus-ku-lo-ap-o-nu-rot'ik) Relating to a muscle and its sheath of connective tissue (aponeurosis).

musculocutaneous (mus-ku-lo-ku-ta'ne-us) Relating to muscle and skin.

musculomembranous (mus-ku-lo-mem'brah-nus) Relating to or composed of muscular and membranous tissues.

musculophrenic (mus-ko-lo-fren'ik) Relating to the muscular portion of the diaphragm.

musculoskeletal (mus-ku-lo-skel'ĕ-tal) Relating to muscles and bones.

musculotropic (mus-ku-lo-trop'ik) Acting upon muscular tissue.

myalgia (mi-al'je-ah) Muscle pain.

myasthenia (mi-as-the'ne-ah) Weakness of muscle.

m. gravis Neuromuscular disorder of autoimmune origin characterized by varying degrees of weakness and fatigability of certain muscle groups, which may progress to paralysis; it frequently begins in the

muscle ■ myasthenia

eyelids, often associated with abnormalities of the thymus. There is evidence that specific antibodies interfere with the action of the neurotransmitter acetylcholine in passing nerve impulses to muscles at the neuromuscular junctions.

myasthenic (mi-as-then'ik) Relating to myasthenia.

myatonia, myatony (mi-ah-to'ne-ah, mi-at'o-ne) Absence of muscle tone. Also called amyotonia.

mylohyoid (mi-lo-hi'oid) Relating to the inner surface of the posterior portion of the mandible and the hyoid bone.

myo- Combining form meaning muscle.

myocardial (mi-o-kar'de-al) Relating to the heart muscle (myocardium).

myocardium (mi-o-kar'de-um) The middle and thickest layer of the heart wall, composed of specialized striated muscle cells and intervening connective tissue.

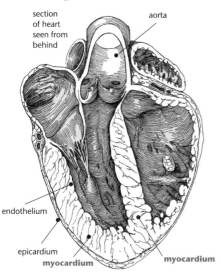

section of heart seen from behind

aorta

endothelium

epicardium

myocardium

myocardium

myofibril (mi-o-fi'bril) One of numerous fine fibrils present in a muscle fiber; each is divided into a series of repeating units (sarcomeres), which are the fundamental structural and functional units of muscle contraction. Also called muscle fibril.

myofilament (mi-o-fil'ah-ment) One of the numerous longitudinally disposed thick and thin microscopic contractile filaments that make up the fibrils of striated muscle; the thick filaments contain the protein myosin, the thin filaments contain the protein actin; both are responsible for cellular contraction of muscle tissue.

myometrium (mi-o-me'tre-um) The smooth muscle forming the middle and main layer of the uterine wall.

myosalpinx (mi-o-sal'pinks) The muscular layer of a uterine (fallopian) tube.

myosin (mi'o-sin) A globulin present in muscle tissue; a type of protein which, combined with actin, forms actomyosin; it is responsible for muscle shortening or contraction.

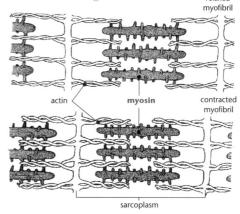

relaxed myofibril

actin

myosin

contracted myofibril

sarcoplasm

myositis (mi-o-si'tis) Inflammation of muscle tissue causing pain and tenderness.

   m. ossificans Formation of bone within muscle tissue; it may be localized secondary to an injury (e.g., after a blow or a tear, especially in a thigh or arm muscle) or, rarely, may be generalized, beginning in childhood and due to unknown causes.

myospasm (mi'o-spazm) Spasmodic contraction of a muscle or group of muscles.

myotactic (mi-o-tak'tik) Relating to the muscular proprioceptive sense; denoting any reflex elicited by tapping the belly or tendon of a muscle.

myotasis (mi-ot'ah-sis) The stretching of a muscle.

myotatic (mi-o-tat'ik) Relating to the stretching of a muscle.

myotonia (mi-o-to'ne-ah) Delayed relaxation of a muscle after voluntary contraction, electrical stimulation, or tapping (percussion) of the muscle.

   m. atrophica See myotonic dystrophy, under dystrophy.

   m. congenita Hereditary condition present at birth, characterized by temporary myotonia whenever a voluntary movement is attempted, often interfering with feeding and causing a "strangled" cry.

myotonic (mi-o-ton'ik) Relating to myotonia.

myotropic (mi-o-trop'ik) Acting upon muscle tissue.

myasthenic ■ myotropic

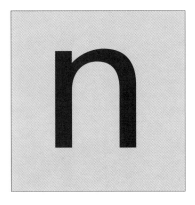

naris (na'ris), pl. na'res Nostril.
    posterior n. See choana.
nasion (na'ze-on) A craniometric point on the middle of the nasofrontal suture. Also called nasal point.

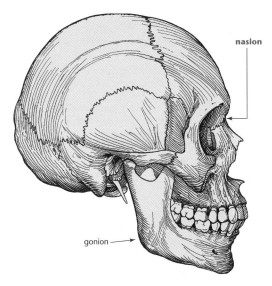

nasoantral (na-zo-an'tral) Relating to the nose and the maxillary sinus.
nasofrontal (na-zo-frun'tal) Relating to the nose (or nasal bone) and the frontal bone.
nasolacrimal (na-zo-lak'rĭ-mal) 1. Relating to the nasal and lacrimal bones. 2. Relating to the nose and the structures producing and conveying tears.
nasopalatine (na-zo-pal'ah-tīn) Relating to the nose and the palate.
nasopharyngeal (na-zo-fah-rin'je-al) Relating to the upper portion of the pharynx (nasopharynx).

nasopharynx (na-zo-far'inks) The nasal part of the pharynx; the uppermost part of the pharynx, located above the level of the soft palate, immediately behind the nasal cavity and above the oral pharynx. Also called rhinopharynx; postnasal space; epipharynx.

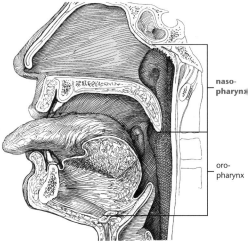

navicular (nah-vik'u-lar) Boat-shaped; applied to certain bones. See also table of bones in appendix I.
neck (nek) 1. The part of the body between the head and trunk. 2. Any relatively narrow area of an anatomic structure.
    anatomic n. of humerus The slightly constricted area separating the head of the humerus from the tuberosities; it affords attachment to the capsule of the shoulder joint. Also called neck of humerus.
    n. of ankle bone See neck of talus.
    n. of condylar process of mandible See neck of mandible.
    n. of femur The short, strong, constricted column of bone connecting the head of the femur to the shaft; in the adult, it is about 5 cm in length forming an obtuse angle of about 128° with the upper end of the shaft, which enables the lower limb to clear the pelvis during movement.
    n. of humerus See anatomic neck of humerus.
    n. of malleus The narrow part of the malleus (ossicle) between the ovoid-shaped head and the enlarged area to which are attached the manubrium, anterior process and lateral process; it affords attachment to the anterior ligament of the malleus.
    n. of mandible The constricted portion of

naris ■ **neck**

the mandible below the knuckle-shaped head; its anterior surface presents a rough depression (pterygoid fovea) that affords attachment to the lateral pterygoid muscle; it is often covered by the parotid gland. Also called neck of condylar process of mandible.

n. of ankle bone See neck of talus.

n. of radius The constricted part of the proximal end of the radius just below the disk-shaped head; its upper part is enlarged by the annular ligament.

n. of scapula The slight narrowing between the glenoid cavity and coracoid process from the rest of the scapula; it affords attachment to the capsule of the shoulder joint.

surgical n. of humerus The narrowest part of the neck of the humerus, just below the tubercles; a common fracture site.

n. of talus A slightly constricted, rough column of bone that connects the body of the talus (ankle bone) to the rounded head; it affords attachment to ligaments; the plantar surface provides a deep groove to accommodate the interosseous talocalcanean and cervical ligaments. Also called neck of ankle bone.

n. of condylar process of mandible See neck of mandible.

n. of tooth The slightly constricted part of a tooth between the crown and the root. Also called dental cervix.

neurocranium (nu-ro-kra'ne-um) The portion of the embryonic skull containing the brain.

neuromuscular (nu-ro-mus'ku-lar) Relating to nerve and muscle.

neuromyasthenia (nu-ro-mi-as-the'ne-ah) Muscular weakness, especially one of emotional origin.

neuromyopathy (nu-ro-mi-op'ah-the) A muscular disorder due to disease of the nerve supplying the muscle.

neuromyositis (nu-ro-mi-o-si'tis) Inflammation of a nerve and the muscle it supplies.

neuroskeleton (nu-ro-skel'ĕ-ton) The part of the skeleton that surrounds the brain and spinal cord.

node (nōd) 1. A circumscribed mass of differentiated tissue. 2. A swelling or protuberance, either normal or abnormal.

atrioventricular n. A small, roughly oval node made of interwoven modified muscle fibers and situated in the right atrial wall of the heart near the orifice of the coronary sinus, just dorsal to the basal attachment of the tricuspid (right atrioventricular) valve.

From the atrium it transmits the cardiac impulse, through the Purkinje fibers, to the ventricular walls. It is slightly smaller than the sinoatrial node. Also called A-V node.

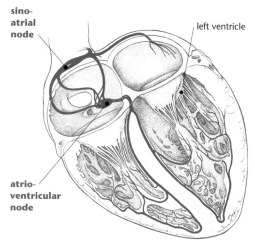

A-V n. See atrioventricular node.

Bouchard's n. A small, hard node located in the proximal interphalangeal joint of a finger; seen in individuals with osteoarthritis. COMPARE Herberden's node.

gouty n. A concretion of sodium biurate generally occurring in the vicinity of joints in certain individuals afflicted with gouty inflammation.

Heberden's n. A pea-sized swelling located in the distal interphalangeal joint of a finger; seen in individuals with osteoarthritis. COMPARE Bouchard's node.

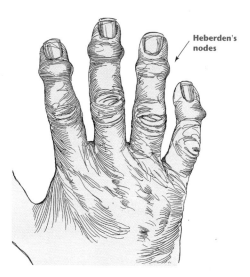

neurocranium ■ node

S-A n. See sinoatrial node.

Schmorl's n. An irregular depression in the margin of the vertebral body, often due to the herniation of the nucleus pulposus of the intervertebral disk into the adjacent vertebra.

sinoatrial n. An elongated ellipical node made of interwoven modified cardiac muscle fibers, situated in the wall of the right atrium near the entance of the superior vena cava; it receives fibers from both the sympathetic and parasympathetic nervous systems and is responsible for initiating each heart beat; often referred to as the pacemaker of the heart. It is slightly larger than the atrioventricular node. Also called S-A node; sinuatrial node; sinus node.

sinuatrial n. See sinoatrial node.

sinus n. See sinoatrial node.

notch (noch) An indentation or depression, usually on a bone, but occasionally applied to an organ.

acetabular n. A notch or gap on the inferior margin of the acetabulum of the hipbone; it is bridged by the transverse acetabular ligament. Also called incisure of acetabulum; cotyloid notch.

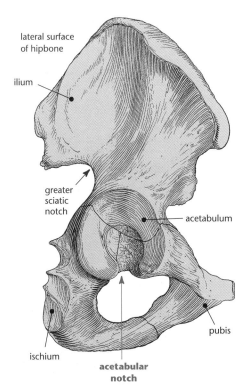

lateral surface of hipbone

ilium

greater sciatic notch

acetabulum

ischium

pubis

acetabular notch

clavicular n. of sternum The indentation on each side of the upper angle of the sternum (breastbone), presenting an oval facet for articulation with the sternal end of the clavicle. Also called clavicular incisure of sternum; clavicular facet.

costal n. of sternum One of the seven indentations or facets on each lateral border of the sternum, for articulation with a costal cartilage. Also called costal incisure of sternum.

cotyloid n. See acetabular notch.

digastric n. See mastoid notch.

ethmoidal n. of frontal bone On the internal surface of the base of the skull, the wide, oblong space between the medial borders of the orbital plates of the frontal bone, in which the cribriform plate of the ethmoid bone is housed. Also called ethmoidal incisure of frontal bone.

fibular n. A smooth concavity on the medial side of the lower end of the tibia articulating with the fibula. Also called fibular incisure of tibia.

frontal n. A small notch on the orbital margin of the frontal bone, just medial to the supraorbital notch; it transmits the supratrochlear nerve and vessels.

Hutchinson's crescentic n. The somewhat semilunar notch on the incisal edge of upper central incisors in Hutchinson's teeth of congenital syphilis; seen also occasionally on other anterior teeth.

interclavicular n. See suprasternal notch.

intercondylar n. A nonarticulating depression between the condyles at the posterior surface of the distal femur; it provides attachment to the cruciate ligaments. Also called intercondylar fossa of femur.

intertragic n. The deep notch in the lower part of the auricle (pinna) just above the lobe, between the tragus and antitragus; it is opened superiorly. Also called intertragic incisure of ear.

jugular n. See suprasternal notch.

jugular n. of temporal bone The large notch on the lower surface of the petrous part of the temporal bone forming the anterior and lateral boundaries of the jugular foramen and accommodating the superior bulb of the internal jugular vein on the lateral side and the vagus, glossopharyngeal, and accsssory nerves on its medial side. Also called jugular incisure of temporal bone.

notch ■ notch

lacrimal n. See lacrimal fossa, under fossa.

mandibular n. The deep semilunar notch on the upper border of the ramus of the mandible, lying between the coronoid process and the articulating condyle; it allows passage of the masseteric vessels and nerve. Also called mandibular incisure.

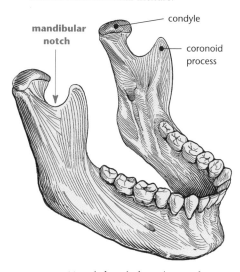

mandibular notch

condyle

coronoid process

mastoid n. A deep indentation on the inner surface of the mastoid process of the temporal bone of the skull; it provides attachment to the posterior belly of the digastric muscle. Also called digastric incisure; digastric notch.

nasal n. The large notch on the margin of the maxilla that forms the lateral and lower boundary of the bony opening of the anterior nasal cavity. Also called nasal notch of maxilla.

nasal n. of maxilla See nasal notch.

parietal n. of temporal bone The notch between the squamous and mastoid parts of the temporal bone, where the squamous and parietomastoid sutures meet; it accommodates the posteroinferior angle of the parietal bone.

popliteal n. A notch in the posterior intercondylar area of the proximal end of the tibia; it affords attachment to the posterior cruciate ligament in the knee joint.

pterygoid n. An angular cleft on the inferior part of the pterygoid process of the sphenoid bone between the medial and lateral pterygoid plates; the margins of the notch articulate with the pyramidal process of the palatine bone. Also called pterygoid incisure; pterygoid fissure.

radial n. of ulna The concavity on the upper end of the lateral surface of the coronoid process of the ulna that articulates with the head of the radius. Also called ulnar incisure of radius; sigmoid cavity of ulna.

scapular n. A semicircular notch on the upper border of the scapula (shoulder blade), at the base of the coracoid process; it is converted into a foramen by the suprascapular ligament, through which the suprascapular nerve passes. Also called incisure of scapula; suprascapular notch.

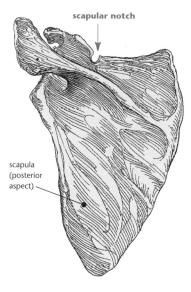

scapular notch

scapula (posterior aspect)

sciatic n.'s Indentations on the posterior border of the hipbone: *Greater sciatic n.*, the deep indentation on the posterior border of the hipbone at the junction of the ilium and ischium, between the posterior inferior iliac spine and the ischial spine; it is converted into the greater sciatic foramen by the sacrospinous and sacrotuberous ligaments. *Lesser sciatic n.*, the notch on the posterior border of the ischium between the ischial spine and the ischial tuberosity; it is converted into the lesser sciatic foramen by the sacrospinous and sacrotuberous ligaments.

sphenopalatine n. A small, round notch between the orbital and sphenoid processes of the palatine bone that permits the passage of the sphenopalatine vessels and nasal nerves from the pterygopalatine fossa to the nasal cavity posterior to the superior meatus; the notch is converted into a foramen (of the same name) by the undersurface of the body

notch ■ notch

of the sphenoid bone that comes in contact with the palatine bone. Also called sphenopalatine incisure.

sternal n. See suprasternal notch.

supraorbital n. A notch or groove (occasionally a foramen) in the superior margin of the orbit, through which pass the supraorbital vessels and nerve.

suprasternal n. The broad indentation on the upper border of the sternum, between the sternal heads of the two sternocleido-mastoid muscles. Also called jugular notch, sternal notch; interclavicular notch.

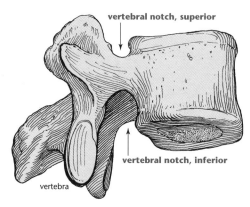

vertebral notch, superior

vertebral notch, inferior

vertebra

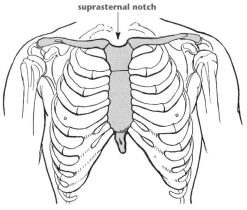

suprasternal notch

vertebral n. One of two deep-pocketed indentations (superior and inferior) above and below the border of the pedicle of a vertebra on each side; the notches of two adjacent vertebrae form an intervertebral foramen, which transmits the spinal nerve and vessels.

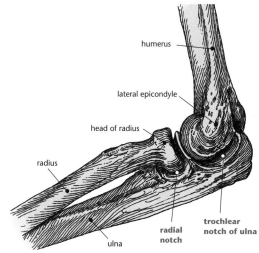

humerus

lateral epicondyle

head of radius

radius

ulna

radial notch

trochlear notch of ulna

trochlear n. of ulna A large concave notch on the anterior surface of the upper end of the ulna, formed by the anterior surface of the olecranon and the superior surface of the coronoid process; it articulates with the trochlea of the humerus at the elbow joint; it is unevenly divided by a smooth longitudinal ridge, which corresponds to the groove of the trochlea. Also called trochlear incisure of ulna; semilunar notch.

ulnar n. A smooth concavity on the medial side of the lower end of the radius that articulates with the head of the ulna.

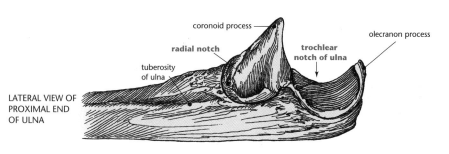

coronoid process

olecranon process

radial notch

trochlear notch of ulna

tuberosity of ulna

LATERAL VIEW OF PROXIMAL END OF ULNA

notch ■ nuchal

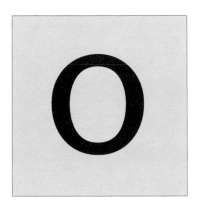

nuchal (nu'kal) Relating to the back of the neck.

obelion (o-be'le-on) A point on the skull where the sagittal suture is crossed by a line connecting the two parietal foramina; a craniometric point.

occipital (ok-sip'ĭ-tal) Relating to the back of the head. See also table of bones in appendix I.

occipitoatloid (ok-sip-ĭ-to-at'loid) Relating to the occipital bone and the first cervical vertebra.

occipitobregmatic (ok-sip-ĭ-to-breg-mat'ik) Relating to the occiput and the bregma (a craniometric point); applied to a measurement of the skull.

occipitofrontal (ok-sip-ĭ-to-fron'tal) Relating to the occiput and the forehead. See also table of muscles in appendix II.

occipitomental (ok-sip-ĭ-to-men'tal) Relating to the back of the head and the chin.

occipitoparietal (ok-sip-ĭ-to-pah-ri'e-tal) Relating to the occipital and parietal bones of the skull.

occipitotemporal (ok-sip-ĭ-to-tem'po-ral) Relating to the occipital and temporal bones of the skull.

occiput (ok'si-put) The lower back part of the head.

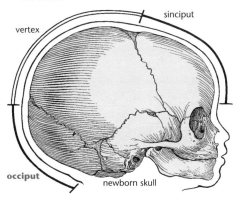

odontoid (o-don'toid) Tooth-shaped (e.g., the odontoid process of the second cervical vertebra).

olecranon (o-lek'rah-non) The bony process of the proximal end of the ulna forming the tip of the elbow; its anterior surface forms part of the trochlear notch. Popularly called point of the elbow; tip of the elbow.

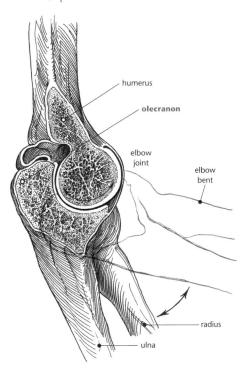

omo- Combining form meaning shoulder.

omoclavicular (o-mo-klah-vik'u-lar) Relating to the shoulder and clavicle.

omohyoid (o-mo-hi'oid) Relating to the shoulder and hyoid bone. See also table of muscles in appendix II.

opistion (o-pis'the-on) The middle point on the posterior margin of the foramen magnum, the large opening at the base of the skull.

opponens (o-po'nenz) Opposing; descriptive term applied to several muscles of the hand or foot whose function is to pull the digit across the palm or sole.

orbit (or'bit) One of two slightly conical cavities in the skull containing the eyeball and associated structures; formed by portions of seven bones: frontal, maxillary, zygomatic, lacrimal, ethmoid, palatine, and sphenoid. Also called orbital cavity; popularly called eye socket.

orbital (or'bĭ-tal) Relating to the orbit.

obelion ■ orbital

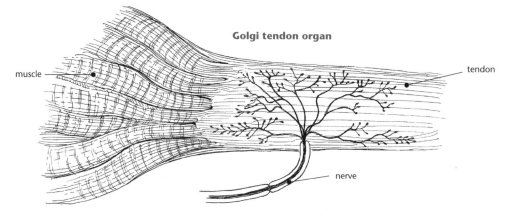

Golgi tendon organ

muscle

tendon

nerve

organ (or'gan) A distinct structural unit of the body that performs specific functions.

    Golgi tendon o. Special neurotendinous endings enclosed in a delicate capsule that ramify chiefly about bundles of collagen fibers of tendons near the junction with muscles. The endings are highly activated by passive stretch of the tendon or by active contraction of the muscle. Also called tendon spindle; Golgi corpuscle.

orifice (or'ĭ-fis) Any entrance or outlet of a body cavity; an opening of a canal. Also called ostium.

    o. of maxillary sinus See maxillary hiatus, under hiatus.

    pharyngeal o. of auditory tube The opening of the auditory tube in the lateral wall of the nasopharynx. Also called pharyngeal orifice of eustachian tube.

    pharyngeal o. of eustachian tube See pharyngeal orifice of auditory tube.

    tympanic o. of auditory tube The opening of the auditory tube in the upper part of the anterior wall of the middle ear chamber. Also called tympanic orifice of eustachian tube; tympanic opening of auditory tube.

    tympanic o. of eustachian tube See tympanic orifice of auditory tube.

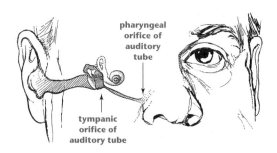

pharyngeal orifice of auditory tube

tympanic orifice of auditory tube

origin (or'ĭ-jin) The site of attachment of a muscle to a bone that is less movable than another bone to which it is inserted.

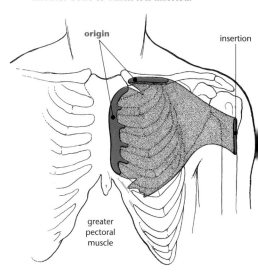

origin

insertion

greater pectoral muscle

oropharynx (o-ro-far'inks) The central portion of the pharynx directly behind the oral cavity, extending from the inferior border of the soft palate to the lingual surface of the epiglottis; it contains the palatine tonsils and the posterior faucial pillars.

orthopedic (or-tho-pe'dik) Relating to orthopedics.

orthopedics (or-tho-pe'diks) The surgically oriented medical specialty concerned with the preservation and restoration of functions of the skeletal system and associated structures. Also spelled orthopaedics.

orthoptics (or-thop'tiks) A method of therapy aimed at achieving coordinated function of the two eyes through a set of exercises; used

organ ■ orthoptics

particularly in treating the muscular imbalance of strabismus.

orthoptist (or-thop'tist) A person who treats those affected with ocular muscle imbalance and faulty visual habits by means of specially designed eye exercises.

orthosis (or-tho'sis), pl. ortho'ses An orthopedic appliance; any mechanical device worn on the body to apply the necessary force to a part; used in the treatment of physical impairment caused either by a congenital defect (e.g., clubfoot, spina bifida, malformation of long bones); by disease (e.g., muscular dystrophy, poliomyelitis, multiple sclerosis); or by trauma (e.g., fractures, spinal cord injuries, tendon tears). Orthoses are generally classified according to the region of the body involved, e.g., ankle-foot orthosis, knee-ankle-foot orthosis, elbow orthosis, wrist orthosis, cervical orthosis, sacroiliac orthosis. Also called orthotic; orthesis. COMPARE prosthesis.

orthotics (or-thot'iks) The science relating to orthoses and their applications.

os (os), pl. os'sa Latin for bone.

osseo- Combining form meaning bone.

osseocartilaginous (os-e-o-kar-tĭ-laj'ĭ-nus) Composed of both bone and cartilage.

osseointegration (os-e-o-in-ter-gra'shun) The growing of bone onto an implanted metal device, such as one that serves as a base for a tooth implant.

osseous (os'e-us) Bony.

ossi- Combining form meaning bone.

ossicle (os'sĭ-kl) A tiny bone, especially of the middle ear.

> **auditory o.'s** The three tiny bones in the middle ear chamber (malleus, incus, stapes), secured to the chamber wall by ligaments;

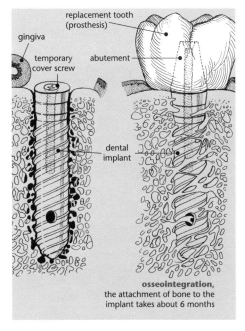

osseointegration,
the attachment of bone to the
implant takes about 6 months

together they form a bony chain across the chamber, from the tympanic membrane (eardrum) to the oval window (adjoining the inner ear). Sound waves striking the tympanic membrane cause the ossicles to vibrate; these vibrations are transmitted to the inner ear where they are converted to

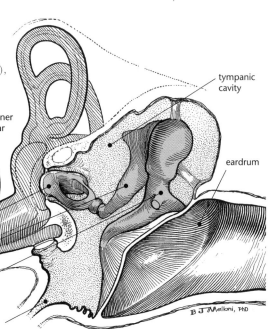

orthoptist ■ ossicle

impulses, which are interpreted by the brain as sound. Also called ear ossicles; ear bones.

ear o.'s See auditory ossicles.

ossicular (os-sik'u-lar) Relating to an ossicle.

ossification (os-ĭ-fi-ka'shun) 1. Replacement of cartilage by bone. 2. Formation of bone.

cartilaginous o. The replacement of a cartilage model by bone.

endochondral o. Ossification that occurs in long bones at the epiphyseal cartilaginous growth plate.

intramembranous o. The development of bone within a connective-tissue membrane without the benefit of a cartilage precursor, as occurs in the calvaria. Also called membranous ossification.

membranous o. See intramembranous ossification.

ossify (os'ĭ-fi) To change into bone.

osteitis (os-te-i'tis) Inflammation of bone.

o. fibrosa cystica Condition characterized by softening and resorption of bone with formation of cysts within the bone marrow and replacement by fibrous tissue; caused by excessive hormone secretion by the parathyroid glands (hyperparathyroidism).

o. pubis Sclerotic changes of the pubic symphysis; often quite painful.

osteo- Combining form meaning bone.

osteoarthritis (os-te-o-ar-thri'tis) The most common form of arthritis, characterized by progressive deterioration and loss of articular cartilage, thickening of underlying bone with formation of spurs near the joint margins, and stiffness of affected joints; may occur at an early age secondary to traumatic, congenital, or systemic disorders. Also called degenerative joint disease; degenerative arthritis; hypertrophic arthritis.

osteoarthropathy (os-te-o-ar-throp'ah-the) Disorder involving bones and joints.

hypertrophic o. Condition marked by periosteal formation of new bone (especially in the distal ends of long bones of the extremities), painful arthritis of adjacent joints, and clubbing of the fingers; it may or may not be secondary to an underlying condition; it most commonly occurs in association with disease of the lungs, especially tumors; also seen in association with heart disease, ulcerative colitis, regional enteritis, and liver disorders.

osteoarticular (os-te-o-ar-tik'u-lar) Relating to both bones and joints.

osteoblast (os'te-o-blast) A bone-forming cell, responsible for the formation of bone matrix.

osteoblastoma (os-te-o-blas-to'mah) A painful noncancerous tumor derived from primitive bone tissue, occurring most frequently on the spine of young individuals. Also called giant osteoid osteoma.

osteochondral (os-te-o-kon'dral) Relating to a bone and its articular cartilage.

osteochondritis (os-te-o-kon-dri'tis) Inflammation of both bone and its cartilage.

o. dissecans The gradual separation of a fragment of cartilage and underlying bone within a joint, most frequently occurring at the knee joint; tends to occur in adolescence; cause is unknown although several possible causes have been suggested, including disruption of blood supply to the bone by injury to a blood vessel.

osteochondrodysplasia (os-te-o-kon-dro-dis-pla'ze-ah) Abnormal development of both cartilage and bone.

osteochondroma (os-te-o-kon-dro'mah) A benign, mushroom-shaped outgrowth of bone capped by growing cartilage; occurs most frequently as a lateral protrusion near the end of a long bone; usually affects individuals from 10 to 20 years of age, often discovered by a chance x-ray finding.

osteochondrosis (os-te-o-kon-dro'sis) Any disorder affecting the ossification centers in the bones of children; characterized by degeneration or death of tissues in the absence of infection.

osteoclasis, osteoclasia (os-te-ok'lah-sis, os-te-o-kla'ze-ah) Surgical or manual fracture or refracture of a deformed bone for the purpose of resetting the bone in a more appropriate position.

osteoclast (os'te-o-klast) A large multinucleated cell formed in bone marrow; it functions in the absorption of bone tissue.

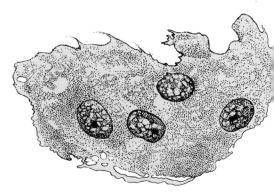

osteoclast

osteocyte (os'te-o-sīt) One of numerous bone cells arising from osteoblasts; it plays a role in maintaining the constituents of bone matrix at normal levels. Also called osseous cell; bone cell; bone corpuscle.

osteodesmosis (os-te-o-des-mo'sis) The abnormal transformation of tendons into bone.

osteodystrophy (os-te-o-dis'tro-fe) Defective bone formation.

osteofibroma (os-te-o-fi-bro'mah) A benign growth composed chiefly of bone and fibrous connective tissue.

osteogen (os'te-o-jen) The inner layer of the bone-covering membrane (periosteum) from which new bone is formed.

osteogenesis (os-te-o-jen'ĕ-sis) The formation of bone.

  o. imperfecta A group of closely related genetic disorders caused by defective bone formation; a common characteristic is bone fragility and susceptibility to fractures; features may also include (depending on degree of genetic defect) deformity of long bones, laxness of ligaments, blueness of scleras, and deafness due to otosclerosis. A rare autosomal recessive variant causes multiple fractures beginning at birth; death usually occurs in the first year of life. Also called brittle bones.

osteogenic, osteogenetic (os-te-o-jen'ik, os-te-o-jĕ-net'ik) Relating to bone formation; derived from bone.

osteoid (os'te-oid) 1. Resembling bone. 2. The soft organic part of intercellular bone matrix that precedes mineralization.

osteology (os-te-ol'o-je) The study of the structure of bones.

osteolysis (os-te-ol'ĭ-sis) Destruction or dissolution of bone tissue.

osteoma (os-te-o'mah) A benign tumor composed of bone tissue, usually protruding from a bone surface; most commonly seen on the facial bones.

  giant osteoid o. See osteoblastoma.

  ostoid o. A painful growth usually about 1 cm in diameter, most commonly occurring near the ends of long bones of the extremities of children and young adults.

osteomalacia (os-te-o-mah-la'she-ah) Softening and deformation of the bones especially those that are weight-bearing; it usually results from impairment of bone mineralization, often due to a deficiency of vitamin D.

osteon (os'te-on) The basic unit of compact bone, composed of a central canal (conveying blood vessels and nerve endings) and several

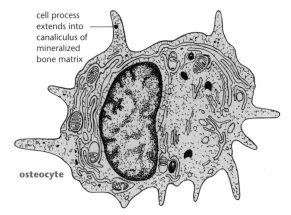

cell process extends into canaliculus of mineralized bone matrix

osteocyte

layers of bony tissue around the canal. Also called haversian system.

osteopetrosis (os-te-o-pe-tro'sis) A rare inherited disease characterized by overgrowth and brittleness of the dense outer (cortical) layer of bones, with reduction of bone marrow, causing frequent fractures and anemia. The ribs, pelvis, and vertebrae are mostly affected. Also called marble bones.

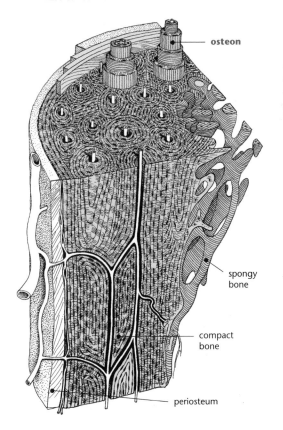

osteon

spongy bone

compact bone

periosteum

osteocyte ■ osteopetrosis

osteoporosis

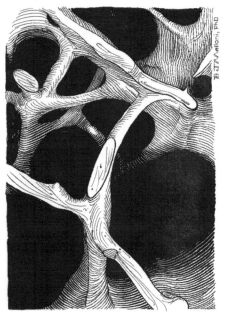

normal bone density

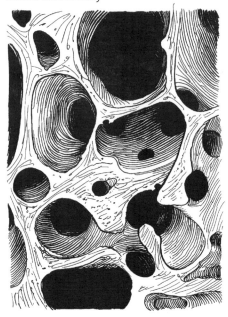

osteoporosis (os-te-o-po-ro'sis) Disease that appears to be the result of increased resorption of bone and diminished bone formation, seen most frequently in the elderly of both sexes, especially postmenopausal women; symptoms include bone pain, reduced height, deformity, and susceptibility to fractures; may be associated with other disorders (e.g., osteomalacia, multiple myeloma, hypopituitarism) or may be caused by certain drug therapies.

osteosarcoma (os-te-o-sar-ko'mah) See osteogenic sarcoma, under sarcoma.

osteosclerosis (os-te-o-skle-ro'sis) Abnormally increased density of bone.

ostial (os'te-al) Relating to an orifice or ostium.

ostium (os'te-um) See orifice.

otosclerosis (o-to-skle-ro'sis) Immobilization of the stapes by an overgrowth of spongy bone along the medial wall of the middle ear chamber; it interferes with conduction of sound waves, leading to hearing impairment.

outlet (owt'let) In anatomy, an opening or passageway that permits an outward movement.

> **pelvic o.** The lower aperture of the pelvis, bounded by the pubic arch, the ischial tuberosities, the sacrotuberous ligaments, and the tip of the coccyx.
>
> **thoracic o.** The outlet of the chest cavity bounded in back by the twelfth thoracic

vertebra, at the sides by the twelfth and eleventh ribs, and in front by the cartilages of the tenth, ninth, eight, and seventh ribs; it is closed by the diaphragm. Also called inferior thoracic aperture.

overextension (o-ver-eks-ten'shun) See hyperextension.

overflexion (o-ver-flek'shun) See hyperflexion.

overriding (o-ver-rīd'ing) Slippage of a fragment of broken bone over the main portion.

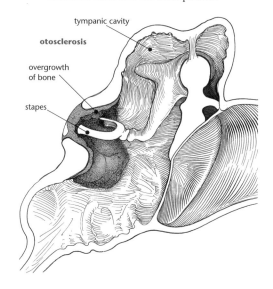

tympanic cavity

otosclerosis

overgrowth of bone

stapes

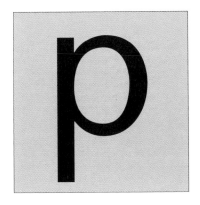

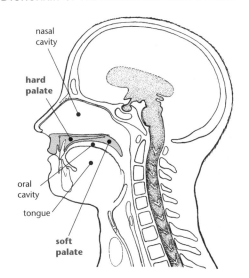

nasal cavity

hard palate

oral cavity

tongue

soft palate

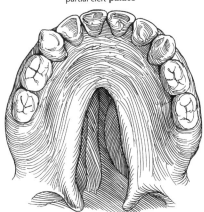

partial cleft **palate**

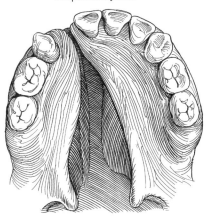

complete cleft **palate**

pachycephaly (pak-e-sef'ah-le) Abnormal thickening of the skull.

pachyperiostitis (pak-e-per-e-os-ti'tis) Inflammatory thickening of periosteum, the membrane that envelops bones.

palate (pal'at) The partition between the nasal and oral cavities. Also called palatum; popularly called roof of mouth.

> **hard p.** The anterior, bony part of the palate.

> **soft p.** The posterior, soft, muscular part of the palate; it extends posteriorly from the posterior margin of the hard palate. Also called velum palatinum.

palatine (pal'ah-ten) Relating to the palate.

palato- Combining form meaning palate.

palatoglossal (pal-ah-to-glos'al) Relating to the palate and tongue.

palatopharyngeal (pal-ah-to-fah-rin'je-al) Relating to the palate and the pharynx.

pan- Combining form meaning complete; all.

panosteitis (pan-os-te-i'tis) Inflammation of all the tissues of a bone, including the periosteum.

panturbinate (pan-ter'bĭ-nat) The entire mucosa and underlying bony tissue of any of the nasal conchae in the nasal cavity.

paramedian (par-ah-me'de-an) Alongside the midline or midplane of a structure.

paramyotonia (par-ah-mi-o-to'ne-ah) Disorder marked by spastic tonicity of muscles.

parasellar (par-ah-sel'ar) Situated near or around the sella turcica of the sphenoid bone in the base of the cranium.

paravertebral (par-ah-ver'tĕ-bral) Adjacent to the vertebral column (spine).

paresis (pah-re'sis) Mild paralysis; weakness of muscles.

paries (pa're-ez) The most superficial part of a structure, such as the wall or boundary of a cavity or organ.

pachycephaly ■ paries

parietofrontal (pah-ri-ĕ-to-fron'tal) Relating to the parietal and frontal bones of the skull. Also called frontoparietal.

parietomastoid (pah-ri-ĕ-to-mas'toid) Relating to the parietal bone and mastoid part of the temporal bone.

parieto-occipital (pah-ri-ĕ-to ok-sip'ĭ-tal) Relating to the parietal and occipital bones of the skull.

parosteal (par-os'te-al) Relating to the outer layer of the periosteum.

pars (parz) Latin for a part.

part (part) A portion.

   abdominal p. of the greater pectoral muscle The abdominal part of the greater pectoral muscle (pectoralis major) originating from the aponeurosis of the external oblique muscle of the abdomen (obliquus externus abdominis).

   alar p. of nasal muscle The dilator muscle of the nose. See also table of muscles in appendix II.

   alveolar p. of mandible The upper part of the body of the mandible containing sockets for the roots of the lower teeth.

   alveolar p. of maxilla The lower part of the maxilla containing sockets for the roots of the upper teeth.

   basilar p. of occipital bone The rectangular part of the occipital bone inclining forward from the foramen magnum to the sphenoid bone where fusion occurs by the twenty-fifth year of life.

   bony p. of auditory tube The part of the auditory (eustachian) tube extending from the front of the middle ear chamber to the petrosquamous junction of the temporal bone, where the cartilaginous part of the auditory tube commences.

   bony p. of nasal septum The nasal septum composed of the perpendicular plate of the ethmoid bone and the vomer.

   buccopharyngeal p. of superior constrictor muscle of pharynx The portion of the superior constrictor muscle of the pharynx that originates from the pterygomandibular raphe.

   cartilaginous p. of auditory tube The part of the auditory (eustachian) tube that is supported by cartilage and extending from the bony part of the auditory tube to the opening (pharyngeal orifice) into the nasopharynx.

   cartilaginous p. of nasal septum The flattened cartilaginous plate of the lower anterior nasal septum; it is quadrilateral in shape; attached posteriorly to the perpendicular plate of the ethmoid bone and the vomer.

   ceratopharyngeal p. of middle constrictor muscle of the pharynx The portion of the

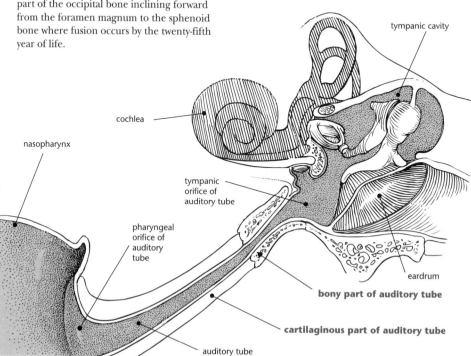

tympanic cavity

cochlea

nasopharynx

tympanic orifice of auditory tube

pharyngeal orifice of auditory tube

eardrum

bony part of auditory tube

cartilaginous part of auditory tube

auditory tube

parietofrontal ■ part

middle constrictor muscle of pharynx that originates from the greater cornu (horn) of the hyoid bone.

chondropharyngeal p. of middle constrictor muscle of pharynx The portion of the middle constrictor muscle of the pharynx that originates from the lesser cornu (horn) of the hyoid bone and the distal part of the stylohyoid ligament.

clavicular p. of the greater pectoral muscle The portion of the greater pectoral muscle (pectoralis major) originating from the medial half of the clavicle.

condylar p. of occipital bone See lateral mass of occipital bone, under mass.

costal p. of diaphragm The part of the respiratory diaphragm that arises from the internal surface of the costal cartilages and adjacent six ribs on either side.

cricopharyngeal p. of inferior constrictor muscle of pharynx The distal part of the inferior constrictor muscle of the pharynx that originates from the lateral side of the cricoid cartilage on either side.

deep p.of external sphincter muscle of anus The ringlike deep part of the external sphincter muscle of the anus; it surrounds the internal anal sphincter muscle at the upper end of the anal canal.

deep p. of masseter muscle The deep, vertical, smaller of the two parts of the masseter muscle; it arises from the lower border of the zygomatic arch and inserts into the outer surface of the coronoid process and the upper half of the ramus of the mandible.

glossopharyngeal p. of superior constrictor muscle of pharynx The portion of the superior constrictor muscle of the pharynx that originates from the side of the root of the tongue.

labial p. of orbicular muscle of mouth The part of the orbicular muscle of mouth (orbicularis oris) that is restricted to the lips.

lacrimal p. of orbicular muscle of eye The part of the orbicular muscle of the eye that originates from the posterior lacrimal crest and crosses the lacrimal sac to become continuous with the palpebral part.

laryngeal p. of pharynx The distal part of the pharynx in the back of the larynx extending from the upper edge of the epiglottis to the lower edge of the cricoid cartilage at which point it continues as the esophagus.

lateral p. of sacrum See sacral crest, under crest.

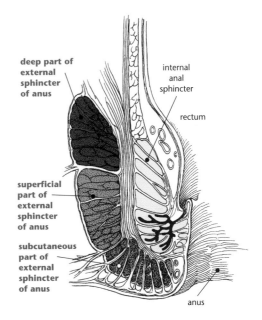

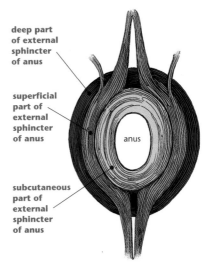

lumbar p. of diaphragm The part of the respiratory diaphragm that originates from the lumbar vertebrae, comprising the right and left diaphragmatic crura; the right crus arising from the first three or four lumbar vertebrae and the left crus from the first two or three lumbar vertebrae. Also called vertebral part of diaphragm.

membranous p. of nasal septum The thickened skin and subcutaneous tissue of the nasal septum at the apex of the nose, immediately under the cartilaginous part of the septum.

part ■ part

mylopharyngeal p. of superior constrictor muscle of pharynx The part of the superior constrictor muscle of the pharynx that originates from the mylohyoid line of the mandible.

nasal p. of frontal bone The central part of the frontal bone that projects downward to articulate with the nasal bones and the frontal processes of the maxillae; it extends back to form part of the roof of the nasal cavity.

oblique p. of cricothyroid muscle The lower of the two parts of the cricothyroid muscle that extends from the cricoid cartilage to the inferior cornu (horn) and inner surface of the thyroid cartilage.

orbital p. of frontal bone The horizontally situated portion of the frontal bone that forms the roof of the orbit, except for a small portion posteriorly; it also serves above as the floor of the anterior cranial fossa. Also called orbital plate of frontal bone.

perpendicular p. of ethmoid bone The thin, flat, quadrilateral bony plate that lies in the midsagittal plane and descends vertically from the crista galli to form the upper third of the nasal septum; inferiorly, the posterior margin articulates with the vomer and superiorly, with the sphenoid crest. Also called perpendicular lamina of ethmoid bone.

petrous p. of temporal bone The dense, pyramidal part of the temporal bone at the base of the skull that houses the inner ear and accommodates part of the internal carotid artery.

pterygopharyngeal p. of superior constrictor muscle of pharynx The part of the superior constrictor muscle of the pharynx that originates from the lower part of the posterior margin and hamulus of the medial pterygoid plate.

squamous p. of temporal bone The thin, scalelike upper part of the temporal bone forming part of the lateral wall of the skull; its lower aspect contains the mandibular fossa for articulation with the lower jaw. Also called temporal squama.

sternal p. of diaphragm The part of the respiratory diaphragm that originates by two muscular slips from the inner aspect of the xiphoid process of the sternum.

sternocostal p. of greater pectoral muscle The part of the greater pectoral muscle (pectoralis major) that arises from the sternum and the ribs.

straight p. of cricothyroid muscle The upper of the two parts of the cricothyroid muscle that extends from the cricoid cartilage upward to the lower margin of the inner surface of the thyroid cartilage.

subcutaneous p. of external sphincter muscle of anus The ringlike band of sphincter muscle that lies around the anal orifice just below the skin.

superficial p. of external sphincter muscle of anus The elliptical superficial part of the external sphincter muscle of the anus that lies between the subcutaneous part and the deep part of the muscle; it surrounds the internal anal sphincter muscle at the lower end of the anal canal.

superficial p. of masseter muscle The superficial, oblique, larger of the two parts of the masseter muscle of the lower jaw; it arises from the lower border of the zygomatic arch and the zygomatic process of the maxilla and is inserted into the lateral surface of the coronoid process and the lower half of the ramus of the mandible.

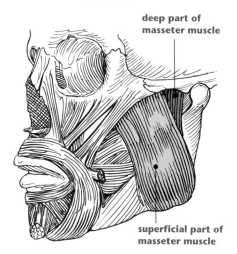

deep part of masseter muscle

superficial part of masseter muscle

thyropharyngeal p. of inferior constrictor muscle of pharynx The part of the inferior constrictor muscle of the pharynx that originates from the inferior cornu (horn) and the oblique line of the thyroid cartilage and inserts into the pharyngeal raphe.

transverse p. of nasal muscle The constrictor muscle of the nose that arises from the maxilla, lateral to the nasal notch and inserts onto the aponeurosis on the nasal cartilage and bridge of nose; it compresses the nostril.

tympanic p. of temporal bone The curved

part ■ part

bony plate of the temporal bone that forms part of the external auditory canal and contains a sulcus that accommodates the tympanic membrane (eardrum).

    vertebral p. of diaphragm See lumbar part of diaphragm.

patella (pah-tel'ah) A flat, triangular sesamoid bone attached at the front of the knee joint, in the combined tendons of the extensor muscles of the leg. Commonly called kneecap.

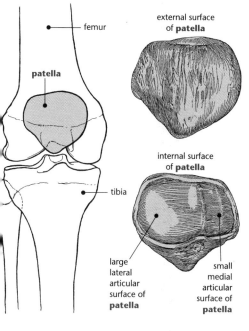

femur

external surface of **patella**

patella

internal surface of **patella**

tibia

large lateral articular surface of **patella**

small medial articular surface of **patella**

patellectomy (pat-ĕ-lek'to-me) Surgical removal of the patella.

pectinate (pek'tĭ-nāt) Comb-shaped; e.g., the comblike pectinate muscles of the auricles of the heart.

pectineal (pek-tin'e-al) Relating to the pubic bone or to any comblike structure.

pectoral (pek'to-ral) Relating to the chest, breast, or thorax.

pectoralis (pek-to-ra'lis) Pectoral; applied especially to the greater and lesser pectoral muscles (pectoralis major and pectoralis minor).

pectus (pek'tus) The anterior wall of the chest cavity.

    p. carinatum See keeled chest, under chest.

    p. excavatum See funnel chest, under chest.

pedicle (ped'ĭ-kl) An anatomic structure resembling a short stem.

    p. of vertebral arch One of two bars of bone extending backward from the bodies of each

vertebra, helping to form the vertebral arch that surrounds the spinal cord.

pediphalanx (ped-ĭ-fa'lanks) A phalanx of a digit of a toe.

pelvi-, pelvo- Combining forms meaning the pelvis.

pelvic (pel'vik) Relating to the pelvis.

pelvicephalometry (pel-ve-sef-ah-lom'ĕ-tre) Comparative measurement of the maternal pelvis and fetal head.

pelvifemoral (pel-ve-fem'o-ral) Relating to the pelvis and the femur.

pelvimetry (pel-vim'ĕ-tre) Measurement of diameters of the female pelvis in pregnancy to determine whether the woman is likely to develop difficult labor due to disproportion between the head of the fetus and maternal pelvis.

    combined p. Pelvimetry made both within the body with the examiner's hand and outside the body with instruments.

    digital p. Pelvimetry determined solely by the examiner's fingers. Also called manual pelvimetry.

    manual p. See digital pelvimetry.

    radiologic p. See x-ray pelvimetry.

    x-ray p. A precise method of assessing the diameters of the vault, midpelvis, and pelvic outlet; performed only if the potential benefit exceeds the risk of radiation to the fetus; usually postponed until near term. Also called radiologic pelvimetry.

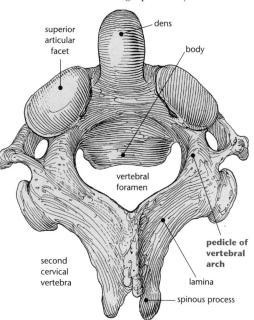

superior articular facet

dens

body

vertebral foramen

second cervical vertebra

pedicle of vertebral arch

lamina

spinous process

male **pelvis**

female **pelvis**

seen from
below

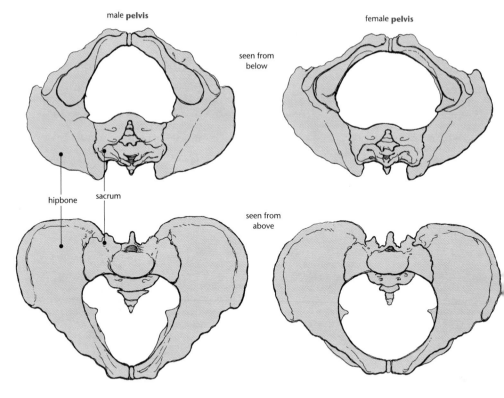

hipbone   sacrum

seen from
above

pelvis (pel'vis), pl. pel'vises, pel'ves 1. The basin-shaped skeletal structure at the lower end of the trunk, composed of the two hipbones and the sacrum and coccyx; it supports the spinal column and rests on the lower limbs. 2. A funnel-like dilatation.

  achondroplastic p. A broad, flattened pelvis, as seen in achondroplastic dwarfs.

  android p. A female pelvis with a wedge-shaped inlet and a narrow anterior segment, characteristics of a typical male pelvis. Also called funnel-shaped pelvis; brachypellic pelvis.

  anthropoid p. A pelvis with a long, narrow, oval inlet; its anteroposterior diameter exceeds its transverse diameter. Also called pithecoid pelvis; dolichopellic pelvis.

  brachypellic p. See android pelvis.

  cordate p. A pelvis with an inlet that is somewhat heart shaped; caused by thrusting forward of the sacrum.

  contracted p. One in which an important diameter of the pelvis is shorter than normal.

  dolichopellic p. See anthropoid pelvis.

  false p. See major pelvis.

  funnel-shaped p. See android pelvis.

  greater p. See major pelvis.

  gynecoid p. A pelvis with an inlet that has a well-rounded oval shape; it represents the average or normal female pelvis.

  kyphotic p. A pelvis that, due to kyphoscoliosis, is contracted transversely and appears funnel shaped with a marked inclination.

  lesser p. See minor pelvis.

  lordotic p. A pelvis that is deformed by an anterior curvature in the lumbar region of the vertebral column.

  major p. The false pelvis; the portion of the pelvis above the oblique plane of the pelvic brim; its cavity is part of the abdomen. Also called false pelvis; greater pelvis.

  minor p. The true pelvis; a narrowed continuation of the major pelvis; it is short, wide and curved and is positioned below and behind the pelvic brim. Also called true pelvis; lesser pelvis.

  p. obtecta A pelvis associated with severe kyphosis, in which the vertebral column extends horizontally across the pelvic inlet.

  pithecoid p. See anthropoid pelvis.

  platypellic p. See platypelloid pelvis.

  platypelloid p. An exceedingly flat, uncommon pelvis; one in which the

pelvis ■ pelvis

transverse diameter of the pelvic inlet is far greater than the anteroposterior diameter. Also called platypellic pelvis.

scoliotic p. An obliquely deformed pelvis, seen in association with scoliosis.

spondylolisthetic p. A pelvis tilted so posteriorly that the body of the fifth lumbar vertebra is situated on a plane in front of the body of the sacrum.

stove-in p. One in which, as a result of a severe compression injury, part of the pelvis is driven into the pelvic cavity.

true p. See minor pelvis.

pelvisacral (pel-vĭ-sa'kral) Relating to the pelvis and sacrum.

pelvospondylitis (pel-vo-spon-dĭ-li'tis) Inflammation of the pelvic portion of the spine, especially the sacroiliac joint.

p. ossificans The presence of bony deposits between the sacroiliac joints or between the sacrum and the adjacent lumbar vertebra.

pennate (pen-āt') Feather-like; similar to a feather in architecture, said especially of muscles in which the fasciculi are oblique to the line of pull (e.g., the rectus muscle of thigh). Also called penniform.

penniform (pen'ĭ-form) See pennate.

periarticular (per-ĭ-ar-tik'u-lar) Situated in the tissues around or near a joint.

perichondral (per-ĭ-kon'dral) Relating to perichondrium.

perichondritis (per-ĭ-kon-dri'tis) Inflammation of cartilage.

perichondrium (per-ĭ-kon'dre-um) The fibrous membrane covering all cartilage except at joint endings; composed of an outer connective tissue layer and an inner one that is responsible for producing new cartilage.

pericranium (per-ĭ-kra'ne-um) The periosteum on the outer surface of the bones of the cranium.

peridesmium (per-ĭ-dez'me-um) The connective tissue covering ligaments.

perimysium (per-ĭ-mis'e-um) Connective tissue separating adjacent bundles (fasciculi) of skeletal muscle fibers.

periodontium (per-e-o-don'she-um) Tissues that surround the teeth, including alveolar bone, cementum, gingiva, and periodontal membrane.

periorbita (per-e-or'bi-tah) The periosteum lining the bones forming the eye socket (orbit); anteriorly, it is continuous with the periosteum on the facial bones and posteriorly, with the outer layer of the dura mater at the superior

orbital fissure and optic foramen. Also called periorbital membrane.

periosteum (per-e-os'te-um) The fibrous membrane covering all bones except in areas of articulation.

periostitis (per-e-os-ti'tis) Inflammation of periosteum.

periosteoma (per-e-os-te-o'mah) A morbid bony growth derived from the periosteum surrounding a bone.

perispondylitis (per-ĭ-spon-dĭ-li'tis) Inflammation of the tissues around a vertebra.

peritendinits (per-ĭ-ten-dĭ-ni'tis) Inflammation of the sheath surrounding a tendon.

perivertebral (per-ĭ-ver'tĕ-bral) Situated around a vertebra or vertebrae.

peroneal (per-o-ne'al) Relating to the fibula, to the fibular (lateral) side of the leg, or to muscles attached to the fibula. See also table of muscles in appendix II.

pes (pes) 1. Latin for foot. 2. Any footlike structure.

p. calcaneus See talipes calcaneus, under talipes.

p. cavus See clawfoot.

p. equinus See talipes equinus, under talipes.

p. planovalgus See talipes planovalgus, under talipes.

p. planus See flatfoot.

p. pronatus See talipes valgus, under talipes.

p. valgus See talipes valgus, under talipes.

p. varus See talipes varus, under talipes.

petrosal (pē-tro'sal) Relating to the petrous part of the temporal bone.

petrous (pet'rus) 1. Hard. 2. Petrosal.

phalangeal (fah-lan'je-al) Relating to a bone in fingers or toes.

phalanx (fa'lanks), pl. phalan'ges Any bone of a finger or toe.

pharyngeal (far-rin'je-al) Relating to the pharynx.

pharyngoglossal (fah-ring-go-glos'al) Relating to the pharynx and the tongue.

pharyngolaryngeal (fah-ring-go-lah-rin'je-al) Relating to the pharynx and the larynx.

pharyngopalatine (fah-ring-go-pal'ah-tīn) Relating to the pharynx and the palate.

pharynx (far'inks) The musculomembranous tubular cavity, lined with mucous membrane, extending from the back of the nasal and oral cavities to the beginning of the trachea and esophagus.

piriform (pir'ĭ-form) Pear-shaped, said especially of the piriform muscle extending from the dorsal sacrum to the greater trochanter of the

pelvisacral ■ piriform

femur. See also table of muscles in appendix II.

pisiform (pi'sĭ-form) Resembling a pea in size and shape, said especially of the pisiform bone of the wrist. See also table of bones in appendix I.

pit (pit) Any normal or abnormal indentation of a surface.

    p. of femoral head See fovea of femoral head, under fovea.

    pterygoid p. See pterygoid fovea, under fovea.

plane (plān) l. A flat or level surface. 2. An imaginary surface formed by extension through two points or an axis.

    auriculo-infraorbital p.
See Frankford plane.

    coronal p. A vertical plane at right angles to the median plane, dividing the head into anterior and posterior portions; named after the cranial suture of that name. Used interchangeably with frontal plane.

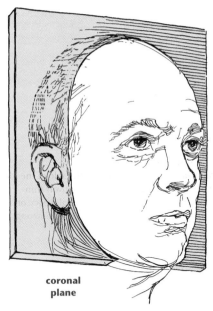

coronal plane

Frankford p., Frankford horizontal p. A craniometric plane of the head represented on an x-ray profile by drawing a line passing through the highest point on the margin of the acoustic meatus and the lowest point on the margin of the orbit. Also called auriculo-infraorbital plane.

    frontal p. A vertical plane passing at right angles to the median plane, dividing the body into anterior and posterior halves. COMPARE coronal plane.

    horizontal p. The plane extending across the long axis of the body separating an upper part from the lower part. Also called transverse plane.

    intercristal p. The horizontal plane passing through the highest points of the iliac crests; it usually lies at the level of the fourth lumbar vertebra.

    interspinous p. A horizontal plane transecting the body at the level of the anterior superior iliac spine of the hipbone.

    intertubercular p. See transtubercular plane.

    lateral rectus sagittal p. The vertical plane passing to the lateral side of the straight muscle of abdomen (rectus abdominis).

    median p. A plane that divides the body vertically into right and left halves. Also called midsagittal plane.

    midclavicular p. The vertical plane passing through the middle of the clavicle.

    midinguinal p. The vertical plane passing through the middle of the inguinal ligament of the hipbone.

    midsagittal p. See median plane.

    p. of occlusion The horizontal plane formed by the occlusal surfaces of the contacting teeth when the jaws are closed.

    parasagittal p. Any vertical plane parallel to the sagittal plane.

    pelvic p. of greatest dimension The roomiest portion of the pelvic cavity extending from the middle of the posterior surface of the pubic symphysis anteriorly to the junction of the second and third sacral vertebrae posteriorly; in the average pregnant woman, the anteroposterior diameter is approximately 12.75 cm and its transverse diameter is around 12.5 cm.

    pelvic p. of inlet The rounded or oval opening of the true (minor) pelvis, bounded anteriorly by the upper border of the pubis, laterally by the iliopectineal line, and posteriorly by the sacral promontory. Also called superior aperture of minor pelvis; superior pelvic strait.

    pelvic p. of least dimension The midpelvis plane, extending from the lower margin of the pubic symphysis through the ischial spines to the apex of the sacrum; in the average pregnant woman, the anteroposterior diameter measures approximately 11.5 cm and its transverse diameter is around 10 cm. Also called pelvic plane of midpelvis.

    pelvic p. of midpelvis See pelvic plane of least dimension.

pisiform ■ plane

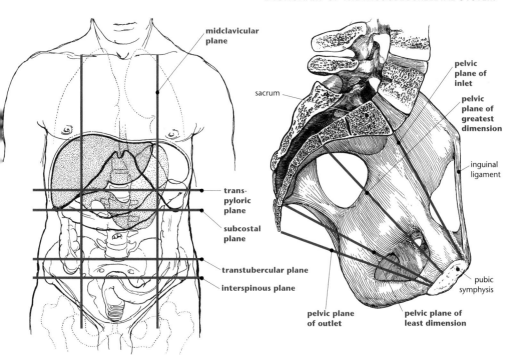

pelvic p. of outlet The plane across the lower opening of the true (minor) pelvis, bounded anteriorly by the pubic symphysis and the sides of the pubic arch, laterally by the ischial tuberosities, and posteriorly by the tip of the coccyx. Also called inferior aperture of minor pelvis; inferior pelvic strait.

p.'s of reference Planes that serve as a guide for the location of specific organs or sites (e.g., the intersection of the transpyloric plane with the right midinguinal plane marks the usual site of the gallbladder's fundus).

sagittal p. A vertical plane extending in an anteroposterior direction. Named after the suture of the cranium of that name.

subcostal p. A horizontal plane passing through the lowest point of the costal margin on each side, usually at the inferior border of the tenth costal cartilage, which is generally at the level of the body of the third lumbar vertebra. Also called subcostal line.

transpyloric p. The horizontal plane passing through the pylorus part of the stomach, which is generally halfway between the suprasternal notch and the pubic symphysis; it passes through the tip of the ninth costal cartilage, the fundus of the gallbladder, the neck of the pancreas, and the body of the first lumbar vertebra.

transtubercular p. The horizontal plane at the level of the tubercles of the iliac crest of the hipbone; usually the same level as the lower part of the fifth lumbar vertebra. Also called intertubercular plane.

transverse p. See horizontal plane.

umbilical p. The horizontal plane passing through the navel (umbilicus).

plantar (plan'tar) Relating to the sole of the foot.

plate (plăt) 1. Any flattened, relatively thin structure. 2. A smooth, flat metal device of uniform thickness, used for approximating fractured bones. 3. A thin, perforated structure for covering defects sustained during injury or surgery.

bone p. A flattened metal bar, with perforations for the insertion of bone screws, for immobilization of fractured bone segments.

cribriform p. of ethmoid bone A perforated strip of a horizontal bony plate that forms a large part of the roof of the nasal cavity; it lodges the olfactory bulbs and provides the numerous perforations that transmit filaments of the olfactory nerve from the bulbs in the calvaria to the olfactory epitheliun lining the medial and lateral walls of the roof of the nasal cavity. The midline of the upper surface of the plate bears a slender elevation, the crista galli. Also called

plantar ■ plate

cribriform lamina of ethmoid bone.

end p. See endplate.

epiphyseal p. The plate or disk of specialized hyaline cartilage interposed between the shaft (diaphysis) and the extremity (epiphysis) of a developing long bone; by its growth, the bone lengthens as it develops to maturity. Also spelled epiphysial plate; also called growth plate; growth cartilage; epiphyseal cartilage.

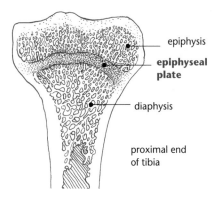

epiphysis

epiphyseal plate

diaphysis

proximal end of tibia

external p. of cranial bone See external cranial lamina, under lamina.

foot p. See footplate.

horizontal p. of palatine bone The horizontal part of the palatine bone forming the back part of the hard palate and the back of the floor of the nasal cavity on either side. Also called horizontal lamina of palatine bone.

internal p. of cranial bone See internal cranial lamina, under lamina.

lateral pterygoid p. The lateral of the two plates forming the pterygoid process, projecting downward from the sphenoid bone; the lateral wall of the pterygoid fossa. Also called lateral pterygoid lamina.

medial pterygoid p. The medial of the two plates forming the pterygoid process, projecting downward from the sphenoid bone; the medial wall of the pterygoid fossa. Also called medial pterygoid lamina.

motor p. The motor end-plate between the expanded terminal of the motor axon and the striated muscle fibers it innervates, forming the neuromuscular junction.

orbital p. of ethmoid bone A vertical, thin plate of bone that forms a large part of the medial wall of the orbit and the lateral wall of the ethmoidal labyrinth on either side; it articulates with the maxilla, and the palatine,

frontal, sphenoid, and lacrimal bones. Also called orbital lamina.

orbital p. of frontal bone See orbital part of frontal bone, under part.

perpendicular p. of ethmoid bone A thin bony plate that descends from the under surface of the cribriform plate of the ethmoid bone to contribute to the formation of the nasal septum. Also called perpendicular lamina of ethmoid bone.

perpendicular p. of palatine bone The thin, flat, vertical portion of the palatine bone, extending from the horizontal lamina and forming part of the lateral wall of the nasal cavity, part of the posterior wall of the maxillary sinus, and the medial wall of the pterygopalatine fossa. Also called perpendicular lamina of palatine bone; vertical plate of palatine bone.

pterygoid p.'s A short, broad lateral plate and a long, narrow medial plate that projects inferiorly from the sphenoid bone; the pterygoid fossa lies between them.

skull p. A thin perforated plate, generally round or oval, that is screwed to the cranium to replace missing bone fragments.

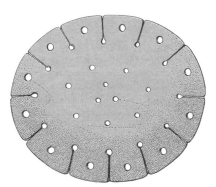

skull plate (oval type)

vertical p. of palatine bone See perpendicular plate of palatine bone.

platysma (plah-tiz′mah) See table of muscles in appendix II.

platyspondylia (plat-e-spon-dil′e-ah) Abnormal flatness of the bodies of vertebrae.

pleonosteosis (ple-on-os-te-o′sis) Abnormally excessive formation of bone tissue.

pneumarthrosis (nu-mar-thro′sis) The presence of air in a joint.

point (point) 1. A minute spot or area. 2. A specific position, condition, or degree. 3. A minute orifice; punctum.

alveolar p. See prosthion.

plate ■ point

contact p. The small area of the interproximal surface of a tooth that is in direct contact with an adjacent tooth. Also called contact area.

craniometric p.'s Fixed standard points on the skull used as landmarks and for measuring the skull. They have special applications in forensic medicine, orthodontics, and plastic surgery.

deaf p.'s Points near the ear where a vibrating tuning fork touching them, cannot be heard by the person being examined.

Galliot's p. A point on the buttock ideally suited for intramuscular injections, located where a horizontal line three to four centimeters above the greater trochanter of the femur intersects a vertical line at the lateral third of the buttock.

p. of maximum impulse The point on the chest wall where the beat of the left ventricle of the heart is felt most intensely; normally felt in the left fifth intercostal space, at the midclavicular line.

midclavicular p. The midpoint of the clavicle (collarbone).

midinguinal p. The point on the inguinal ligament halfway between the pubic symphysis and the anterior superior iliac spine.

nasal p. See nasion.

occipital p. The most posterior point of the occipital bone, situated in the median plane at the tip of the external occipital protuberance. The plane formed by a line between the occipital point and the glabella represents the maximum anteroposterior length of the skull; the opisthocranion.

p. of ossification The point or center in a cartilage where the earliest bone formation (ossification) occurs.

pressure-arresting p. The point or area of the skin at which exerted pressure elicits relief of spasm of underlying muscles.

sylvian p. See pterion.

polyarthritis (pol-e-ar-thri'tis) Simultaneous inflammation of more than one joint (e.g., rheumatoid arthritis).

polychondritis (pol-e-kon-dri'tis) Inflammation involving several cartilages, such as those of the larynx, trachea, and joint cartilages.

popliteal (pop-lit'e-al) 1. Relating to the area behind the knee. 2. A muscle on the posterior surface of the knee. See also table of muscles in appendix II.

posterior (pos-tēr'e-or) 1. Situated behind a structure. 2. Relating to the back or dorsal

aspect of the body or part.

postero- Combining form meaning back, posterior.

posteroanterior (pos-ter-o-an-tēr'e-or) From the back to the front.

posterolateral (pos-ter-o-lat'er-al) Behind and to one side.

posteromedial (pos-ter-o-me'de-al) Behind and toward the middle.

prehyoid (pre-hi'oid) Situated anterior to the hyoid bone.

premaxillary (pre-mak'sĭ-ler-e) Situated in front of the maxilla.

prepatella (pre-pah-tel'ah) Situated in front of the patella (kneecap).

prevertebral (pre-ver'te-bral) In front of a vertebra or of the vertebral column (spine).

process (pros'es) A marked prominence extending from an anatomic structure, usually a bony extension for the attachment of muscles and ligaments.

acromial p. See acromion.

articular p. of sacrum One of two rounded processes projecting upwardly from the top surface of the sacrum, bearing the hyaline-coated concave joint surface for articulation with the inferior articular facet of the fifth lumbar vertebra.

articular p. of vertebra One of the small projections on the upper and lower surfaces of the vertebra, on either side: *Inferior articular p. of vertebra*, one of a pair of downward projections from the lamina of a vertebra, bearing the hyaline-coated facet for articulation with the vertebra below. *Superior articular p. of vertebra*, one of a pair of upward projections from the junction of the pedicle and lamina, bearing the hyaline-coated facet for articulation with the vertebra above.

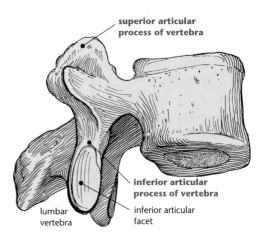

superior articular process of vertebra

inferior articular process of vertebra

lumbar vertebra

inferior articular facet

point ■ process

clinoid p. One of three pairs of extensions from the sphenoid bone of the skull: *Anterior clinoid p.*, one of a pair of tips directed medially, from the posterior border of the lesser wing of the sphenoid bone; it provides attachment for the anterior end of the free border of the tentorium cerebelli. *Posterior clinoid p.*, one of a pair of processes situated at the anterosuperior border of the dorsum sellae in the back of the hypophyseal fossa; it provides attachment for the fixed margin of the tentorium cerebelli.

condylar p. A rounded projection on the surface of a bone.

condylar p. of mandible The projection from the upper part of the posterior margin of the ramus of the lower jaw; composed of a constricted, slightly flattened neck and an expanded head bearing a knuckle-shaped condyle. The process can be felt in front of the tragus of the ear.

coracoid p. of scapula A thick, strong, curved bony process arising from the superior border of the scapula, partly overhanging the glenoid fossa; it provides attachment for the short head of the biceps muscle of arm, coracobrachial muscle, and the smaller (lesser) pectoral muscle (pectoralis minor); it also provides attachment to the conoid and coracoacromial ligaments. The process can be felt below the lateral third of the clavicle.

coronoid p. of mandible The flattened triangular process at the upper anterior part of the ramus of the lower jaw; it provides attachment for most of the fibers of the temporal muscle.

coronoid p. of ulna A wide bracketlike projection from the front of the proximal end of the ulna at the elbow joint, just below the olecranon; it forms the lower boundary of the trochlear notch.

costal p. of cervical vertebra The rounded anterior bar of the transverse process of a cervical vertebra in front of the transverse foramen; it corresponds to the vertebral end of a rib.

ethmoidal p. of inferior nasal concha A small, thin, bony plate projecting upward from the top margin of the inferior nasal concha in the nasal cavity to articulate with the uncinate process of the ethmoid bone across the opening of the maxillary sinus.

frontal p. of maxilla The process of the maxilla extending upward to articulate with the frontal, nasal and lacrimal bones; it

forms the medial boundary of the orbit.

frontal p. of zygomatic bone The process of the zygomatic bone extending upward to articulate with the frontal bone and behind with the greater wing of the sphenoid bone; it forms the lateral boundary of the orbit.

hamular p. of sphenoid bone See pterygoid hamulus, under hamulus.

p.'s of incus Processes projecting from the incus, the middle auditory ossicle: *lenticular p. of incus*, the rounded projection extending at a right angle from the long process of the incus of the middle ear chamber; it articulates with the head of the stapes. *Long p. of incus*, a slender process projecting downward from the body of the incus; its lower end bends and terminates in a bulbous form (the lenticular process) for articulation with the head of the stapes, smallest auditory ossicle. *Short p. of incus*, a conical-shaped process that projects posteriorly from the body of the incus; it is attached to the wall of the middle ear chamber by small ligaments.

inferior articular p. of vertebra One of a pair of bony projections extending downward from the lamina of a vertebra, bearing the facet for articulation with the facet on the superior articular process of the vertebra below.

intercondylar p. of tibia See intercondylar eminence of tibia, under eminence.

intrajugular p. of occipital bone A bony spicule that projects into the jugular notch of the occipital bone, dividing it into a lateral and a medial part.

intrajugular p. of temporal bone A bony spicule that projects into the jugular notch of the petrous part of the temporal bone, dividing it into a lateral and a medial part.

jugular p. of occipital bone The quadrilateral bony plate projecting laterally from the occipital condyle and forming the posterior border of the jugular notch; it articulates with the petrous part of the temporal bone.

lateral p. of calcaneus A bony process projecting downward from the lower lateral portion of the calcaneal tuberosity, providing partial attachment to muscle.

lateral p. of talus The lateral process of the talus that articulates with the lateral malleolus of the fibula.

long p. of incus See crus of incus, under crus.

long p. of malleus See manubrium of malleus, under manubrium.

p.'s of malleus Processes projecting from

process ■ process

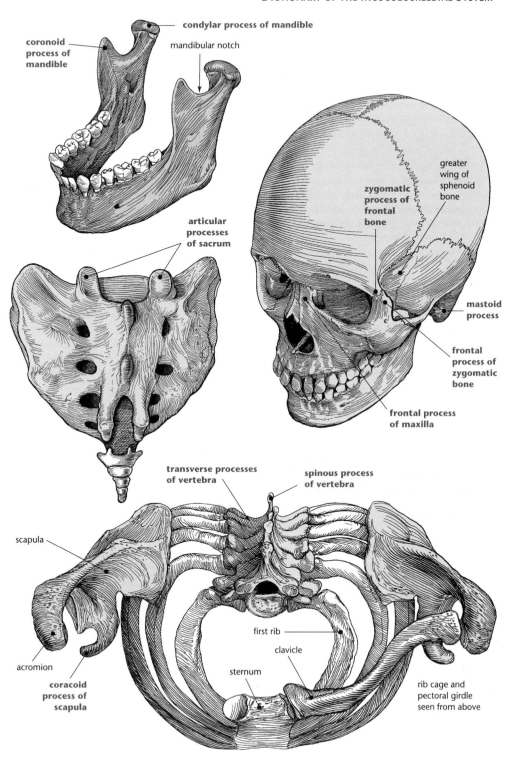

coronoid process of mandible

condylar process of mandible

mandibular notch

articular processes of sacrum

zygomatic process of frontal bone

greater wing of sphenoid bone

mastoid process

frontal process of zygomatic bone

frontal process of maxilla

transverse processes of vertebra

spinous process of vertebra

scapula

first rib

clavicle

acromion

sternum

coracoid process of scapula

rib cage and pectoral girdle seen from above

process ■ process

the malleus, the largest auditory ossicle: *Anterior p. of malleus*, a slender bony spicule directed anteriorly from just below the neck of the malleus toward the petrotympanic fissure, where it is connected by small ligaments. *Lateral p. of malleus*, a blunt lateral process that projects from the root of the handle (manubrium) of the malleus, attaching to the upper part of the tympanic membrane (eardrum), thereby dividing the tympanic membrane into a small upper flaccid part (pars flaccida), and a large lower taut part (pars tensa). *Long p. of malleus*, see manubrium of malleus, under manubrium.

mamillary p. of lumbar vertebrae A rough elevation on the posterior border of each superior articular process of the lumbar vertebrae; it affords attachment to the multifidus and the medial intertransverse lumbar muscles.

mastoid p. A downward conical projection of the mastoid part of the temporal bone of the skull; situated behind the ear with its apex on a level with the middle of the ear lobe; it contains the mastoid air cells and its lateral surface provides attachment for the sternocleidomastoid muscle and the splenius and longissimus muscles of the head.

maxillary p. of inferior nasal concha The thin, irregular plate descending from the middle of the upper border of the inferior nasal concha and articulating with the maxilla and partially constricting the orifice of the maxillary sinus; it attaches the concha to the lateral wall of the nasal cavity while contributing to the medial wall of the maxillary sinus.

medial p. of calcaneus A large bony process projecting downward from the lower medial portion of the calcaneal tuberosity; separated from the smaller lateral process by a notch and providing attachment to the flexor retinaculum, plantar aponeurosis and some muscles.

odontoid p. of axis A toothlike process, or dens, of the second cervical vertebra that protrudes sharply upward from the vertebral body to articulate with the first cervical vertebra; in the adult, it is about 1.5 cm in length.

orbital p. of palatine bone The irregular, upward and lateral projection from the perpendicular plate of the palatine bone, articulating with the ethmoid, sphenoid, and maxillary bones at the back of the orbit; it is separated from the sphenoidal process of the palatine bone by the sphenopalatine notch.

posterior p. of talus The posterior projection on the back of the talus affording attachment to the posterior talofibular ligament; it is divided by the incisure (groove) of the talus for the tendon of the long flexor of the big toe (flexor hallucis longus) into medial and lateral tubercles.

pterygoid p. A long bony mass extending downward from the base of the skull, at the junction of the body of the sphenoid bone and the greater wing, on either side; it consists of parallel medial and lateral plates, the upper anterior parts of which are fused together, while the posterior parts diverge to form the pterygoid fossa.

pyramidal p. of palatine bone A triangular bony process projecting backward and laterally from the lower part of the palatine bone to articulate with the margins of the pterygoid notch.

sphenoid p. of palatine bone The smaller of the two processes at the upper extremity of the perpendicular plate of the palatine bone; it articulates with the sphenoid concha and the medial pterygoid plate.

spinous p. of vertebra The elongated process that projects backward from the junction of the laminae of the vertebral arch; it provides attachment for ligaments and muscles of the back. See also vertebral spine, under spine.

styloid p. of fibula A process extending upward on the posterolateral surface of the upper end of the fibular head; it provides attachment for the arcuate popliteal ligament of the knee joint and for the tendon of the biceps muscle of the thigh (biceps femoris muscle). Also called apex of head of fibula.

styloid p. of radius A downward-directed blunt conical process on the lateral surface of the lower end of the radius; can be felt through the skin when the overlying tendons are relaxed.

styloid p. of temporal bone A slender, tapering process of variable length, extending downward and slightly forward from the base of the skull; it provides attachment for the stylopharyngeus, styloglossus, and stylohyoid muscles and for the stylomandibular and stylohyoid ligaments.

styloid p. of ulna A short, rounded, non-articular process at the lower end of the posteromedial surface of the ulna; its tip can

process ■ process

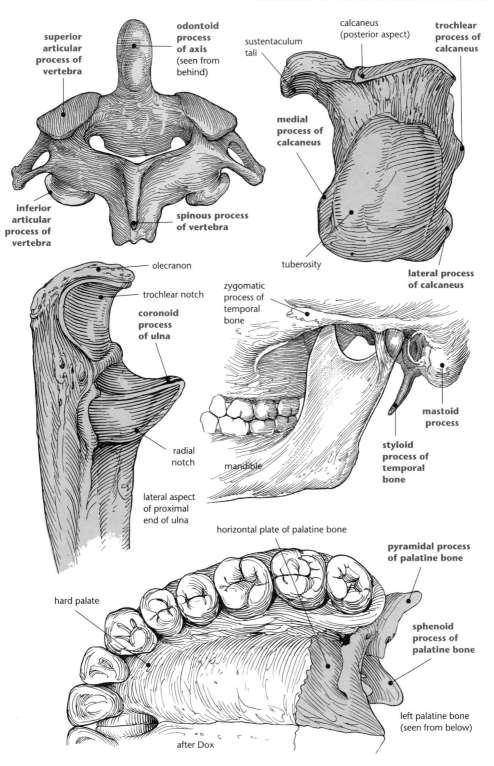

superior articular process of vertebra

odontoid process of axis (seen from behind)

inferior articular process of vertebra

spinous process of vertebra

sustentaculum tali

calcaneus (posterior aspect)

trochlear process of calcaneus

medial process of calcaneus

tuberosity

lateral process of calcaneus

olecranon

trochlear notch

coronoid process of ulna

radial notch

lateral aspect of proximal end of ulna

zygomatic process of temporal bone

mastoid process

styloid process of temporal bone

mandible

horizontal plate of palatine bone

pyramidal process of palatine bone

hard palate

sphenoid process of palatine bone

left palatine bone (seen from below)

after Dox

process ■ process

be felt through the skin on the posteromedial aspect of the wrist.

superior articular p. of vertebra One of a pair of bony projections extending upward from the junction of the pedicle and lamina of a vertebra, bearing the facet for articulation with the facet on the inferior articular process of the vertebra above.

temporal p. of zygomatic bone The posterior prolongation of the zygomatic bone that articulates with the zygomatic process of the temporal bone to form the zygomatic arch.

transverse p. of vertebra The bony process projecting laterally from each side of the arch of a vertebra, providing attachment to muscles and ligaments; in the thoracic area it has facets that articulate with ribs.

trochlear p. of calcaneus A small ridgelike projection from the lateral side of the heel bone (calcaneus) that separates the tendons of the long and short peroneal muscles; located approximately one inch below the lateral malleolus.

uncinate p. of ethmoid bone An irregular bony plate extending from the labyrinth of the ethmoid bone at the front of the orbital plate and curving downward to articulate with the inferior nasal concha to form the medial boundary of the semilunar hiatus (semilunar opening of ethmoid bone).

xiphoid p. The small, flat, pointed process connected to the lower end of the body of the sternum; it is cartilaginous in youth and ossifies with passing age; it provides attachment for the thoracic and abdominal muscles; so called because of its sword shape. Also called xiphoid cartilage.

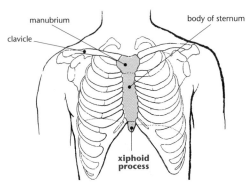

zygomatic p. of frontal bone The strong and prominent process of the frontal bone directed downward at the lateral end of the supraorbital margin, on either side, to articulate with the zygomatic bone to form the lateral margin of the orbit.

zygomatic p. of maxilla The broad, rough, pyramidal projection from the anterior surface of the maxilla that articulates with the zygomatic bone.

zygomatic p. of temporal bone The narrow prolongation of the temporal bone projecting anteriorly to articulate with the temporal process of the zygomatic bone to form the zygomatic arch. .

profunda (pro-fun'da) Latin (feminine) for deep; applied to certain anatomic structures.

profundus (pro-fun'dus) Latin (masculine) for deep; applied to certain anatomic structures.

prognathism (prog'nah-thizm) Abnormal forward projection of one or both jaws.

prominence (prom'ĭ-nens) A projection or elevation.

canine p. See cuspid eminence, under eminence.

laryngeal p. The subcutaneous projection at the front of the neck formed by the prominence of the thyroid cartilage; it enlarges in males at puberty. Also called Adam's apple; laryngeal protuberance.

p. of malleus A small projection on the upper inner surface of the tympanic membrane (eardrum), seen on otoscopic examination, and produced by the underlying lateral process of the first ear ossicle (malleus); it separates the small flaccid part of the tympanic membrane from the larger taut portion.

promontory (prom'on-to-re) A projecting part.

pronator (pro-na'tor) Any muscle involved in turning a part into the prone position.

proprioceptor (pro-pre-o-sep'tor) A sensory nerve ending, mainly located within muscles and tendons, that collects information relating to sensations of the body's movements and position.

muscle p. See muscle spindle, under spindle.

prosthion (pros'the-on) A craniometric point at the midpoint of the alveolar rim of the maxilla; it is the most anterior projection, between the two central incisors. Also called alveolar point.

protuberance (pro-tu'ber-ans) A prominence or bulge, usually rounded or blunt.

p. of chin See mental protuberance.

external occipital p. A prominence on the back of the skull, at the middle of the outer surface of the occipital bone, midway between the foramen magnum and the summit of the bone, to which the nuchal ligament is attached.

process ■ protuberance

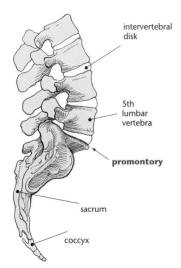

intervertebral disk

5th lumbar vertebra

promontory

sacrum

coccyx

Relating to the pterygoid process of the sphenoid bone and the mandible (lower jaw).

pterygomaxillary (ter-ĭ-go-mak'sĭ-ler-e) Relating to the pterygoid process of the sphenoid bone and the maxilla (upper jaw).

pterygopalatine (ter-ĭ-go-pal'ah-tin) Relating to the pterygoid process of the sphenoid bone and the hard palate.

pubic (pu'bik) Relating to the pubic bone or area.

pubis (pu'bis) 1. The pubic bone. 2. The region over the pubic bone.

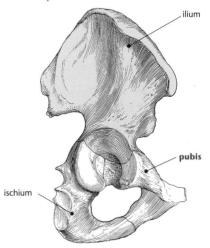

ilium

pubis

ischium

frontal p. See frontal eminence, under eminence.

internal occipital p. A prominence at the midpoint of the inner surface of the occipital bone next to the confluence of the sinuses; it divides the bone into four fossae.

laryngeal p. See laryngeal prominence, under prominence.

mental p. The prominence of the chin formed at the midline of the lower border of the body of the mandible. Also called protuberance of chin.

parietal p. See parietal eminence, under eminence.

tubal p. The cartilaginous projection of the posterior lip of the pharyngeal opening of the auditory (eustachian) tube, to which the salpingopharyngeal muscle is attached.

proximal (prok'sĭ-mal) 1. Nearest the center, midline, or point of origin. 2. The surface of a tooth that is nearest an adjacent tooth, on either side.

pseudarthrosis (su-dar-thro'sis) An abnormal joint formed on the shaft of a long bone, at the site of an ununited fracture. Also called false joint.

pseudofracture (su-do-frak'tūr) An x-ray image of periosteal thickening and new bone formation in an area of injury that gives the appearance of an incomplete fracture.

psoas (so'as) See table of muscles in appendix II.

pterion (te're-on) A craniometric point on either side of the skull at the junction of four bones: frontal, sphenoid, parietal, and temporal. Also called sylvian point.

pterygoid (ter'ĭ-goid) Wing-shaped, applied to various anatomic structures, such as the pterygoid process of the sphenoid bone.

pterygomandibular (ter-ĭ-go-man-dib'u-lar)

pump (pump) A device that propels a fluid to move in a desired direction.

muscle p. The contracting calf muscles act as a pump to propel peripheral venous blood up from the lower extremity toward the heart.

pyarthrosis (pi-ar-thro'sis) Purulent joint infection as seen in acute suppurative arthritis.

pyloromyotomy (pi-lo-ro-mi-ot'o-me) A surgical muscle-splitting incision of the pylorus (up to the mucosal layer) for the relief of hypertrophic pyloric stenosis, a condition occasionally seen in newborn infants.

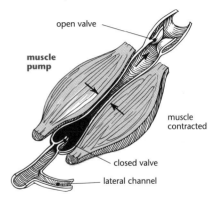

open valve

muscle pump

muscle contracted

closed valve

lateral channel

proximal ■ pyloromyotomy

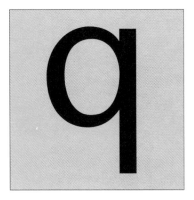

quadrate (kwod'rāt) A four-sided structure; especially used to describe four-sided muscles. See also table of muscles in appendix II.

quadriceps (kwod'rĭ-seps) Having four heads; applied to certain muscles, especially the quadriceps muscle of the thigh (quadriceps femoris), the large muscle of the anterior thigh.

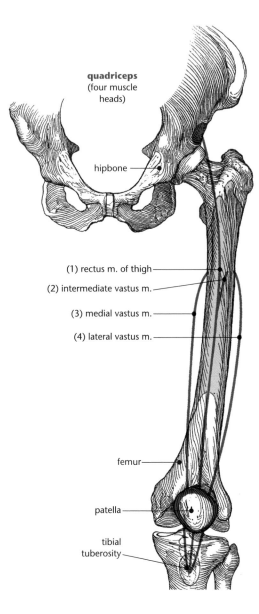

quadriceps
(four muscle
heads)

hipbone

(1) rectus m. of thigh

(2) intermediate vastus m.

(3) medial vastus m.

(4) lateral vastus m.

femur

patella

tibial
tuberosity

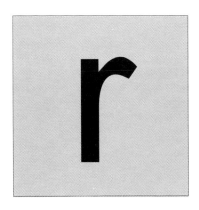

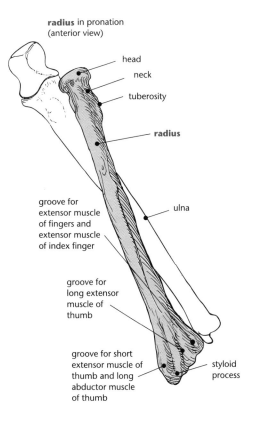

radius in pronation
(anterior view)

head

neck

tuberosity

radius

groove for
extensor muscle
of fingers and
extensor muscle
of index finger

ulna

groove for
long extensor
muscle of
thumb

groove for short
extensor muscle of
thumb and long
abductor muscle
of thumb

styloid
process

radial (ra'de-al) 1. Relating to a bone in the forearm (radius) or to the side of the forearm in which the radius is positioned. 2. Diverging in several directions from a central point.

radicular (rah-dik'u-lar) Relating to the root of an anatomic structure (e.g., of a tooth).

radiocarpal (ra-de-o-kar'pal) Relating to the radius and the wrist bones (carpus), especially the joint between the lower end of the radius and the proximal row of wrist bones. Also called cubitocarpal.

radiohumeral (ra-de-o-hu'mer-al) Relating to two bones, the radius (in the forearm) and the humerus (in the arm).

radiopalmar (ra-de-o-pal'mar) 1. Relating to the radial (lateral) side of the palm. 2. Relating to the radius and the palm.

radioulnar (ra-de-o-ul'nar) Relating to the two bones of the forearm, radius and ulna.

radius (ra'de-us) The shorter of the two bones of the forearm, situated on the side of the thumb. See also table of bones in appendix I.

ramus (ra'mus), pl. ra'mi 1. A branch; the term is commonly used to describe branches or subdivisions of nerves, but is applicable to other anatomic structures. 2. A slender part of an irregularly shaped bone that angles away from the main body of the bone.

    ischiopubic r. The bony bar formed by the conjoined ramus of the ischium and the inferior ramus of the pubis on each side, contributing to the formation of the pubic arch.

    r. of ischium The ramus that projects from the tuberosity of the ischium in an upward medial direction to fuse with the inferior ramus of the pubic bone.

    r. of mandible The broad quadrilateral bony process projecting upward from the posterior part of the mandible on either side; it affords attachment on its lateral surface to

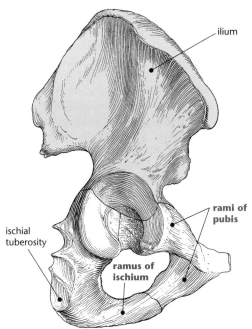

ilium

rami of
pubis

ischial
tuberosity

ramus of
ischium

radial ■ ramus

muscles of mastication.

rami of pubis The two rami that project from the body of the pubic bone at the anteroinferior portion of the hipbone; the superior ramus projects from the body in an upward posterolateral direction to fuse with the ilium and the ischium to form part of the acetabulum; the inferior ramus projects from the body in a downward postero-lateral direction to fuse with the ramus of the ischium.

raphe (ra'fe) A ridge or line marking the union of two similar structures.

r. of pharynx A strong fibrous seam extending downward from the base of the skull along the midline plane of the posterior wall of the pharynx, and affording attachment to the constrictor muscles of the pharynx of the two sides.

pterygomandibular r. A narrow tendinous band extending from the pterygoid hamulus of the skull to the inner surface of the lower jaw at the level of the third molar; it provides attachment anteriorly to the buccinator muscle (of the cheek) and posteriorly to the superior constrictor muscle of the pharynx.

recess (re'ses) A small shallow cavity or indentation; a depression.

epitympanic r. The portion of the middle ear chamber situated above the level of the tympanic membrane (eardrum); it contains the head of the malleus and the body of the incus.

piriform r. An elongated recess in the laryngopharynx on each side of the opening of the larynx, bounded medially by the aryepiglottic fold and laterally by the thyrohyoid membrane and the lamina of the thyroid cartilage. Also called piriform fossa.

sacciform r. of distal radioulnar articulation The bulging of the articular capsule of the elbow joint, caused by an extension of the cavity of the radioulnar articulation.

sphenoethmoidal r. A narrow cleftlike fossa at the most superior and posterior part of the nasal cavity, bounded above by the cribriform plate of the ethmoid bone and the body of the sphenoid bone and below by the superior concha in the lateral wall of the nasal cavity into which the sphenoidal sinus opens.

subpopliteal r. See bursa of popliteal tendon, under bursa.

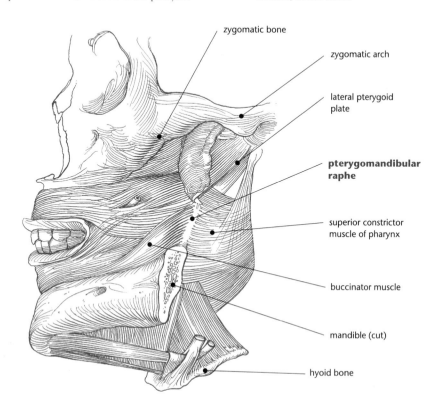

zygomatic bone

zygomatic arch

lateral pterygoid plate

pterygomandibular raphe

superior constrictor muscle of pharynx

buccinator muscle

mandible (cut)

hyoid bone

raphe ■ recess

reflex (re'fleks) l. An involuntary and immediate response to a stimulus. 2. Turned backward.

abdominal r. Contraction of the abdominal wall musculature elicited by light stroking of the overlying skin.

Achilles r. Contraction of the calf muscles with resulting plantar flexion of the foot, elicited by a sharp tap on the Achilles (calcaneal) tendon. Also called Achilles tendon reflex; ankle reflex; ankle jerk; calcaneal tendon reflex; Achilles jerk.

Achilles tendon r. See Achilles reflex.

acquired r. See conditioned reflex.

acromial r. Contraction of the biceps muscle of the arm (biceps brachii) with flexion of the forearm upon sharply striking the acromion of the scapula.

adductor r. of thigh Adduction of the abducted thigh upon tapping the tendon of the great adductor muscle (adductor magnus) near its lowest point of insertion onto the adductor tubercle of the distal femur.

ankle r. See Achilles reflex.

Babinski r. See extensor plantar reflex.

biceps r. The normal contraction of the biceps muscle of the arm (biceps brachii) with further flexion of the partially bent elbow on tapping its tendon of insertion in the antecubital fossa. Also called biceps jerk.

bladder r. See micturition reflex.

brachioradial r. Contraction of the brachioradialis muscle when tapping the lower end of the radius in a partially pronated forearm, causing flexion and partial rotation of the forearm and hand (supination). Also called radioperiosteal reflex; supinator jerk; supinator jerk reflex.

calcaneal tendon r. See Achilles reflex.

conditioned r. A reflex that is developed through association with, and repetition of, a stimulus. Also called acquired reflex; trained reflex.

coordinated r. Reflex involving several muscles.

cremasteric r. Retraction of the testicle upon gently scratching the inner aspect of the upper thigh of the same side.

crossed r. A muscular contraction on one side of the body elicited by a sharp tap on the opposite side.

crossed adductor r. Inward rotation of the leg upon tapping of the sole.

crossed extension r. Response elicited from a newborn infant indicating integrity of the spinal cord; placing the child in the supine position, the examiner extends and presses down on one of the child's legs and stimulates the sole of the foot; this causes the free leg to flex, adduct, and then extend.

crossed knee r. Contraction of the anterior muscles of the thigh in response to a sharp tap on the patellar ligament of the opposite knee. Also called crossed knee jerk.

deep r. Any of a group of reflexes characterized by a sudden brief stretching and then immediate contraction of a muscle, elicited by a sharp tap on the muscle or its tendon. Also called myotatic reflex; deep tendon reflex; tendon reflex; stretch reflex; tendon jerk.

deep tendon r. See deep reflex.

elbow r. See triceps reflex.

extensor plantar r. Abnormal reflex characterized by extension of the big toe with fanning of the small toes upon scratching the sole of the foot. Also called Babinski reflex. COMPARE plantar reflex.

extensor plantar reflex

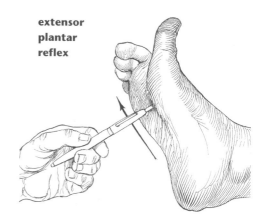

femoral r. Extension of the knee and plantar flexion of the toes induced by stroking the upper anterior part of the thigh. Also called Remak's reflex.

Gordon r. Abnormal reflex characterized by extension of the big toe elicited by firm squeezing of the calf muscles.

interscapular r. Striking the back of the body between the two scapulas usually causes contraction of the rhomboid muscles and approximation of the scapulas.

knee r. See patellar reflex.

knee-jerk r. See patellar reflex.

mandibular r. Brisk closure of the mouth caused by a spasmodic contraction of the muscles of mastication following a downward

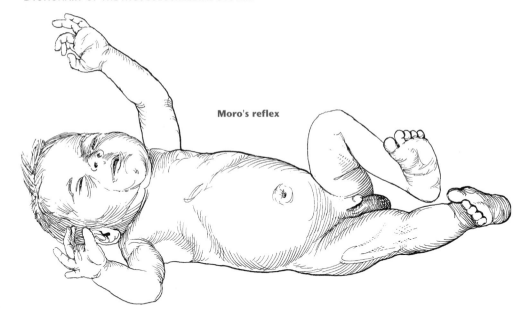

Moro's reflex

tap on the chin while the lower jaw hangs loosely open. Also called jaw jerk.

micturition r. Any of the reflexes controlling effortless urination and the subconscious ability to retain urine within the bladder. Also called bladder reflex; urinary reflex; vesical reflex.

Moro's r., Moro's embrace r. A normal reflex of newborn infants in response to loud noises or sudden changes in position; characterized by tensing of muscles, a wide embracing motion of the arms, and extension of the thighs, legs, and fingers, except the thumb and index finger, which remain in a "C" position. Also called startle reflex.

myotatic r. See deep reflex.

olecranon r. Flexion of the forearm when the olecranon is tapped.

oral r. Normal reflex elicited when the corner of the mouth of a newborn infant is touched; the bottom lip lowers on the same side and the tongue moves forward and toward the examiner's finger.

patellar r. Extension of the leg upon tapping of the patellar tendon while the leg hangs loosely at right angles to the thigh. Also called knee jerk; knee-jerk reflex; knee reflex; patellar tendon reflex; quadriceps reflex; quadriceps jerk.

patellar tendon r. See patellar reflex.

plantar r. Flexion of the toes upon scratching of the sole of the foot; a normal

response. Also called sole reflex. COMPARE extensor plantar reflex.

primitive r. Any of the reflexes occurring naturally in the newborn; an indication of normal neuromuscular development; it occurs in the adult only in certain degenerative disorders.

pronator r. Pronation and adduction of the hand in response to striking the styloid process of the distal ulna. Also called ulnar reflex.

proprioceptive r. Any of various reflexes brought about by stimulation of sensory nerve endings (proprioceptors), which respond to stimuli relating to movements

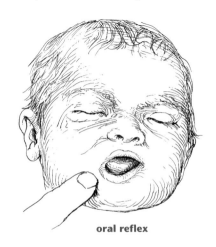

oral reflex

and position of the body.

quadriceps r. See patellar reflex.

radial r. Flexion of the forearm upon tapping of the lower end of the radius.

radioperiosteal r. See brachioradial reflex.

Remak's r. See femoral reflex.

scapulohumeral r. Adduction and lateral rotation of the arm due to contraction of the subscapular muscle when the vertebral border of the scapula is struck.

sole r. See plantar reflex.

startle r. See Moro's reflex.

stretch r. See deep reflex.

superficial r. Any reflex elicited by stimulation of the skin and mucous membranes.

supinator jerk r. See brachioradial reflex.

suprapatellar r. The patella rises when contraction of the quadriceps is induced by percussing sharply a finger placed along the upper border of the patella; a variation of the patellar reflex.

tendon r. See deep reflex.

trained r. See conditioned reflex.

triceps r. A sudden extension of the forearm on tapping of the triceps tendon at the elbow while the forearm hangs loosely at a right angle to the arm. Also called elbow reflex; elbow jerk.

ulnar r. See pronator reflex.

urinary r. See micturition reflex.

vesical r. See micturition reflex.

region (re'jun) l. An arbitrary division, or continuous area on the surface of the body, with more or less definite boundaries. 2. A bodily part having a special function.

abdominal r.'s The nine regions into which the abdomen is divided by imaginary planes, namely the right and left hypochondriac, epigastric, right and left lumbar, umbilical, right and left inguinal, and pubic.

cubital r. A region around the elbow: *Anterior cubital r.*, the front part of the elbow; *Posterior cubital r.*, the back part of the elbow.

femoral r. The region of the thigh.

frontal r. The region of the forehead, overlying the frontal bone of the skull.

gluteal r. The region of the buttock, overlying the gluteal muscles.

infraclavicular r. The region of the chest, just below the clavicle.

nuchal r. The region of the back of the neck.

occipital r. The part of the scalp in the back of the head overlying the occipital bone.

patellar r. The part of the leg in front of the knee.

perineal r. The region overlying the pelvic outlet; it is divided into two triangles by a transverse line connecting the ischial tuberosities; a triangle of the anal region posteriorly and a triangle of the urogenital region (perineum) anteriorly.

popliteal r. The region in the back of the knee.

pubic r. The lowest midabdominal region, between the inguinal regions.

sacral r. The region of the lower back overlying the sacrum.

sacrococcygeal r. The region of the lower back overlying the sacrum and coccyx.

supraclavicular r. The hollow above the collarbone (clavicle), on each side.

suprasternal r. The hollow in the midline of the front of the neck, just above the suprasternal notch.

umbilical r. The central part of the abdomen surrounding the navel (umbilicus); situated above the transtubercular plane and below the transpyloric plane.

zygomatic r. The part of the face on either side, over the zygomatic (cheek) bone.

retinaculum (ret-ĭ-nak'u-lum), pl. retinac'ula A fascial band that retains a structure in place.

extensor r. of ankle Strong fascial band overlying the ankle joint: *Inferior extensor r. of ankle*, a retinaculum of deep fascia shaped like the letter Y, with the stem extending from the lateral wall of the upper part of the calcaneus, passing medially as two segments;

abdominal regions

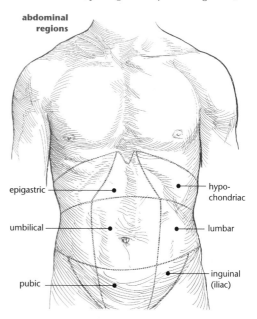

epigastric

umbilical

pubic

hypo-chondriac

lumbar

inguinal (iliac)

region ■ retinaculum

the upper segment attaches to the medial malleolus of the tibia and the lower segment descends to the plantar aponeurosis; the retinaculum overrides the tendons of the extensor muscles (anterior tibial muscle, long extensor muscle of big toe, long extensor muscle of toes, and third peroneal muscle) and helps to keep them in their proper place. *Superior extensor r. of ankle,* a thickening of deep fascia anchored to the lower part of the tibia and fibula of the leg; it extends from the anterior border of the tibia transversely to the anterior border of the fibula and overrides the tendons of the extensor muscles (anterior tibial muscle, long extensor muscle of big toe, long extensor muscle of toes, and third peroneal muscle).

extensor r. of hand See extensor retinaculum of wrist.

extensor r. of wrist A strong band extending obliquely across the back of the wrist; it retains in position the extensor tendons of the fingers. Also called extensor retinaculum of hand.

fibular patellar r.
See patellar retinaculum, lateral.

flexor r. of ankle A thickened band of fascia in back of the ankle joint passing from the bottom of the medial malleolus of the tibia, to the medial side of the calcaneus as well as to the plantar aponeurosis; it overrides the tendons of various muscles (posterior tibial muscle, long flexor muscle of toes, long flexor muscle of big toe) as they make their way to the sole of the foot.

flexor r. of hand
See flexor retinaculum of wrist.

flexor r. of wrist A strong, transverse fibrous band (about 2.5 by 3 cm) that spans the hollow area of the front of the wrist bones (carpus) creating the carpal tunnel, which conveys the median nerve and the flexor tendons of the fingers; a superficial slip projects from it to cross the ulnar vessels and nerve before blending with the rest of the retinaculum. Also called flexor retinaculum of hand.

patellar r. Fibrous bands superficial to the knee joint capsule: *Lateral patellar r.,* a downward tendinous expansion of the lateral vastus muscle blending with the knee joint capsule and extending to the margin of the kneecap (patella), patellar ligament, and condyle of the tibia; it is strengthened by the overlying iliotibial tract. Also called fibular

patellar retinaculum. *Medial patellar r.,* a downward tendinous expansion of the medial vastus muscle blending with the knee joint capsule and extending to the margin of the kneecap (patella), patellar ligament, and condyle of the tibia. Also called tibial patellar retinaculum.

peroneal r. Fibrous slings that hold the peroneal tendons in place as they curve around the lateral side of the ankle: *Inferior peroneal r.,* a band that extends from the stem of the Y-shaped inferior extensor retinaculum to the lateral side of the heel bone (calcaneus). *Superior peroneal r.,* A band that extends from the lower part of the lateral malleolus of the fibula to the lateral side of the calcaneus.

tibial patellar r.
See patellar retinaculum, medial.

retromandibular (re-tro-man-dib'u-lar)
Behind the lower jaw.

retromastoid (re-tro-mas'toid) Posterior to the mastoid process of the temporal bone, especially relating to the posterior mastoid air cells.

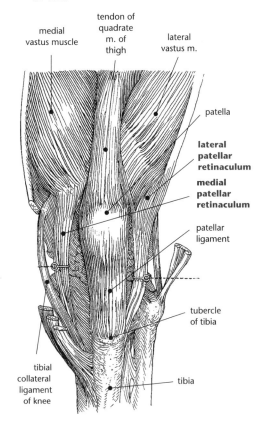

tendon of quadrate m. of thigh

medial vastus muscle

lateral vastus m.

patella

lateral patellar retinaculum

medial patellar retinaculum

patellar ligament

tubercle of tibia

tibial collateral ligament of knee

tibia

retinaculum ■ retromastoid

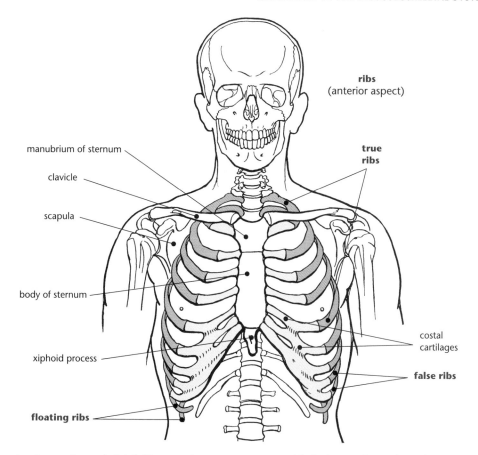

ribs
(anterior aspect)

manubrium of sternum

clavicle

scapula

body of sternum

xiphoid process

floating ribs

true ribs

costal cartilages

false ribs

retropharynx (re-tro-far'inks) The posterior part of the pharynx.

retrospondylolisthesis (re-tro-spon-dĭ-lo-lis-the'sis) Posterior displacement or slippage of a vertebra.

retrosternal (re-tro-ster'nal) Behind the sternum.

rhinion (rin'e-on) The lowest end of the union of the two nasal bones; a craniometric point.

rhomboid (rom'boid) Shaped like a kite, said especially of the rhomboid muscles. See also table of muscles in appendix II.

rib (rib) One of a series of long, thin, rather elastic, curved bones that articulates posteriorly with a thoracic vertebra and extends anteriorly to join the costal cartilage in forming the major part of the thoracic cage; normally there are 12 ribs on each side.

   cervical r. An abnormal extra rib connected to the seventh cervical vertebra, with an anterior end that may be free, or joined to the first rib or costal cartilage, rarely, if ever, to the sternum; it may interfere

with the innervation and vascularization to the arm by compressing the brachial plexus and the axillary artery. Also called pleurapophysis.

   false r. One of the five lower pairs of ribs that does not articulate through its costal cartilage directly with the sternum. Also called vertebrochondral rib; spurious rib.

   floating r. One of the two lower pairs of false ribs that is free at the anterior end. Also called vertebral rib.

   slipping r. Recurrent dislocation of a rib's costal cartilage.

   spurious r. See false rib.

   sternal r. See true rib.

   true r. One of the seven pairs of upper ribs that is connected anteriorly, through the costal cartilage, to the lateral surface of the sternum. Also called vertebrosternal rib; sternal rib.

   vertebral r. See floating rib.

   vertebrochondral r. See false rib.

   vertebrosternal r. See true rib.

retropharynx ■ rib

rickets (rik'ets) A disease primarily of infants and young children, caused by vitamin D deficiency, resulting in defective bone growth.

ridge (rij) A linear elevation (e.g., on a bone or a tooth).

   alveolar r. The bony ridge of the jaw containing sockets (alveoli) which accommodate the roots of teeth.

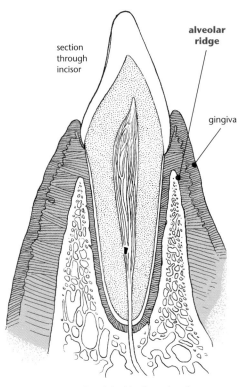

section through incisor

alveolar ridge

gingiva

deltoid r. See deltoid tuberosity of humerus, under tuberosity.

   dental r. Any linear elevation on the surface of a tooth, forming the border of a cusp or the margin of a crown.

   gluteal r. of femur See gluteal tuberosity of femur, under tuberosity.

   interarticular r. of head of rib See crest of head of rib, under crest.

   intertrochanteric r. See trochanteric crest, under crest.

   lateral supracondylar r. of humerus A prominent, curved ridge on the distal sharp portion of the lateral margin of the humerus, providing attachment in front to the long radial extensor muscle of wrist (extensor carpi radialis longus) and the brachioradial muscle. Also called lateral supracondylar crest of humerus.

   medial supracondylar r. of humerus A prominent, curved ridge on the distal sharp portion of the medial margin of the humerus, providing attachment to the brachial muscle in front and to the medial head of the triceps muscle of arm (triceps brachii) behind. Also called medial supracondylar crest of humerus.

   mylohyoid r. See mylohyoid line, under line.

   oblique r. A variable ridge running across the chewing surface of an upper molar.

   palatine r. One of four or six transverse ridges on the anterior region of the hard palate.

   Passavant's r. The prominence formed in the posterior wall of the pharynx by the contraction of the superior constrictor muscle during the act of swallowing.

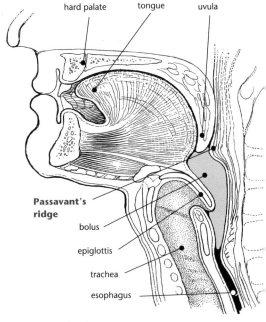

hard palate   tongue   uvula

Passavant's ridge

bolus

epiglottis

trachea

esophagus

   supinator r. See supinator crest, under crest.

   supraorbital r. The curved elevation of the frontal bone forming the upper border of the eye socket.

   temporal r.'s See temporal lines, under line.

   transverse r. of sacrum See transverse line of sacrum, under line.

rima (ri'mah) A cleft, fissure, slit, or elongated opening.

   r. glottidis See fissure of glottis,

under fissure.

r. vestibuli
See fissure of false glottis, under fissure.

ring (ring) A circular band of tissue surrounding an opening.

abdominal r. See deep inguinal ring.

common tendinous r. See common annular tendon, under tendon.

deep inguinal r. The oval orifice in the transverse fascia of the external oblique muscle marking the deep opening of the inguinal canal. Also called abdominal ring; internal inguinal ring.

external inguinal r.
See superficial inguinal ring.

femoral r. The abdominal or superior oval opening of the conical femoral canal underlying the inguinal ligament at the groin; it is bounded posteriorly by the pectineus muscle, medially by the lacunar ligament and laterally by the femoral vein. It is normally filled with extraperitoneal fatty and lymphoid tissues and is a potential site of hernia.

internal inguinal r. See deep inguinal ring.

subcutaneous inguinal r.
See superficial inguinal ring.

superficial inguinal r. The orifice in the aponeurosis of the external oblique muscle forming the external opening of the inguinal canal. Also called external inguinal ring; subcutaneous inguinal ring.

tracheal r.'s
See tracheal cartilages, under cartilage.

tympanic r. An incomplete bony ring at the medial end of the cartilaginous external auditory canal that supports the tympanic membrane in the fetus and newborn; it develops into the tympanic part of the temporal bone.

umbilical r. The opening in the abdominal connective tissue (linea alba) of the fetus through which pass the umbilical arteries and veins.

roof (roof) Any structure functioning as the cover of a cavity.

r. of mouth See palate.

r. of skull See calvaria.

root (root) 1. The attachment by which an anatomic structure is secured to its base. 2. The embedded part of a structure, as of a tooth or hair.

anatomic r. The root of a tooth extending from the cervical line to its apical extremity and normally contained in the bony socket of the jaw; the part of the tooth covered by cementum.

clinical r. The portion of the tooth below the gingival crest, which is not visible in the mouth.

lingual r. The back part of the tongue, behind the V-shaped furrow (terminal sulcus of tongue).

r. of nose The upper part of the nose adjoining the forehead, between the two orbits.

rotator (ro'ta-tor) Any muscle that rotates a body part around a specified axis.

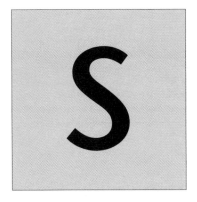

sac (sak) A pouchlike anatomic structure.

    endolymphatic s. The blind extremity of the endolymphatic duct of the inner ear, situated under the dura mater on the back surface of the petrous part of the temporal bone.

    synovial s. A closed pouch of synovial membrane extending beyond the normal confines of the joint; it contains a thick, viscous, lubricating fluid (similar to the white of an egg) that facilitates movement of the joint.

sacrad (sa′krad) Toward the sacrum.

sacral (sa′kral) Relating to the sacrum.

sacro-, sacr- Combining forms meaning sacrum.

sacrococcygeal (sa-kro-kok-sij′e-al) Relating to the sacrum and the coccyx.

sacrococcyx (sa-kro-kok′siks) The sacrum and the coccyx considered as a unit.

sacroiliac (sa-kro-il′e-ak) Relating to the sacrum and ilium.

sacrosciatic (sa-kro-si-at′ik) Relating to the sacrum and the ischium.

sacrospinal (sa-kro-spi′nal) See sacrovertebral.

sacrovertebral (sa-kro-ver′tĕ-bral) Relating to the sacrum and the rest of the vertebral column. Also called sacrospinal.

sacrum (sa′krum) A slightly curved, triangular bone composed of five fused vertebrae, forming the back of the pelvis; it articulates on each side with the corresponding ilium and with the last lumbar vertebra above, and the coccyx below.

    assimilation s. A condition in which the last lumbar vertebra is fused to the sacrum or the last sacral vertebra is fused to the first coccygeal body.

    tilted s. A forward displacement of the sacrum resulting from separation of the sacroiliac joints.

sagittal (saj′ĭ-tal) In an anteroposterior direction; i.e., occurring or situated in the median plane of the body or in a plane parallel to it.

sarcoma (sar-ko′mah) Cancerous tumor composed of connective tissue.

    Ewing's s. An uncommon malignant tumor of bone, affecting predominantly long tubular and pelvic bones; occurs in children and young adults. Also called Ewing's tumor.

    osteogenic s. A malignant primary tumor of bone composed of a malignant connective tissue stroma with strong indications of malignant bone or cartilage formation. Also called osteosarcoma.

    synovial s. A highly malignant tumor arising from synovial epithelial cells; seen most commonly around joints rather than within (e.g., in relation to bursae and tendon sheath); seen also around the pharynx and in the abdominal wall. Also called malignant synovioma.

sarcostosis (sar-ko-sto′sis) Ossification of muscle tissue.

sarcous (sar′kus) Relating to muscle tissue.

saucerization (saw-ser-i-za′shun) A flat, disk-shaped defect formed along the shaft of a long bone; it contains microscopic calcifications and is considered typical of a fibrosarcoma with bone involvement.

scala (ska′lah), pl. sca′lae An anatomic structure resembling a winding staircase; applied especially to some passages of the cochlea (in the inner ear).

    s. media See cochlear duct, under duct.

    s. tympani The perilymph-filled canal, about 36 mm in length, within the cochlea; it is continuous with the scala vestibuli through the helicotrema, a small opening at the apex of the cochlea; it spirals about $2^3/_4$ turns and increases gradually in diameter

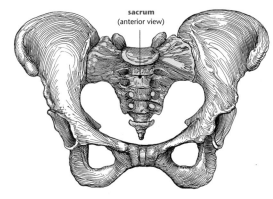

sacrum
(anterior view)

from the apex to the base; it ends blindly near the round window (fenestra cochleae) where it is separated from the middle ear chamber by the secondary tympanic membrane. Also called tympanic canal of cochlea.

s. vestibuli The perilymph-filled canal, about 36 mm in length, within the cochlea; it is continuous with the scala tympani through the helicotrema, a small opening at the apex of the cochlea; it spirals about $2^3/_4$ turns and diminishes gradually in diameter from the base to the apex. The canal begins near the inside of the oval window (fenestra vestibuli) where it is separated from the middle ear chamber by the base or footplate of the smallest ear ossicle (stapes), which occludes the window. Also called vestibular canal of cochlea.

scalene (ska'lēn) A triangle with sides of unequal length; applied to certain muscles. See also table of muscles in appendix II.

scapha (ska'fah) See scaphoid fossa, under fossa.

scaphoid (skaf'oid) Boat-shaped; applied to certain bones. See also table of bones in appendix I.

scapula (skap'u-lah), pl. scap'ulas, scap'ulae Either of two large, flat, triangular bones overlying the upper part of the ribs, and forming the back of the shoulder; it articulates laterally with the humerus and medially with the clavicle. Also called shoulder blade.

alar s. See winged scapula.

Graves' s. See scaphoid scapula.

scaphoid s. A scapula in which the vertebral (medial) border is slightly concave. Also called Graves' scapula.

winged s. A scapula having a prominent vertebral (medial) border that stands out from the thorax; generally caused by paralysis of the anterior serratus muscle. Also called alar scapula.

scapular (skap'u-lar) Relating to the scapula (shoulder blade).

scapuloclavicular (skap-u-lo-klah-vik'u-lar) Relating to the scapula and the clavicle.

scapulohumeral (skap-u-lo-hu'mer-al) Relating to the scapula and the humerus.

schindylesis (skin-dĭ-le'sis) A fibrous joint in which the sharp edge of one bone fits into a groove of the other (e.g., the articulation between the vomer and the rostrum of the sphenoid bone in the skull).

sciatic (si-at'ik) Relating to the hip or to the ischium.

scolio- Combining form meaning crooked.

scoliokyphosis (sko-le-o-ki-fo'sis) Associated scoliosis and kyphosis, i.e., both lateral (scoliotic) and posterior (kyphotic) abnormal curvature of the spine.

scoliolordosis (sko-le-o-lor-do'sis) Associated scoliosis and lordosis, i.e., both lateral (scoliotic) and anterior (lordotic) abnormal curvature of the spine.

scoliosis (sko-le-o'sis) An abnormal, lateral curvature of the spine.

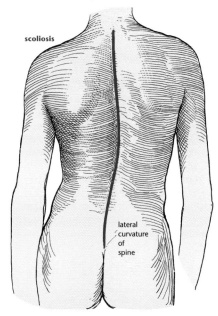

scoliosis

lateral curvature of spine

congenital s. Scoliosis present at birth attributed to congenital anomalies of the vertebrae.

coxitic s. Scoliosis in the lumbar spine attributed to tilting of the pelvis; caused by hip-joint disease.

fixed s. Lateral curvature of the spine that cannot be corrected by suspension or manipulation, often due to deformities of muscles and bones.

habit s. Lateral curvature of the spine resulting from persistent poor posture.

idiopathic s. Scoliosis of unknown cause.

inflammatory s. Lateral curvature of the spine due to vertebral disease associated with acute inflammation.

myopathic s. Scoliosis due to weakness or paralysis of spinal muscles. Also called paralytic scoliosis.

neuromuscular s. Scoliosis caused by any of various diseases affecting the motor nerve cells.

scalene ■ scoliosis

osteopathic s. Scoliosis caused by disease of the vertebrae (e.g., tuberculosis, osteomalacia, tumors, rickets).

paralytic s. See myopathic scoliosis.

static s. Lateral curvature of the spine attributed to difference in the length of the legs.

scute (skut) A thin scalelike plate.

tympanic s. The thin bony plate separating the upper part of the middle ear chamber from the mastoid air cells.

sella (sel'ah) See sella turcica.

sella turcica (sel'ah tur'si-kah) A depression with two prominences (anterior and posterior) on the upper surface of the sphenoid bone in the middle cranial fossa at the base of the skull; it resembles a Turkish saddle and houses the pituitary (hypophysis). Frequently called sella.

semiflexion (sem-e-flek'shun) The position of a limb midway between extension and flexion.

semipenniform (sem-e-pen'ĭ-form) Shaped like a feather on one side only; applied to certain muscles. Also called unipennate.

semitendinous (sem-e-ten'dĭ-nus) Partly tendinous; applied to certain muscles.

sensorimuscular (sen-so-re-mus'ku-lar) Denoting reflex action of muscles in response to a sensory stimulus.

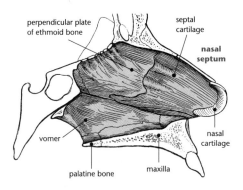

perpendicular plate of ethmoid bone

septal cartilage

nasal septum

vomer

nasal cartilage

palatine bone   maxilla

septum (sep'tum), pl. sep'ta A thin wall or partition between two cavities or masses of soft tissue.

alveolar s. See interalveolar septum.

atrial s. See interatrial septum.

femoral s. The delicate layer of connective tissue that closes the femoral ring (anulus femoralis) at the base of the femoral canal; it is perforated by lymphatic vessels.

interalveolar s. The thin alveolar bone that separates the tooth sockets. Also called alveolar septum.

interatrial s. The partition between the right and left atria of the heart. Also called atrial septum.

intermuscular s. A fascial sheet that separates adjacent muscles of the limbs or groups of muscles.

interradicular s. The thin alveolar bone that separates the sockets of a multirooted tooth.

interventricular s. The musculomembranous partition dividing the right and left ventricles of the heart. Also called ventricular septum.

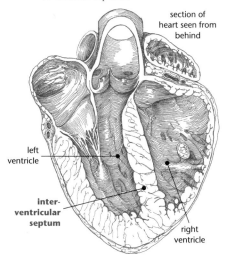

section of heart seen from behind

left ventricle

inter-ventricular septum

right ventricle

nasal s. The thin median wall dividing the nasal cavity into right and left halves; composed posteriorly of bone (vomer, perpendicular plate of ethmoid, nasal crests of the maxilla and palatine bones) and anteriorly of cartilage (septal cartilage).

ventricular s. See interventricular septum.

serosynovitis (se-ro-sin-o-vi'tis) Inflammation of the lining membrane of a joint cavity with effusion of serum into the cavity.

serrate, serrated (ser'āt, ser'āt-ed) Notched.

sesamoid (ses'ah-moid) 1. Resembling a sesame seed; nodular. 2. Denoting a small, ovoid bone that is embedded within a tendon or a capsule of a joint to facilitate sliding over a hard structure, such as bone; it is found mainly within the tendons of the extremities; the kneecap (patella) is the largest such bone in the body.

shaft (shaft) An elongated or rodlike structure, such as the portion of the long bone between the epiphyses.

s. of femur The main cylindrical part of the femur that extends distally from the tuberosities to the condyles; it is fortified by a strong ridge (linea aspera) that divides into the lateral and medial supracondylar ridges at the lower part of the humerus.

s. of fibula The main part of the fibula that extends from the head of the fibula proximally to the lateral malleolus distally.

s. of humerus The main part of the humerus that extends from the surgical neck proximally to the epicondyles distally.

s. of radius The main part of the radius that extends distally from the tuberosity to the lower end of the bone.

s. of tibia The elongated or main part of the tibia that extends from the proximal end at the knee with the two condyles to the distal end at the ankle with the medial malleolus.

s. of ulna The elongated or main part of the ulna that extends from the hook-like proximal end at the elbow to the distal end at the wrist.

shank (shangk) The anterior part of the human leg, from the knee to the ankle.

sheath (shēth) An enveloping structure, usually composed of connective tissue that surrounds a structure, such as a muscle or tendon.

common s. of extensor digitorum longus and peroneus tertius The common synovial sheath around the tendons of the long extensor muscle of the toes (extensor digitorum longus) and the third peroneal muscle (peroneus tertius), situated mostly under the inferior retinaculum on the dorsum of the foot.

common synovial s. of digital flexors A large common synovial sac around the tendons of the deep and superficial flexor muscles of the fingers (flexor digitorum profundus and flexor digitorum superficialis); it extends from the distal part of the forearm, traverses the flexor retinaculum, ending in the palm halfway along the metacarpal bones, where often it is continuous with the synovial sheath of the little finger.

common s. of tendons of peroneal muscles A common synovial sheath around the tendons of the long peroneal muscle and the short peroneal muscle (the lateral group of muscles that are evertors of the foot) stretching across the lateral side of the ankle, below the peroneal trochlea.

crural s. See femoral sheath.

femoral s. A downward funnel-shaped sheath, about 1.25 cm in length, located behind and just below the inguinal ligament of the groin, and derived from the intra-abdominal fascia; it is divided into three compartments: the lateral compartment contains the femoral artery, the middle one contains the femoral vein, the medial one (femoral canal) contains lymphatic vessels and a lymph node. Also called crural sheath.

synovial s. A thin, double-layered sheath commonly found around tendons (tendon synovial sheath) where it lies in contact with bone; it passes under a ligamentous band, through a fascial sling, or osseofibrous tunnel. The intervening space of the sheath contains a capillary mucuslike film of synovial fluid to facilitate the gliding of the tendon. Also called synovial sheath of tendon.

synovial s. of abductor pollicis longus and extensor pollicis brevis The common synovial sheath for the tendons of the long abductor muscle of the thumb (abductor pollicis longus) and the short extensor muscle of the thumb (extensor pollicis brevis); it commences just proximal to the extensor retinaculum, which it traverses, and ends by bifurcating at the base of the 1st metacarpal bone.

synovial s. of extensor carpi radialis longus and brevis The common synovial sheath for the long radial extensor muscle of the wrist (extensor carpi radialis longus) and the short radial extensor muscle of the wrist (extensor carpi radialis brevis); it commences just proximal to the extensor retinaculum and ends at the dorsal surface of the base of the 2nd and 3rd metacarpal bones; after passing under the extensor retinaculum, it often communicates with the overlying synovial sheath of the extensor pollicis longus.

synovial s. of extensor carpi ulnaris The synovial sheath around the tendon of the ulnar extensor muscle of the wrist (extensor carpi ulnaris); it commences proximal to the extensor retinaculum, which it traverses, and ends at the insertion of the tendon at the base of the 5th metacarpal bone.

synovial s. of extensor digiti minimi The synovial sheath around the tendon of the extensor muscle of the little finger (extensor digiti minimi); it extends from the lower end of the forearm to the middle of the 5th metacarpal bone; it is partially covered by the extensor retinaculum.

synovial s. of extensor hallucis longus The synovial sheath around the tendon of the

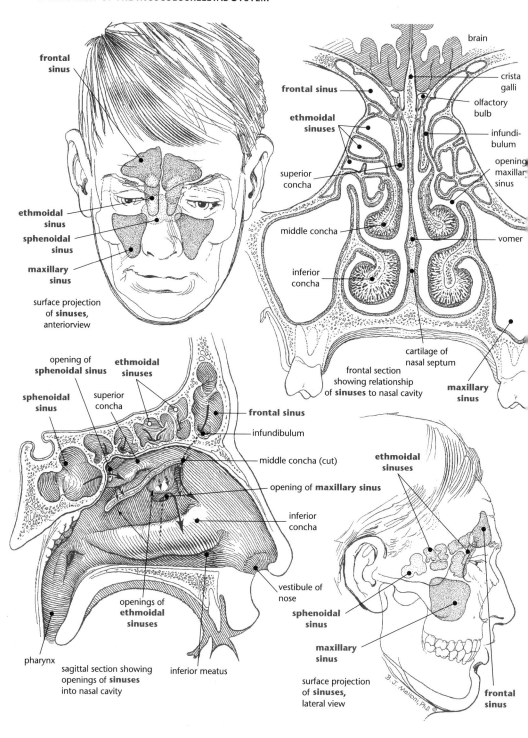

frontal sinus

ethmoidal sinus

sphenoidal sinus

maxillary sinus

surface projection
of **sinuses**,
anterior view

brain

frontal sinus

ethmoidal sinuses

superior concha

middle concha

inferior concha

crista galli

olfactory bulb

infundibulum

opening maxillary sinus

vomer

cartilage of nasal septum

frontal section
showing relationship
of **sinuses** to nasal cavity

maxillary sinus

opening of **sphenoidal sinus**

ethmoidal sinuses

sphenoidal sinus

superior concha

frontal sinus

infundibulum

middle concha (cut)

opening of **maxillary sinus**

inferior concha

vestibule of nose

openings of **ethmoidal sinuses**

pharynx

sagittal section showing
openings of **sinuses**
into nasal cavity

inferior meatus

ethmoidal sinuses

sphenoidal sinus

maxillary sinus

surface projection
of **sinuses**,
lateral view

frontal sinus

B. J. Melloni, Ph.D. ©

sinus ■ sinus

long extensor muscle of the toes (extensor digitorum longus) extending from the lower leg just above the inferior extensor retinaculum to the dorsum of the foot near the proximal end of the metatarsal bones.

synovial s. of extensor pollicis longus The synovial sheath around the tendon of the long extensor muscle of the thumb (extensor pollicis longus); it commences from just proximal to the extensor retinaculum, which it traverses, and ends at the dorsal surface of the base of the 1st metacarpal bone.

synovial s. of flexor carpi radialis The synovial sheath around the tendon of the radial flexor muscle of the wrist (flexor carpi radialis) as it passes through a tunnel created by the lateral splitting of the flexor retinaculum and the groove on the trapezium.

synovial s. of flexor pollicis longus A long synovial sheath around the tendon of the long flexor muscle of the thumb (flexor pollicis longus), extending from the lower forearm about 2.5 cm proximal to the flexor retinaculum, which it traverses, to the insertion on the distal phalanx of the thumb. Also called radial bursa.

synovial s. of superior oblique muscle See bursa of superior oblique muscle of eyeball, under bursa.

synovial s. of tendon See synovial sheath.

synovial s. for tendons of extensor digitorum and extensor indicis The common synovial sheath on the back of the wrist for the tendons of the extensor muscle of the fingers (extensor digitorum) and extensor muscle of the index finger (extensor indicis) over the lower end of the radius and carpus; the sheath extends from just above the overlying extensor retinaculum to the proximal part of the metacarpus.

synovial s. for tendon of flexor digitorum longus The synovial sheath around the tendon of the long flexor muscle of the toes (flexor digitorum longus), extending from behind the medial malleolus, slipping under the flexor retinaculum, to reach the undersurface of the navicular bone.

synovial s. for tendon of flexor hallucis longus The synovial sheath around the tendon of the long flexor muscle of the big toe (flexor hallucis longus); it extends from the lower end of the posteromedial surface of the tibia, just above the proximal margin of the flexor retinaculum, to the sole of the foot.

tendon s. of anterior tibial muscle A synovial sheath around the tendon of the anterior tibial muscle; it extends from just above the proximal margin of the superior extensor retinaculum to the gap between the diverging limbs of the inferior extensor retinaculum at the level of the talonavicular joint.

tendon s. of posterior tibial muscle A synovial sheath around the tendon of the posterior tibial muscle; it extends from just above the medial malleolus to the inside of the foot at the level of the navicular bone.

shin (shin) The anterior portion of the leg, below the knee.

saber s. An anteriorly bowed tibia; a characteristic bone complication of syphilis.

shinbone (shin'bōn) The tibia.

shin-splints (shin' splints) Pain and inflammation of the extensor muscles of the leg (lower lateral area) caused by overextension and overexercise of the muscles.

sinciput (sin'sĭ-put) The upper frontal surface of the head.

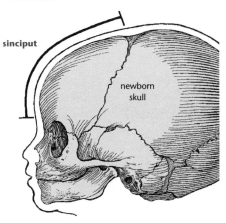

sinciput

newborn skull

sinus (si'nus) Any cavity within a bone normally filled with air.

ethmoidal s. One of the honeycomblike air spaces situated in the ethmoid bone, medial to the orbit, and draining into the upper part of the nasal cavity on either side; grouped into anterior, middle and, posterior divisions.

frontal s. One of the two air spaces in the frontal bone, just above the eyebrows, that opens into the upper part of the nasal cavity on either side.

mastoid s. One of the many honeycomblike air spaces in the mastoid process of the temporal bone; those located

sheath ■ sinus

SKELETON

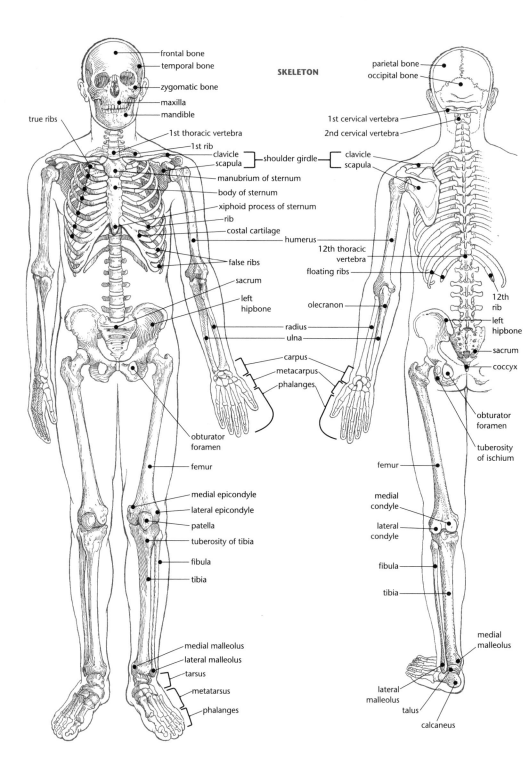

frontal bone
temporal bone
zygomatic bone
maxilla
mandible
true ribs
1st thoracic vertebra
1st rib
clavicle
scapula — shoulder girdle
manubrium of sternum
body of sternum
xiphoid process of sternum
rib
costal cartilage
false ribs
sacrum
left hipbone
obturator foramen
femur
medial epicondyle
lateral epicondyle
patella
tuberosity of tibia
fibula
tibia
medial malleolus
lateral malleolus
tarsus
metatarsus
phalanges

parietal bone
occipital bone
1st cervical vertebra
2nd cervical vertebra
clavicle
scapula — shoulder girdle
humerus
12th thoracic vertebra
floating ribs
olecranon
radius
ulna
carpus
metacarpus
phalanges
12th rib
left hipbone
sacrum
coccyx
obturator foramen
tuberosity of ischium
femur
medial condyle
lateral condyle
fibula
tibia
medial malleolus
lateral malleolus
talus
calcaneus

skeleton ■ skeleton

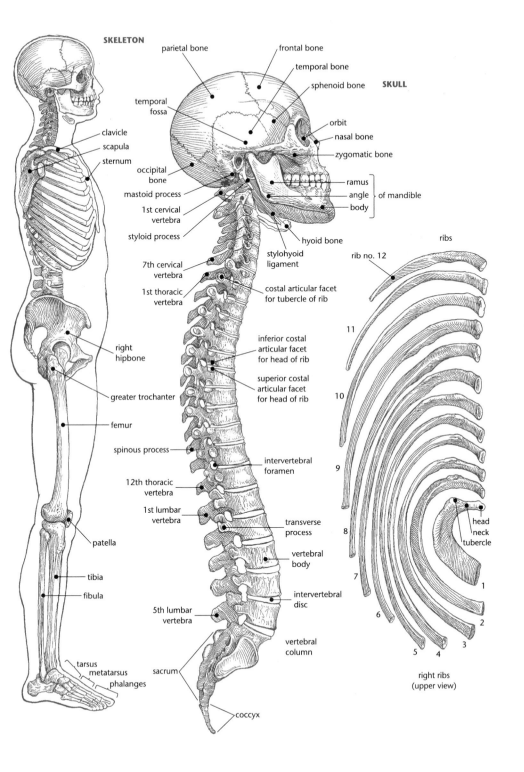

SKELETON

parietal bone

frontal bone

temporal bone

sphenoid bone

SKULL

temporal fossa

orbit

nasal bone

zygomatic bone

clavicle

scapula

sternum

occipital bone

ramus

angle } of mandible

body

mastoid process

1st cervical vertebra

styloid process

hyoid bone

ribs

stylohyoid ligament

rib no. 12

7th cervical vertebra

1st thoracic vertebra

costal articular facet for tubercle of rib

11

inferior costal articular facet for head of rib

right hipbone

superior costal articular facet for head of rib

10

greater trochanter

femur

spinous process

intervertebral foramen

9

12th thoracic vertebra

1st lumbar vertebra

transverse process

8

vertebral body

patella

head

neck

tubercle

7

1

tibia

fibula

intervertebral disc

5th lumbar vertebra

6

2

vertebral column

3

tarsus

metatarsus

phalanges

sacrum

5

4

right ribs (upper view)

coccyx

skeleton ■ skeleton

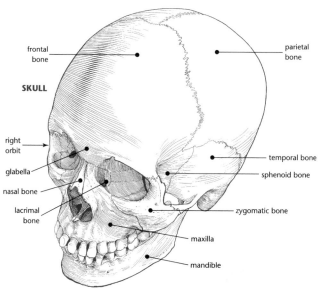

frontal
bone

parietal
bone

SKULL

right
orbit

glabella

nasal bone

lacrimal
bone

temporal bone

sphenoid bone

zygomatic bone

maxilla

mandible

at the apex of the mastoid process contain some bone marrow. Also called tympanic antrum.

maxillary s. One of two large air cavities within the upper jaw (maxilla), under the cheek bone, on either side of the nasal cavity, into which it opens. Also called maxillary antrum.

nasal s.'s See paranasal sinuses.

paranasal s.'s The air chambers (frontal, maxillary, ethmoidal, sphenoidal) situated within the bones of the face; they surround, and open into, the nasal cavity and are lined with mucous membrane that is continuous with that of the nasal cavity. Also called nasal sinuses.

sphenoidal s. One of a paired collection of irregular air spaces situated within the sphenoid bone, behind and above the nasal cavity, and separated from its fellow by a thin bony plate at the midline. It opens into the upper part of the nasal cavity.

tarsal s. A sinus or groove situated between the talus (ankle bone) and calcaneus (heel bone); it contains the interosseous talocalcaneal ligament. Also called tarsal canal.

skeletal (skel′ĕ-tal) Relating to the skeleton.

skeleton (skel′ĕ-ton) 1. The internal framework of vertebrates composed of bones and cartilages, serving to support the soft tissues. 2. The bones of the body considered as a whole.

appendicular s. The bones of the limbs and of the shoulder and pelvic girdles.

axial s. The skull and vertebral column.

skull (skul) The bony framework of the head; includes the bones encasing the brain and the bones of the face. Also called cranium.

skullcap (skul′kap) See calvaria.

socket (sok′et) A cavity or hollow into which a compatible or corresponding part fits, such as the socket of the eye, tooth, joint, or stump.

dry s. A condition sometimes occurring after extraction of a tooth in which the blood clot in the socket disintegrates, leading to a dry appearance of the exposed bone socket, followed by secondary infection; it is more prevalent after traumatic extractions and is often accompanied by severe pain.

eye s. See orbit.

hip s. See acetabulum.

tooth s. The elongated cavity in the alveolar bone of the jaw in which the root of

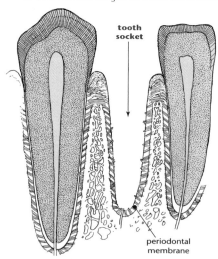

tooth
socket

periodontal
membrane

a tooth is embedded; it can vary in size, shape, and depth according to the tooth it accommodates. In the adult, there are 16 sockets in the mandible (lower jaw) and 16 sockets in the maxilla (upper jaw).

space (spās) Any bodily area or volume between specified boundaries; a delimited three-dimensional area.

anticubital s.
See cubital fossa, under fossa.

cartilage s.
See cartilage lacuna, under lacuna.

epidural s. The space between the dura mater of the spinal cord and the periosteum of the vertebral canal (foramen); it contains loose areolar and fibrous tissue, as well as a plexus of veins.

epitympanic s. The upper portion of the middle ear chamber above the level of the upper part of the eardrum (tympanic membrane); it contains the head of the malleus and the body of the incus, two of the three middle ear ossicles.

haversian s.'s
See haversian canals, under canal.

hypothenar s. See palmar space.

intercostal s. The intervening space between adjoining ribs; the breadth is greater on the ventral surface and also between the upper ribs, in contrast to the lower ones.

interradicular s. The space between the roots of a multirooted tooth, occupied by bony septum and the periodontal membrane.

joint s. The space in a joint between two articulating surfaces.

lumbar s.'s a) *Superior lumbar s.* see Grynfelt-Lesshaft's triangle, under triangle. b) *Inferior lumbar s.* see lumbar triangle, under triangle.

marrow s. See medullary space.

medullary s. The marrow-containing central cavity in trabecular (spongy) bone. Also called marrow space.

palmar s. A large fascial space in the hand between the thenar and hypothenar eminences, divided by a fibrous septum into middle palmar space (toward the little finger) and the thenar space (toward the thumb). Also called hypothenar space.

paraxial s. The space within the capsule of a muscle spindle containing intrafusal muscle fibers and accompanying nerve endings.

perilymphatic s. The perilymph-containing space in the inner ear that separates the membranous labyrinth from the bony labyrinth.

pharyngeal s. The space within the pharynx (i.e., within the nasopharynx, oropharynx, and laryngopharynx).

pharyngomaxillary s. The space located between the lateral wall of the pharynx, the medial pterygoid muscle and the cervical vertebrae.

plantar s.'s Four spaces between fascial layers of the foot; they help to control the spread of infection to other parts of the foot.

popliteal s.
See popliteal fossa, under fossa.

postnasal s. See nasopharynx.

pterygomandibular s. The space between the pterygoid process of the sphenoid bone and the inner surface of the mandibular ramus.

suprasternal s. A narrow space created when the deep cervical fascia divides and the superficial part attaches to the front margin of the manubrium while the deep part attaches to the back margin.

spasm (spazm) An involuntary, abrupt contraction of a muscle or of a group of muscles.

carpopedal s. Spasm of the hands and feet, characteristic of tetany and calcium deficiency.

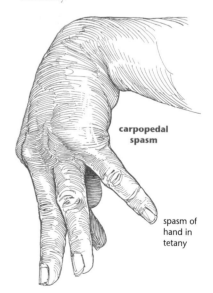

carpopedal
spasm

spasm of
hand in
tetany

clonic s. A spasm characterized by alternate rigidity and relaxation of muscles.

tonic s. Spasm in which the muscular contraction is persistent.

space ■ spasm

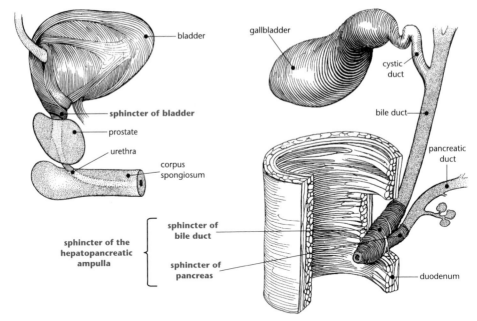

bladder

gallbladder

cystic duct

sphincter of bladder

bile duct

prostate

urethra

pancreatic duct

corpus spongiosum

sphincter of the hepatopancreatic ampulla

sphincter of bile duct

sphincter of pancreas

duodenum

sphenion (sfe'ne-on) A craniometric point located at the tip of the sphenoid angle of the parietal bone.

spheno- Combining form meaning shaped like a wedge.

sphenobasilar (sfe-no-bas'ā-lar) Relating to the sphenoid bone and the basilar part of the occipital bone.

sphenoid (sfe'noid) Wedge-shaped; applied to a large wedge-shaped bone at the base of the skull. See also table of bones in appendix I.

sphenopalatine (sfe-no-pal'ah-tin) Relating to the sphenoid and palatine bones.

sphenoparietal (sfe-no-pah-ri'ě-tal) Relating to the sphenoid and parietal bones.

sphenopetrosal (sfe-no-pe-tro'sal) Relating to the sphenoid bone and the petrous portion of the temporal bone.

sphenorbital (sfe-nor'bi-tal) Relating to the sphenoid bone and the orbit, or the portion of the sphenoid bone forming part of the orbit.

sphenosquamosal (sfe-no-skwa-mo'sal) Relating to the sphenoid bone and the squamous portion of the temporal bone.

sphincter (sfingk'ter) 1. Any circular muscle that normally maintains constriction of a natural body opening and that is capable of relaxing in order to permit passage of substances through the opening. 2. A portion of a tubular structure that functions as a sphincter.

  s. of bile duct A sphincter of smooth muscle around the lower part of the bile duct within the wall of the duodenum, from the

duodenal entrance to its junction with the pancreatic duct; it regulates the bile flow and, retrogressively, the filling of the gallbladder. Also called sphincter choledochus.

  s. of bladder A thickening of the middle circular layer of the muscular fibers of the bladder surrounding the internal urethral opening at the neck of the bladder; it is composed of nonstriated (smooth) muscle and is not under voluntary control. Along with the sphincter of the urethra, it controls the outflow of urine from the bladder. Also called sphincter vesicae; vesicular sphincter.

  s. choledochus See sphincter of bile duct.

  external anal s. A flat band of muscular fibers, elliptical in shape, encircling the anal opening; consists of three parts: subcutaneous, superficial and deep; it closes the anal canal and anus.

  s. of the hepatopancreatic ampulla The sphincter of smooth circular muscle fibers around the terminal part of the main pancreatic duct and bile duct, including the duodenal ampulla (papilla of Vater); it constricts both the lower part of the bile duct and the main pancreatic duct so that reflux cannot occur. Also called sphincter of Oddi.

  ileocecal s.
See ileocecal valve, under valve.

  internal anal s. A muscular ring formed of the thickened inner circular coat at the caudal end of the bowel, surrounding about

sphenion ■ sphincter

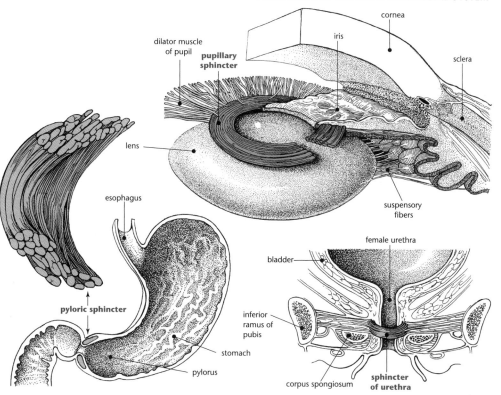

Labels: cornea, iris, sclera, dilator muscle of pupil, pupillary sphincter, lens, esophagus, suspensory fibers, female urethra, bladder, pyloric sphincter, inferior ramus of pubis, stomach, pylorus, corpus spongiosum, sphincter of urethra

2.5 cm of the anal canal; it is in contact with, but separate from, the external anal sphincter; it closes the anal canal and anus.

lower esophageal s. A high pressure zone in the distal portion of the esophagus where resting pressure is usually higher than pressure in the fundus of the stomach; cannot be identified anatomically but its pressure can be determined; normally it straddles the diaphragm extending 1 to 3 cm below to 1 to 2 cm above the diaphragmatic hiatus; it acts as a barrier preventing the reflux of gastric contents.

s. of Oddi See sphincter of hepatopancreatic ampulla.

s. of pancreas A sphincter of smooth circular muscle fibers around the terminal (intraduodenal) part of the main pancreatic duct where it joins the bile duct before entering into the duodenum; it constricts the terminal part of the main pancreatic duct. Also called sphincter of pancreatic duct.

s. of pancreatic duct See sphincter of pancreas.

s. of pupil See pupillary sphincter.

pupillary s. A circular, flattened band of muscle slightly less than 1 mm in width, in the pupillary margin of the iris; it regulates the size of the pupil. Also called sphincter of pupil.

pyloric s. A muscular ring formed by a thickening of the circular layer of the stomach at the pyloric orifice; it acts as a valve to close the pyloric lumen.

s. of urethra A flat striated muscle that closely surrounds the membranous portion of the urethra in the male and the terminal part of the urethra in the female; along with the vesicular sphincter, it controls the outflow of urine from the urinary bladder by compressing the urethra; it is under voluntary control after early infancy. Also called sphincter urethrae.

s. urethrae See spincter of urethra.

s. vesicae See sphincter of bladder.

vesicular s. See sphincter of bladder.

spicule (spik'ūl) A small needle-shaped structure.

spina (spi'nah) 1. The vertebral column. 2. Any sharp bony projection.

s. bifida Congenital defect of the vertebral column in which the posterior portion (vertebral arch) of one or several vertebrae fails to develop; the resulting gap allows spinal membranes and sometimes the spinal

sphincter ■ spicule

cord and nerve roots to protrude. Also called cleft spine.

s. bifida occulta Spina bifida without protrusion of the spinal cord or its membranes.

spinal (spi'nal) 1. Relating to a spine. 2. Relating to the vertebral column.

spindle (spin'dl) Any spindle-shaped or fusiform anatomic structure; an elongated form with a thick central portion and tapered extremities.

intermediate muscle s. A muscle spindle possessing a single secondary nerve ending as well as the primary nerve ending.

muscle s. A specialized sensory organ in voluntary muscle that consists of a small bundle of delicate muscle fibers (intrafusal fibers) invested in a multilaminar fibrous capsule within which the sensory nerve fibers terminate; it is positioned parallel to the extrafusal fibers, varies in length from 0.8 to 5 mm, and has a fusiform appearance. Also called neuromuscular spindle; muscle proprioceptor.

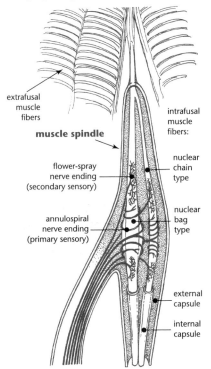

extrafusal muscle fibers

muscle spindle

flower-spray nerve ending (secondary sensory)

annulospiral nerve ending (primary sensory)

intrafusal muscle fibers:

nuclear chain type

nuclear bag type

external capsule

internal capsule

neuromuscular s. See muscle spindle.

simple muscle s. A muscle spindle that contains only a primary nerve ending.

tendon s. See Golgi tendon organ, under organ.

spine (spīn) 1. A sharp-pointed projection of bone. 2. The vertebral column; see under column. 3. A short projection.

anterior nasal s. The pointed median projection of bone of the maxilla situated on the lower margin of the bony external nares.

bamboo s. See poker spine.

basal s. See pharyngeal spine.

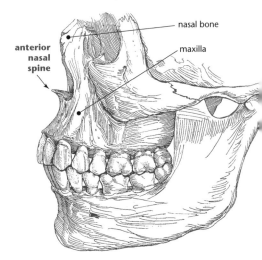

anterior nasal spine

nasal bone

maxilla

cervical s. The seven cervical vertebrae considered as a whole.

cleft s. See spina bifida.

s. of greater tubercle of humerus A bony projection on the greater tubercle of the humerus, at the shoulder, forming the lateral border of the intertubercular groove.

s. of smaller tubercle of humerus A bony projection on the smaller (lesser) tubercle of the humerus, at the shoulder, forming the medial border of the intertubercular groove.

s. of helix The small pointed projection on the anterior border of the auricular cartilage of the ear where the helix bends upward.

iliac s. Any of the four spines of the ilium (part of hipbone): *Anterior inferior iliac s.*, the spine (blunt projection) on the front border of the ilium just above the anterior part of the acetabulum; it provides attachment to the rectus muscle of the thigh (rectus femoris muscle) and to the iliofemoral ligament; *Anterior superior iliac s.*, the spine forming the front end of the crest of the ilium; it provides attachment to the lateral end of the inguinal ligament and just below to the sartorius muscle. It lies at the lateral end of the fold of the groin and is easily felt.

spinal ■ spine

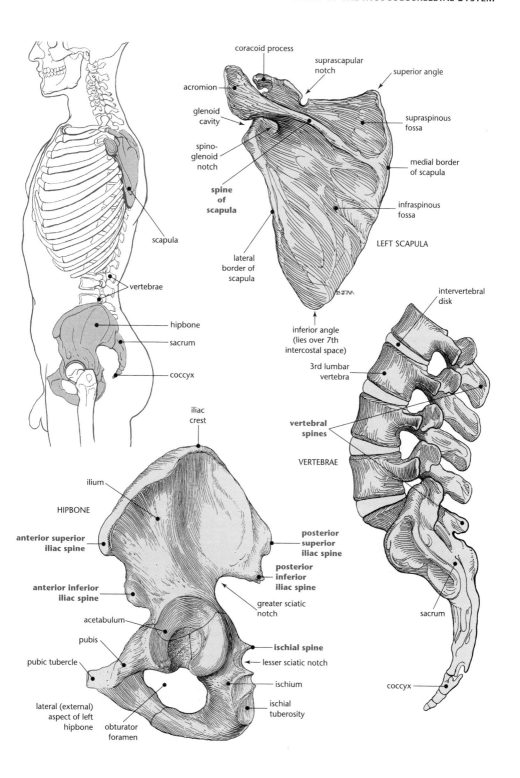

coracoid process

suprascapular notch

superior angle

acromion

glenoid cavity

spino-glenoid notch

spine of scapula

supraspinous fossa

medial border of scapula

infraspinous fossa

LEFT SCAPULA

scapula

vertebrae

hipbone

sacrum

coccyx

lateral border of scapula

inferior angle (lies over 7th intercostal space)

intervertebral disk

3rd lumbar vertebra

vertebral spines

VERTEBRAE

iliac crest

ilium

HIPBONE

anterior superior iliac spine

posterior superior iliac spine

posterior inferior iliac spine

greater sciatic notch

anterior inferior iliac spine

acetabulum

pubis

ischial spine

lesser sciatic notch

ischium

pubic tubercle

lateral (external) aspect of left hipbone

obturator foramen

ischial tuberosity

sacrum

coccyx

spine ■ spine

DICTIONARY OF THE MUSCULOSKELETAL SYSTEM

Posterior inferior iliac s., the spine (wide projection) at the lower end of the posterior border of the ilium, where it makes a sharp bend forward to form the upper border of the greater sciatic notch; it provides attachment to the piriform muscle. *Posterior superior iliac s.*, the spine forming the back end of the crest of the ilium; it provides attachment to the sacrotuberal ligament and the dorsal (posterior) sacroiliac ligament. Usually, the spine cannot be felt, but its position is indicated by a prominent dimple about 4 cm lateral to the second spinous tubercle of the sacrum.

ischial s. A bony spine situated on the posterior aspect of the ischium (part of hipbone) near the posteroinferior border of the acetabulum; it provides attachment to the sacrospinal ligament. Also called sciatic spine.

kissing s.'s Abnormal contact between the tips of the spinous processes of adjacent vertebrae (usually between any two lumbar vertebrae or between the fifth lumbar and the first sacral) resulting in midline lower back pain that intensifies on extension of the spine.

lumbar s. The five lumbar vertebrae considered as a unit.

mental s.'s
See genial tubercles, under tubercle.

nasal s. of frontal bone A sharp median spine projecting downward from the nasal part of the frontal bone and articulating in front with the upper part of the nasal bone, and behind with the ethmoid bone; it forms part of the roof of the nasal cavity as well as a small part of the nasal septum.

nasal s. of palatine bone
See posterior nasal spine.

peroneal s. of calcaneus
See peroneal trochlea, under trochlea.

pharyngeal s. A small midline elevation on the inferior surface of the basilar part of the occipital bone, about 1 cm in front of the foramen magnum; it provides attachment to the fibrous raphe of the pharynx. Also called basal spine; pharyngeal tubercle; basilar crest of occipital bone.

poker s. The spine characteristic of ankylosing spondylitis, sometimes called bamboo spine because of its resemblance to a rigid bamboo shoot (lipping of vertebral margins) on x-ray film. Also called rigid spine; bamboo spine.

posterior nasal s. A small, sharp bony spine projecting backward from the median end of the posterior border of the horizontal plate of the palatine bone; it provides attachment to the muscle of the uvula. Also called nasal spine of palatine bone.

pubic s.
See pubic tubercle, under tubercle.

rigid s. See poker spine.

s. of scapula The somewhat triangular shelf of bone projecting from the back of the scapula, extending from the vertebral border laterally across to the shoulder joint where it bears the acromion; it is covered by skin and superficial fascia and provides attachment to the supraspinous and infraspinous muscles.

sciatic s. See ischial spine.

s. of Spix
See lingula of mandible, under lingula.

thoracic s. The twelve thoracic vertebrae considered as a unit.

tibial s. See intercondylar eminence of tibia, under eminence.

vertebral s. The spinous process of vertebrae projecting backward from the vertebral arch (junction of laminae), providing attachment to muscles of the back which extend and rotate the vertebral column. It can vary in shape, size and direction from the short, bifid process of some cervical vertebrae to the large, thick quadrangular process seen in lumbar vertebrae. The vertebral spine of the seventh cervical vertebra is very prominent; it is long and ends in a tubercle that is easily palpable at the lower end of the nuchal furrow; the vertebral spine of the first thoracic vertebra is equally prominent, while the typical thoracic vertebral spines are not outstanding and simply slant backward and downward. The first cervical vertebra does not have a vertebral spine.

spinocostalis (spi-no-kos-ta'lis) The superior and inferior serratus muscles considered as a unit.
spinous (spi'nus) Relating to the spine.
spondylarthritis (spon-dil-ar-thri'tis) Arthritis of the joints of the vertebral column.
spondylitis (spon-dī-li'tis) Inflammation of one or more of the vertebral bodies.
spondylo-, spondyl- Combining forms meaning a relationship to a vertebra or to the vertebral column.
spondyloarthropathy (spon-dī-lo-ar-throp'ah-the) Any disease affecting the joints of the vertebral column.
spondylolisthesis (spon-dī-lo-lis'the-sis) Forward slippage of one vertebra over the

spine ■ spondylolisthesis

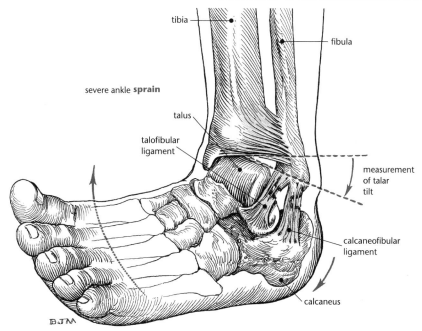

tibia

fibula

severe ankle **sprain**

talus

talofibular
ligament

measurement
of talar
tilt

calcaneofibular
ligament

calcaneus

B.J.M

vertebra below, usually of the fifth lumbar over
the sacrum or, less often, of the fourth lumbar
over the fifth lumbar; causing low-back pain,
limitation of movement, and protrusion of the
involved spinous process; generally manifested
in late childhood and adolescence. Also called
spondyloptosis.

spondylomalacia (spon-dĭ-lo-mah-la'she-ah)
Softening of the vertebra.

spondyloptosis (spon-dĭ-lop-to'sis) See
spondylolisthesis.

spondylosis (spon-dĭ-lo'sis) Abnormal
thickening and immobility of a vertebral joint.

sprain (sprān) Injury to the fibrous band
(ligament) joining two bones of a joint, usually
occurring when the joint is wrenched or twisted
beyond its normal range of motion, which tears
fibers but leaves the integrity of the ligament
intact.

spur (sper) An abnormal spinelike projection
from a bone or a horny outgrowth from
the skin.

    calcaneal s. A projection from the plantar
surface of the calcaneus (heel bone); often
causes pain when walking. Also called
heel spur.

    elbow s. See olecranon spur.

    heel s. See calcaneal spur.

    olecranon s. A benign bony protuberance
on the olecranon at the insertion of the
triceps muscle of the arm (triceps brachii).

Also called elbow spur.

squama (skwa'mah), pl. squa'mae 1. A thin,
expanded plate of bone, especially in the wall
of the cranial cavity. 2. A scalelike structure.

    frontal s. The broad and curved part of
the frontal bone above the supraorbital
margins forming the anterior part of the
calvaria and the forehead.

    occipital s. The squamous part of the
occipital bone extending from the back edge
of the foramen magnum upward to the
lambdoid suture.

    temporal s. See squamous part of the
temporal bone, under part.

squamomastoid (skwa-mo-mas'toid) Relating to
the squamous and mastoid parts of the
temporal bone.

squamoparietal (skwa-mo-pah-ri'ĕ-tal) Relating
to the squamous part of the temporal bone and
to the parietal bone.

squamopetrosal (skwa-mo-pe-tro'sal) Relating
to the squamous and petrous parts of the
temporal bone.

squamosa (skwa-mo'sah) The platelike portion
of the temporal bone.

stapediovestibular (stah-pe-de-o-ves-tib'u-lar)
Relating to both the stapes of the middle ear
chamber and vestibule of the inner ear.

stapedius (stah-pe'de-us) See table of muscles in
appendix II.

stapes (sta'pēz) The smallest and innermost of

spondylomalacia ■ stapes

the three movable ossicles of the middle ear chamber; it articulates by its head with the incus (middle ossicle) and its base (footplate) is inserted and attached to the margin of the oval window; the smallest bone in the body, it resembles a stirrup and is sometimes called by that name. See also table of bones in appendix I.

staphylion (stah-fil'e-on) A craniometric landmark; the midpoint of the posterior edge of the hard palate.

stenion (sten'e-on) A craniometric point located at each end of the shortest transverse diameter of the head in the temporal fossa.

stephanion (ste-fa'ne-on) A craniometric point at the intersection of the coronal suture and the inferior temporal line.

sternad (ster'nad) Toward or in the direction of the sternum.

sternal (ster'nal) 1. Relating to the sternum. 2. See table of muscles in appendix II.

sterno-, stern- Combining forms meaning sternum.

sternoclavicular (ster-no-klah-vik'u-lar) Relating to the sternum and the clavicle. Also called sternocleido.

sternocleidomastoid (ster-no-kli-do-mas'toid) Relating to the sternum, clavicle, and the mastoid process; applied to the neck muscle that has its origin and insertion on these bones. See also table of muscles in appendix II.

sternocostal (ster-no-kos'tal) 1. Relating to the sternum and the ribs. 2. See table of muscles in appendix II.

sternohyoid (ster-no-hi'oid) Relating to the sternum and the hyoid bone.

sternum (ster'num) A long, flat bone forming the middle part of the anterior wall of the thoracic cage; composed of three parts: manubrium, body, and xiphoid process; it articulates with the clavicles and the cartilages of the first seven pairs of ribs.

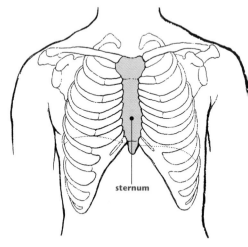

sternum

strain (strān) 1. Tearing of a muscle or its tendon caused by extreme pulling, pushing, or overstretching of the muscle or tendon insertion, as in lifting a heavy weight or bearing an external force (usually a traction force). 2. To produce such an injury.

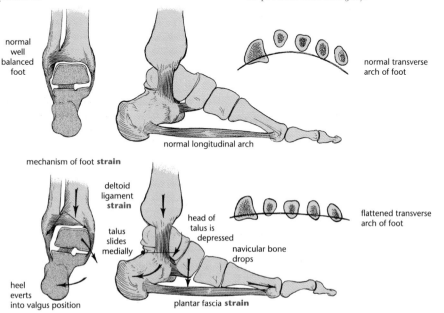

normal well balanced foot

normal transverse arch of foot

normal longitudinal arch

mechanism of foot **strain**

deltoid ligament **strain**

head of talus is depressed

flattened transverse arch of foot

talus slides medially

navicular bone drops

heel everts into valgus position

plantar fascia **strain**

staphylion ■ strain

strait (strāt) A narrow passage or space.

    inferior pelvic s.
    See pelvic plane of outlet, under plane.

    superior pelvic s.
    See pelvic plane of inlet, under plane.

stratum (stra'tum) See layer.

stria (stri'ah) See line.

stylo- Combining form meaning styloid.

styloglossus (sti-lo-glos'us) Relating to the styloid process of the temporal bone of the skull and the tongue; applied to certain structures (e.g., a muscle). See also table of muscles in appendix II.

stylohyoid (sti-lo-hi'oid) Relating to the styloid process on the inferior surface of the temporal bone and to the hyoid bone.

styloid (sti'loid) Shaped like a peg; applied to certain bony processes.

stylomastoid (sti-lo-mas'toid) Relating to the styloid and mastoid processes of the temporal bone.

subacetabular (sub-as-ĕ-tab'u-lar) Situated beneath the acetabulum of the hipbone.

subacromial (sub-ah-kro'me-al) Situated beneath the acromion of the scapula.

subclavicular (sub-klah-vik'u-lar) Beneath the clavicle.

subcostal (sub-kos'tal) Beneath the ribs.

subcranial (sub-kra'ne-al) Below the skull.

subluxation (sub-luk-sa'shun) Partial dislocation of a body part, especially of a joint.

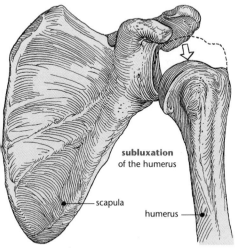

subluxation
of the humerus

scapula

humerus

submandibular (sub-man-dib'u-lar) Beneath the mandible (lower jaw).

submaxillary (sub-mak'sĭ-ler-e) Beneath the maxilla (upper jaw).

submental (sub-men'tal) Under the chin.

subnasion (sub-na'ze-on) The point at the junction of the nasal septum and the upper lip.

suboccipital (sub-ok-sip'ĭ-tal) Below the occipital bone or the back of the head (occiput).

suborbital (sub-or'bĭ-tal) See infraorbital.

subpubic (sub-pu'bik) Situated beneath the pubic arch or pubic symphysis.

subscapular (sub-skap'u-lar) Beneath or below the scapula (shoulder blade).

substance (sub'stans) Matter; material of a specified constitution.

    cortical s. of bone
    See compact bone, under bone.

    ground s. An amorphous viscous gel that, along with fibers (collagen, reticulum, and elastin), make up the extracellular matrix of connective tissue; it is the non-fibrous element of matrix in which cells and other components are embedded. Also called interstitial substance.

    interstitial s. See ground substance.

    spongy s. of bone
    See trabecular bone, under bone.

substernal (sub-ster'nal) Beneath the sternum (breastbone).

sulcus (sul'kus), pl. sul'ci
A groove, furrow, or depression.

    arterial sulci Grooves on the internal surface of the skull that house the meningeal arteries and their branches. Also called arterial grooves.

    s. of auditory tube A furrow on the internal surface of the base of the skull between the posterior border of the greater wing of the sphenoid bone and the petrous part of the temporal bone. Also called groove for auditory tube.

    s. of calcaneus The broad, deep, transverse groove on the top surface of the calcaneus (heel bone), located between the medial and posterior articular facets; in association with a corresponding groove on the talus (ankle bone), it forms the tarsal sinus, which contains the interosseous talocalcaneal ligament.

    carotid s. of sphenoid bone See carotid groove of sphenoid bone, under groove.

    carpal s. The broad, deep concavity on the front (volar surface) of the wrist (carpus) formed by the arching carpal bones; it transmits the flexor tendons and the median nerve to the palm of the hand. Also called carpal groove.

    chiasmatic s. A transverse groove on the upper surface of the sphenoid bone just in front of the hypophyseal fossa; it accommodates the optic chiasma and is

strait ■ sulcus

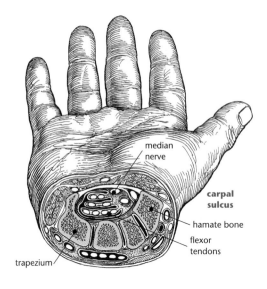

continuous with the optic canal. Also called optic groove.

coronary s. A sulcus encircling the outside surface of the heart between the atria and ventricles, and lodging the coronary blood vessels. Also called atrioventricular groove.

costal s. See costal groove, under groove.

ethmoidal s. of nasal bone See ethmoidal groove, under groove.

intertubercular s. of humerus A deep longitudinal groove that runs down the anterior surface of the upper humerus, between the lesser tubercle and the greater tubercle; it accommodates the tendon of the long head of the biceps muscle of the arm (biceps brachii) and affords attachment to the latissimus dorsi muscle. Also called bicipital groove of humerus.

interventricular s. See interventricular groove, under groove.

lateral bicipital s. See lateral bicipital groove, under groove.

malleolar s. A broad vertical groove on the posterior surface of the medial malleolus of the lower tibia; it accommodates the tendons of the posterior tibial muscle and the long flexor muscle of the toes (flexor digitorum longus muscle). Also called malleolar groove.

medial bicipital s. See medial bicipital groove, uner groove.

median s. of tongue A slight, median, longitudinal depression running forward on the dorsal surface of the tongue from the foramen cecum; it divides the tongue into symmetrical halves.

s. of middle temporal artery See groove for middle temporal artery, under groove.

mylohyoid s. of mandible See mylohyoid groove, under groove.

s. of nail The cutaneous groove formed by the infolding of skin in which the proximal and lateral borders of the nail are embedded. Also called nail groove.

nasolabial s. The depression extending downward and laterally from the side of the nose to the angle of the mouth; the junction between the cheek and the lips. Also called nasolabial groove.

obturator s. of pubis See obturator groove, under groove.

s. of occipital artery See groove for occipital artery, under groove.

occlusal s. A sulcus on the occlusal surface of a tooth.

preauricular s. See preauricular groove of ilium, under groove.

s. of pterygoid hamulus See hamular groove, under groove.

pulmonary s. of thorax The broad, deep vertical groove lying on either side of the

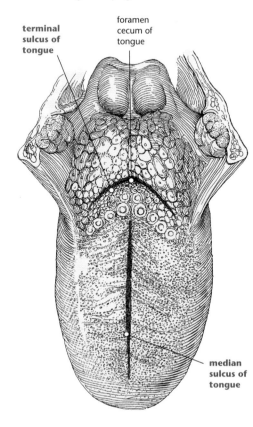

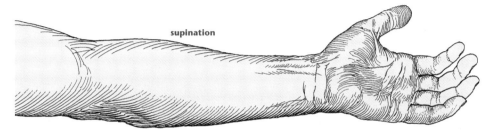
supination

vertebral column in the thorax, resulting from the posterior curvature of the ribs; it accommodates the posterior, bulky part of the lung.

s. of radial nerve See groove for radial nerve, under groove.

s. of sigmoid sinus See groove for sigmoid sinus, under groove.

s. of spinal nerves A groove on the upper surface of the transverse processes of the third through the sixth cervical vertebrae, accommodating the emerging anterior rami of the spinal nerves.

s. of subclavian artery
See subclavian grooves, under groove.

s. of subclavian vein
See subclavian grooves, under groove.

s. of superior sagittal sinus See groove for superior sagittal sinus, under groove.

s. tali See sulcus of talus.

s. of talus The broad, deep, transverse groove on the bottom of the talus (ankle bone), located between the medial and posterior articular facets; in association with a corresponding groove on the calcaneus (heel bone), it forms the tarsal sinus which contains the interosseous talocalcaneal ligament. Also called sulcus tali.

s. of tendon of long flexor muscle of big toe See groove for tendon of long flexor muscle of big toe, under groove.

terminal s. of tongue A shallow V-shaped groove on the tongue running laterally and forward from the foramen cecum; it marks the separation between the oral part of the tongue (anterior two-thirds) from the pharyngeal part of the tongue (posterior third).

s. of transverse sinus See groove for transverse sinus, under groove.

s. of ulnar nerve See groove for ulnar nerve, under groove.

superextension (soo-per-eks-ten'shun) See hyperextension.

superflexion (soo-per-flek'shun) See hyperflexion.

superior (su-pe're-or) Above; higher; (in

humans, upright posture) near the top of the head.

supination (su-pĭ-na'shun) 1. The act of lying on the back. 2. Rotation of the arm so that the palm of the hand faces forward or upward.

supinator (su-pĭ-na'tor) A muscle that supinates the forearm. See also table of muscles in appendix II.

supine (su'pīn) Lying on the back.

supraclavicular (su-prah-klah-vik'u-lar) Above the clavicle (collarbone).

supracondylar (su-prah-kon'dĭ-lar) Above a condyle.

supracostal (su-prah-kos'tal) Above the ribs.

supradiaphragmatic (su-prah-di-ah-frag-mat'ik) Above the respiratory diaphragm.

suprahyoid (su-prah-hi'oid) Above the hyoid bone.

supralumbar (su-prah-lum'bar) Above the lumbar area.

supramandibular (su-prah-man-dib'u-lar) Above the mandible.

supramental (su-prah-men'tal) Above the chin.

supraorbital (su-prah-or'bi-tal) Above the orbit (eye socket).

suprapubic (su-prah-pu'bik) Above the pubic arch or pubic symphysis.

suprascapular (su-prah-skap'u-lar) Above or in the upper part of the scapula (shoulder blade).

suprasellar (su-prah-sel'ar) Above the sella turcica which lodges the hypophysis.

supraspinous (su-prah-spi'nus) Above a spine, especially of the vertebra.

suprasternal (su-prah-ster'nal) Above the sternum (breastbone).

supratympanic (su-prah-tim-pan'ik) Above the middle ear chamber.

surface (sur'fis) 1. The outer boundary or outermost aspect of an object. 2. The surface of a structure that faces in a specific direction.

articular s.
The surface of an articulating joint.

articular s. of acetabulum The horseshoe-shaped articular portion of the acetabulum that articulates with the head of the femur in the hip joint.

superextension ■ surface

buccal s. The surface of premolars and molars facing the cheek.

distal s. a) The surface of a structure that is farther from the point of reference. b) The proximal or contact surface of a tooth facing away from the midline of the dental arch.

facial s. See vestibular surface.

labial s. The surface of incisors and cuspids facing the lip.

lateral s. a) The surface facing the direction of the side of the body. b) The contact surface of the incisor or cuspid tooth facing away from the midline of the dental arch.

lingual s. The surface of a tooth facing the tongue.

medial s. The surface of a structure that is closer to the point of reference. Also called mesial surface.

mesial s. a) See medial surface. b) The proximal or contact surface of the incisor or cuspid tooth facing the midline of the dental arch.

occlusal s. The grinding surface of a posterior tooth that comes in contact with one in the opposing jaw during occlusion; the working part of a tooth during mastication.

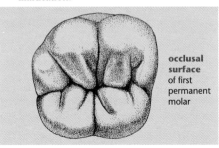

occlusal surface of first permanent molar

patellar articulating s. The upper posterior surface of the patella (kneecap), divided by a vertical median ridge into two smooth surfaces that articulate with both condyles of the femur.

proximal s. a) The surface that is nearer to a point of reference. b) The surface of a tooth facing an adjacent tooth in the same dental arch.

tooth s.'s The five surfaces of a tooth: occlusal (O), buccal (B), lingual (L), distal (D), and mesial (M).

vestibular s. The surface of a tooth facing outwardly toward the vestibule of the mouth, comprising the labial, buccal, or combined labiobuccal surface. Also called facial surface.

suture (su'chur) 1. An immovable fibrous joint uniting the bones of the cranium. 2. Stitch or stitches used in surgery to unite two surfaces.

apposition s. A stitch or a number of stitches for securing two tissue edges in exact anatomic approximation. Also called coaptation suture.

coaptation s. See apposition suture.

coronal s. The line of junction on top of the skull, between the posterior border of the frontal bone and the anterior borders of the two parietal bones.

cranial s. A type of immovable fibrous articulation between two bones of the cranium.

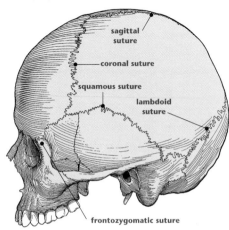

sagittal suture

coronal suture

squamous suture

lambdoid suture

frontozygomatic suture

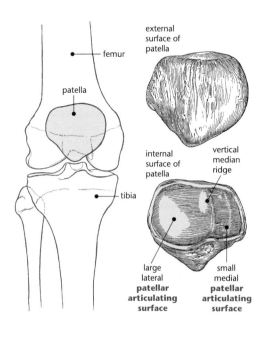

femur

patella

tibia

external surface of patella

internal surface of patella

vertical median ridge

large lateral patellar articulating surface

small medial patellar articulating surface

surface ■ suture

cruciform s. A suture of the hard (bony) palate formed by the intermaxillary and interpalatine sutures in the median plane, crossed by the palatomaxillary suture in the coronal plane.

denticulate s. An articulation between two bones in which the bone margins are small toothlike projections that often widen toward the free ends; it provides a highly effective interlocking mechanism.

ethmoid maxillary s. The line of junction in the inferomedial part of the eye socket (orbit), between the lower margin of the orbital plate of the ethmoid bone and the orbital margin of the maxilla.

false s. Articulation between contiguous complementary bone surfaces without interlocking or fibrous union. Also called plane suture; flat suture.

flat s. See false suture.

frontal s. The suture between the two halves of the developing frontal bone, commonly seen in newborns and infants prior to complete ossification into one bone; ossification usually is active from the second year of life to about the eighth year when the process is completed.

frontolacrimal s. The line of junction between the orbital part of the frontal bone and the uppermost border of the lacrimal bone.

frontomaxillary s. The suture between the frontal bone and the frontal process of the maxilla.

frontonasal s. The line of junction on the front of the skull between the frontal bone and the uppermost border of the nasal bones. Also called nasofrontal suture.

frontosphenoid s.
See sphenofrontal suture.

frontozygomatic s. The line of junction on the lateral border of the orbit, between the zygomatic process of the frontal bone and the frontal process of the zygomatic bone. Also called zygomaticofrontal suture.

internasal s. The line of junction between the medial margins of the two nasal bones.

interpalatine s. The suture between the apposing horizontal plates of the two palatine bones, located on the median plane at the posterior part of the hard palate (on the roof of the mouth); it is continuous anteriorly with the intermaxillary suture and forms the posterior part of the cruciform suture. Also called middle palatine suture.

intermaxillary s. The suture between the apposing maxillae, located on the median plane at the anterior part of the hard palate (on the roof of the mouth); it is continuous posteriorly with the interpalatine suture and forms the anterior part of the cruciform suture.

lacrimomaxillary s. The line of junction on the medial wall of the orbit (eye socket), between the lacrimal bone and the maxilla.

lambdoid s. The line of junction at the back of the skull, between the occipital and parietal bones; it resembles the Greek letter lambda (λ). Also called parietooccipital suture.

middle palatine s. See interpalatine suture.

nasofrontal s. See frontonasal suture.

nasomaxillary s. The line of junction between the lateral border of the nasal bone and the anterior border of the frontal process of the maxilla.

occipitomastoid s. The line of junction on the posterolateral surface of the skull, between the occipital bone and the posterior margin of the temporal bone; it is a continuation of the lambdoid suture.

palatomaxillary s. The suture between the maxillary bone and the palatine bone; it forms the coronal part of the cruciform suture.

parietomastoid s. The line of junction on the lateral surface of the skull, between the posterior inferior angle of the parietal bone and the mastoid bone; it is a continuation of the lambdoid suture.

parietooccipital s. See lambdoid suture.

plane s. See false suture.

sagittal s. The median suture between the upper serrated margins of the two parietal bones located at the top of the skull.

serrate s. A suture in which the bone margins are highly complex and irregular, with spikes and recesses intimately interdigitated.

sphenofrontal s. A suture in the internal surface of the base of the skull, between the posterior border of the orbital part of the frontal bone and the sphenoid bone on either side of the skull. Also called frontosphenoid suture.

sphenoparietal s. The suture in the temporal fossa (at the pterion, an important craniometric point), between the upper tip of the greater wing of the sphenoid bone and the anterior part of the lower border of the parietal bone.

sphenosquamosal s. The suture between

the posterior margin of the greater wing of the sphenoid bone and the anterior margin of the squamous part of the temporal bone.

sphenozygomatic s. A suture between the anterior border of the greater wing of the sphenoid bone and the orbital surface of the zygomatic bone. Also called zygomaticosphenoid suture.

squamosoparietal s. The suture on the side of the skull, between the squamous part of the temporal bone and the parietal bone.

squamous s. A type of suture in which one bone margin overlaps its apposing bone margin, as the suture between the temporal and parietal bones.

temporozygomatic s. See zygomatico-temporal suture.

vomero-ethmoidal s. The suture of the thin bony nasal septum between the vomer and the overriding perpendicular plate of the ethmoid bone. The vomer forms the lower and posterior part of the nasal septum while the perpendicular plate of the ethmoid bone forms the upper and anterior part of the septum and is continuous above with the cribriform plate. When the nasal septum is deviated, the defect usually occurs at the line of the vomero-ethmoidal suture.

zygomaticofrontal s. See frontozygomatic suture.

zygomaticomaxillary s. A suture between the maxillary border of the zygomatic bone and the zygomatic process (upper oblique surface) of the maxilla.

zygomaticosphenoid s. See zygomatic spheno suture.

zygomaticotemporal s. A suture between the zygomatic process of the temporal bone and the temporal process of the zygomatic bone; easily palpable where the cheek and temple meet each other. Also called temporozygomatic suture.

swayback (swa'bak) See lordosis.

symphyseal. symphysial (sim-fiz'e-al) Relating to the symphysis.

symphysis (sim'fi-sis), pl. sym'physes 1. A type of articulation in which two opposing surfaces of bones are covered with a thin layer of hyaline cartilage and united by fibrocartilage. 2. In pathology, the abnormal fusion of two surfaces.

mandibular s. The midline fibrocartilaginous union of the two halves of the lower jaw, forming the prominence of the chin; it becomes ossified during the first year after birth.

manubriosternal s. The joint at the sternal angle uniting the manubrium with the body of the sternum; beginning as a temporary cartilaginous joint, it eventually develops into a symphysis and frequently by the age of 30 years it is completely ossified.

pubic s. The symphysis between the pubic bones where they meet at the median plane of the pelvis; the bones are connected by an interpubic disk of fibrocartilage, and by the superior pubic ligament above and the arcuate pubic ligament below.

synarthrosis (sin-ar-thro'sis), pl. synarthro'ses

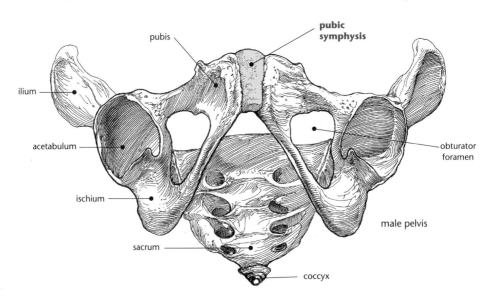

male pelvis

pubis — pubic symphysis — ilium — acetabulum — ischium — sacrum — coccyx — obturator foramen

suture ■ synarthrosis

See fibrous joint, under joint.

synchondrosis (sin-kon-dro'sis), pl. synchondro'ses The union of two bones by cartilage; usually the cartilage is replaced by bone (e.g., the junction between skull bones of the newborn infant).

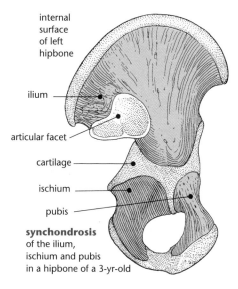

internal surface of left hipbone
ilium
articular facet
cartilage
ischium
pubis

synchondrosis of the ilium, ischium and pubis in a hipbone of a 3-yr-old

xiphisternal s. The cartilaginous union between the xiphoid process and the body of the sternum; it eventually ossifies, frequently by the age of 30 years.

syndesmo- Combining form meaning ligament.

syndesmosis (sin-des-mo'sis), pl. syndesmo'ses A type of fibrous articulation in which the fibrous tissue between the bones forms a membrane or ligament, as the articulation between the tibia and fibula or the union of the footplate of the stapes to the oval window. Also called ligamentous joint.

synostosis (sin-os-to'sis) Abnormal fusion of the bones forming a joint by proliferation of bony tissue. Also called true ankylosis; bony ankylosis.

synovia (sĭ-no've-ah) The clear, thick lubricating fluid in a joint, bursa, or tendon sheath that is lined by synovial membrane; it is secreted by the membrane.

synovial (sĭ-no've-al) Relating to synovia.

synovianalysis (sĭ-no-ve-ah-nal'ĭ-sis) The microscopic examination, crystal identification, and cell count of synovial fluid (synovia) drawn from a joint. Five categories can be distinguished: normal, noninflammatory, inflammatory-immunologic, inflammatory-crystalline, and inflammatory-infectious.

synovitis (sin-o-vi'tis) Inflammation of the membrane lining a joint.

traumatic s. See traumatic tenosynovitis, under tenosynovitis.

syssarcosis (sis-sar-ko'sis) A muscular articulation; the union of bones by muscle (e.g., the connection between the hyoid bone and the lower jaw).

system (sis'tem) A functionally related group of parts or organs (e.g., a group of organs united in a common function, as the muscular system).

cardiovascular s. The heart and blood vessels through which blood is pumped and circulated throughout the body.

syssarcosis

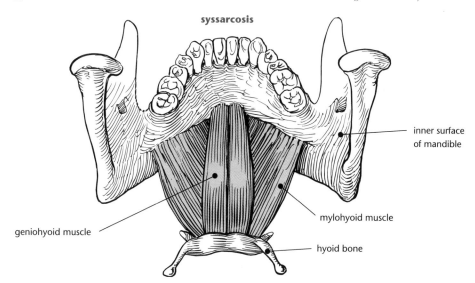

inner surface of mandible
geniohyoid muscle
mylohyoid muscle
hyoid bone

synchondrosis ■ system

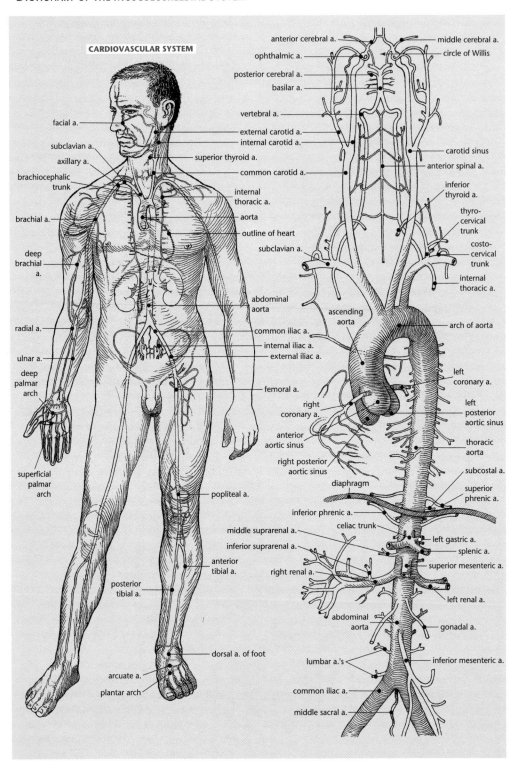

CARDIOVASCULAR SYSTEM

anterior cerebral a.
ophthalmic a.
posterior cerebral a.
basilar a.
vertebral a.
external carotid a.
internal carotid a.
superior thyroid a.
common carotid a.
internal thoracic a.
aorta
outline of heart
subclavian a.
abdominal aorta
common iliac a.
internal iliac a.
external iliac a.
femoral a.
popliteal a.
middle suprarenal a.
inferior suprarenal a.
anterior tibial a.
posterior tibial a.
dorsal a. of foot
arcuate a.
plantar arch

facial a.
subclavian a.
axillary a.
brachiocephalic trunk
brachial a.
deep brachial a.
radial a.
ulnar a.
deep palmar arch
superficial palmar arch

middle cerebral a.
circle of Willis
carotid sinus
anterior spinal a.
inferior thyroid a.
thyro-cervical trunk
costo-cervical trunk
internal thoracic a.
arch of aorta
left coronary a.
left posterior aortic sinus
thoracic aorta
subcostal a.
superior phrenic a.
left gastric a.
splenic a.
superior mesenteric a.
left renal a.
gonadal a.
inferior mesenteric a.

ascending aorta
right coronary a.
anterior aortic sinus
right posterior aortic sinus
diaphragm
inferior phrenic a.
celiac trunk
right renal a.
abdominal aorta
lumbar a.'s
common iliac a.
middle sacral a.

MUSCULOSKELETAL SYSTEM

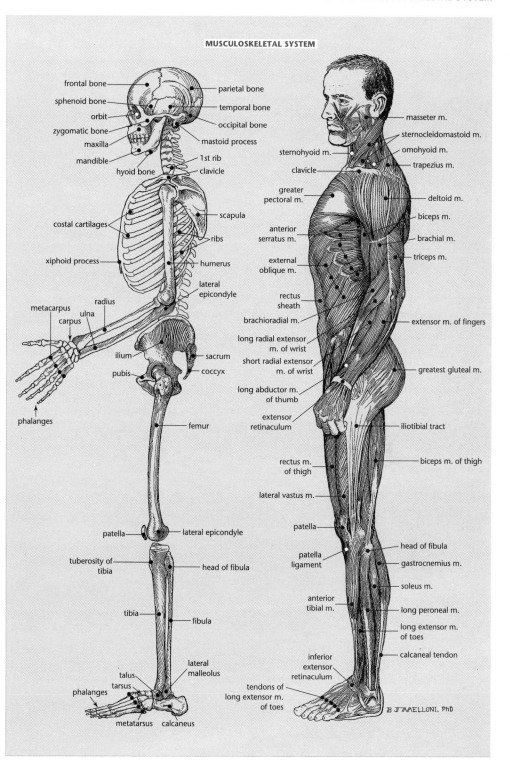

frontal bone
sphenoid bone
orbit
zygomatic bone
maxilla
mandible
hyoid bone

parietal bone
temporal bone
occipital bone
mastoid process
1st rib
clavicle

costal cartilages
xiphoid process

scapula
ribs
humerus
lateral epicondyle

metacarpus
carpus
radius
ulna

ilium
pubis

sacrum
coccyx

phalanges

femur

patella
tuberosity of tibia

lateral epicondyle
head of fibula

tibia

fibula

talus
tarsus
phalanges

lateral malleolus

metatarsus   calcaneus

masseter m.
sternocleidomastoid m.
omohyoid m.
trapezius m.
deltoid m.
biceps m.
brachial m.
triceps m.

sternohyoid m.
clavicle
greater pectoral m.
anterior serratus m.
external oblique m.
rectus sheath
brachioradial m.
long radial extensor m. of wrist
short radial extensor m. of wrist
long abductor m. of thumb
extensor retinaculum

extensor m. of fingers
greatest gluteal m.
iliotibial tract
biceps m. of thigh

rectus m. of thigh
lateral vastus m.
patella
patella ligament
anterior tibial m.
inferior extensor retinaculum
tendons of long extensor m. of toes

head of fibula
gastrocnemius m.
soleus m.
long peroneal m.
long extensor m. of toes
calcaneal tendon

B. JMELLONI, PhD

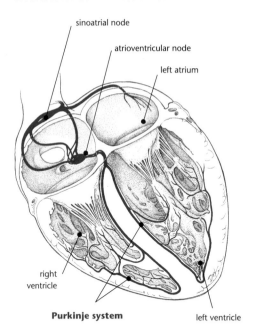

sinoatrial node

atrioventricular node

left atrium

right ventricle

Purkinje system

left ventricle

conducting system of heart

conducting s. of heart The tracts and network of various cell types (nodal, transitional, and Purkinje's myocytes) that are responsible for the conduction of impulses through the heart; they cause the heart to beat about 60 to 100 cycles per minute, maintaining perfusion of blood through the pulmonary and systemic tissues.

haversian s. See osteon.

hematopoietic s. The blood-producing tissues concerned with the formation of blood and its cellular constituents.

muscular s. The muscles of the body considered collectively.

musculoskeletal s. All the muscles and bones of the body and their connecting structures considered collectively.

neuromuscular s. The nerves and the muscles they innervate.

Purkinje s. The specialized system of modified muscle fibers in the heart concerned with conduction of impulses.

systremma (sis-trem'ah) A muscular cramp, especially of the calf muscles of the leg (chiefly the bellies of the gastrocnemius and soleus muscles); the contracted muscles form a hard bulge.

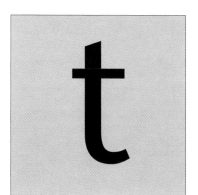

talar (ta'lar) Relating to the talus.

talipes (tal'ĭ-pez) General term that denotes a deformity involving the talus (ankle bone) and the foot, which results in an abnormal shape and position.

t. calcaneovalgus A relatively common congenital disorder in which the ankle joint is dorsiflexed and the foot is everted; believed to be caused by the position of the fetus in the uterus; the opposite of clubfoot (talipes equinovarus).

t. calcaneovarus A deformity of the ankle and foot with combined features of talipes calcaneus and talipes varus.

t. calcaneus Foot deformity characterized by an elevated forefoot and a depressed heel placing the weight of the body on the heel; generally the result of calf muscle paralysis. Also called pes calcaneus.

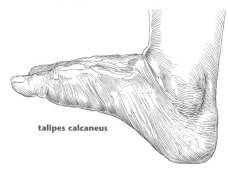

talipes calcaneus

t. cavus An exaggerated longitudinal arch of the foot due to contraction of the plantar fascia; may also be caused by a deformed bony arch. Also called cavus; equinocavus.

t. equinovalgus Foot deformity in which the characteristics of talipes equinus and talipes valgus are present, with weight borne on the metatarsophalangeal joints; the heel is elevated and turned outward from the body's midline. Also called equinovalgus.

t. equinovarus Congenital deformity of the foot in which only the outer portion of the foot touches the ground; with the ankle plantar flexed, the foot is inverted, and the anterior half of the foot is directed toward the middle. Also called clubfoot; equinovarus.

t. equinus A deformity characterized by fixed plantar extension of the foot, causing the weight of the body to rest on the ball of the foot or the metatarsophalangeal joints; the ankle joint is plantar flexed. Also called pes equinus; equinus.

t. planovalgus A deformity of the foot in which the characteristics of both talipes planus (flatfoot) and talipes valgus are present, with body weight distributed along the medial edge of the everted foot; the heel is turned outward and the foot's outer border is more elevated than the inner border; it may be congenital (permanent) or caused by reflex spasm of the muscles controlling the foot. Also called pes planovalgus.

t. planus See flatfoot.

t. valgus Outward turning of the foot, causing only the inner side of the sole to touch the ground; accompanied by flattening of the longitudinal arch. Also called pes valgus; pes pronatus.

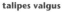

talipes valgus

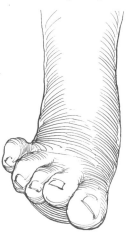

t. varus Deformity considered to be an incomplete form of clubfoot (talipes equinovarus); characterized by a turning inward of the foot, causing only the outer

talar ■ talipes

talipes varus

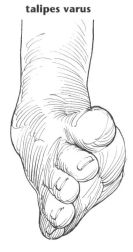

part of the sole to touch the ground; accompanied by increased height of the longitudinal arch. Also called pes varus.

talo- Combining form meaning the talus (ankle bone).

talocalcaneal, talocalcanean (ta-lo-kal-ke'ne-al, ta-lo-kal-ka'ne-an) Relating to the talus (ankle bone) and calcaneus (heel bone).

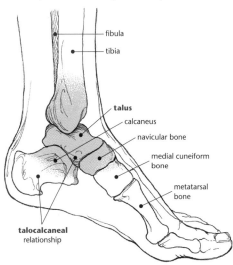

fibula
tibia
talus
calcaneus
navicular bone
medial cuneiform bone
metatarsal bone
talocalcaneal relationship

talocrural (ta-lo-kroo'ral) Relating to the ankle joint or to both the talus and bones of the leg.

talofibular (ta-lo-fib'u-lar) Relating to the ankle bone and the thin bone of the leg, the fibula.

talonavicular (ta-lo-nah-vik'u-lar) Relating to the talus (ankle bone) and the navicular bone (in the foot), especially its articulation.

talotibial (ta-lo-tib'e-al) Relating to the talus (ankle bone) and the tibia (shinbone).

talo ■ temporo-

talus (ta'lus) The large bone at the ankle articulating with the two leg bones (tibia and fibula) to form the ankle joint; it is the second largest bone of the tarsus. Popularly called ankle bone; formerly called astragalus. See also table of bones in appendix I.

tarsal (tahr'sal) Relating to the bones forming the tarsus, the posterior portion of the foot.

tarso- Combining form meaning tarsus.

tarsometatarsal (tahr-so-met-ah-tahr'sal) Relating to the tarsus and metatarsus.

tarsus (tahr'sus) The skeleton of the posterior part of the foot between the leg and the metatarsus; it consists of seven bones: the talus and calcaneus in the proximal row and the medial, intermediate, and lateral cuneiform bones and the cuboid bone in the distal row, with the navicular bone interposed between the rows.

tear (tār) 1. To rip or pull apart. 2. A rip or break of continuity of a structure.

    bowstring t. A longitudinal split of a meniscus, a semilunar cartilage within the knee joint; the anterior and posterior portions of the cartilage remain attached to the joint capsule while the free split inner border becomes displaced across the joint like a bowstring.

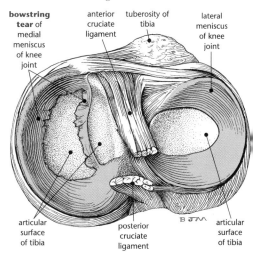

bowstring tear of medial meniscus of knee joint
anterior cruciate ligament
tuberosity of tibia
lateral meniscus of knee joint
articular surface of tibia
posterior cruciate ligament
articular surface of tibia

tegmen (teg'men) Rooflike structure that covers a part.

    t. tympani The bony roof of the middle ear chamber.

temporal (tem'po-ral) 1. Relating to the temple or to the lateral side of the head above the zygomatic arch. 2. Not permanent.

temporo- Combining form meaning the temple.

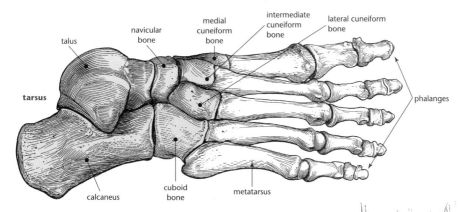

talus, navicular bone, medial cuneiform bone, intermediate cuneiform bone, lateral cuneiform bone, tarsus, phalanges, calcaneus, cuboid bone, metatarsus

temporomandibular (tem-po-ro-man-dib'u-lar) Relating to the temporal bone and mandible (e.g., a joint connecting the mandible to the skull).

temporo-occipital (tem-po-ro-oks-ĭp'ĭ-tal) Relating to the temporal and occipital bones of the skull.

temporoparietal (tem-po-ro-pah-ri'ĕ-tal) Relating to the temporal and the parietal bones, at the sides and upper part of the head.

tendinitis (ten-dĭ-ni'tis) Inflammation of a tendon, the fibrous tissue attaching muscle to bone or to another muscle, most frequently caused by repeated or severe trauma, strain, or excessive unaccustomed exercise; usually accompanied by inflammation of the membrane enveloping the tendon. Also spelled tendonitis. See also tenosynovitis.

   calcific t. Tendinitis resulting from deposition of calcium salts in a tendon, causing pain that may be sudden and severe.

   suppurative t. Tendinitis with pus formation frequently occurring in the fingers, causing swelling and tenderness, with flexion of the digit and pain on extension.

   traumatic ossifying t. Trauma-induced areas of ossification in tendons.

tendo calcaneus (ten'do kal-ka'ne-us) See calcaneal tendon, under tendon.

tendon (ten'dun) Fibrous band attaching a muscle to a bone.

   Achilles t. See calcaneal tendon.

   calcaneal t. The common tendon attaching the gastrocnemius and soleus muscles of the calf to the calcaneus (heel bone). Also called Achilles tendon; tendo calcaneus; tendo Achillis; heel tendon.

   central t. of diaphragm A fibrous aponeurotic sheath occupying the center of

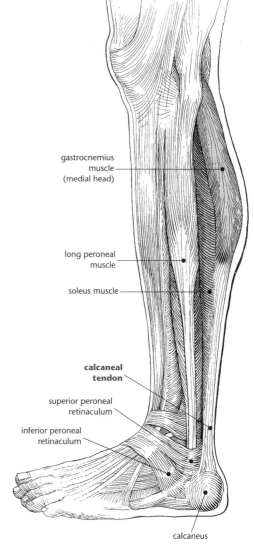

gastrocnemius muscle (medial head), long peroneal muscle, soleus muscle, **calcaneal tendon**, superior peroneal retinaculum, inferior peroneal retinaculum, calcaneus

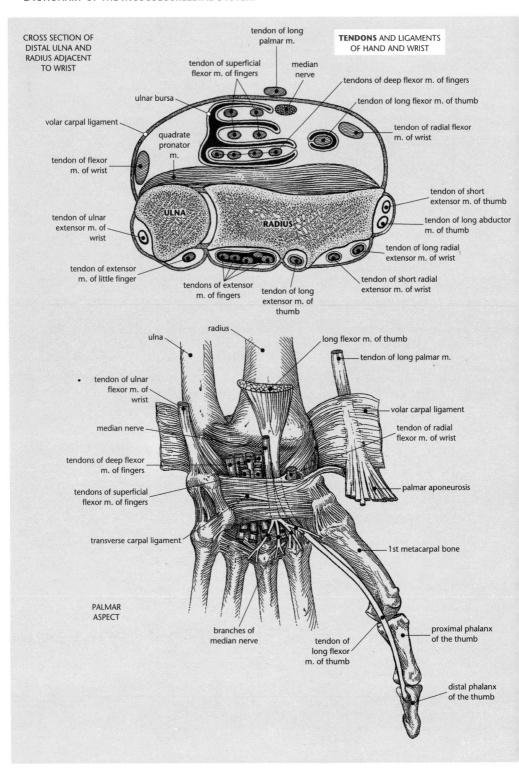

CROSS SECTION OF DISTAL ULNA AND RADIUS ADJACENT TO WRIST

tendon of long palmar m.

TENDONS AND LIGAMENTS OF HAND AND WRIST

tendon of superficial flexor m. of fingers

median nerve

tendons of deep flexor m. of fingers

ulnar bursa

tendon of long flexor m. of thumb

volar carpal ligament

quadrate pronator m.

tendon of radial flexor m. of wrist

tendon of flexor m. of wrist

tendon of short extensor m. of thumb

ULNA

RADIUS

tendon of ulnar extensor m. of wrist

tendon of long abductor m. of thumb

tendon of long radial extensor m. of wrist

tendon of extensor m. of little finger

tendons of extensor m. of fingers

tendon of long extensor m. of thumb

tendon of short radial extensor m. of wrist

radius

ulna

long flexor m. of thumb

tendon of long palmar m.

tendon of ulnar flexor m. of wrist

median nerve

volar carpal ligament

tendon of radial flexor m. of wrist

tendons of deep flexor m. of fingers

tendons of superficial flexor m. of fingers

palmar aponeurosis

transverse carpal ligament

1st metacarpal bone

PALMAR ASPECT

branches of median nerve

tendon of long flexor m. of thumb

proximal phalanx of the thumb

distal phalanx of the thumb

tendon ■ tendon

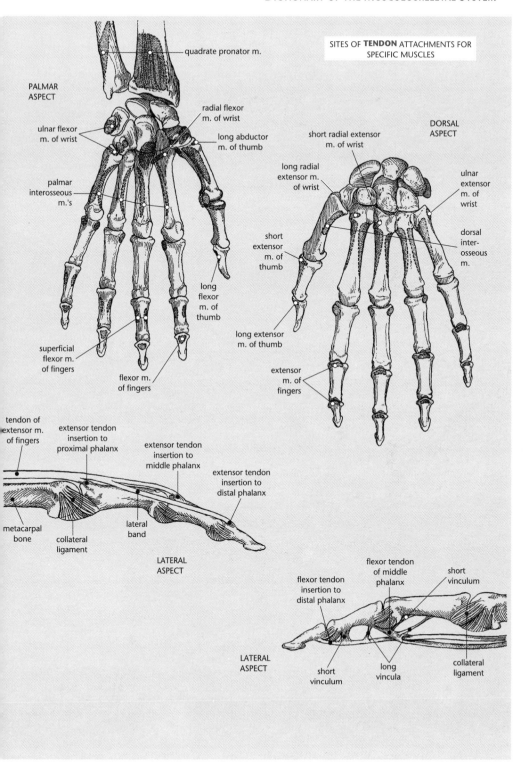

SITES OF **TENDON** ATTACHMENTS FOR SPECIFIC MUSCLES

PALMAR ASPECT

quadrate pronator m.

radial flexor m. of wrist

ulnar flexor m. of wrist

long abductor m. of thumb

palmar interosseous m.'s

superficial flexor m. of fingers

flexor m. of fingers

long flexor m. of thumb

DORSAL ASPECT

short radial extensor m. of wrist

long radial extensor m. of wrist

ulnar extensor m. of wrist

dorsal interosseous m.

short extensor m. of thumb

long extensor m. of thumb

extensor m. of fingers

tendon of extensor m. of fingers

extensor tendon insertion to proximal phalanx

extensor tendon insertion to middle phalanx

extensor tendon insertion to distal phalanx

metacarpal bone

collateral ligament

lateral band

LATERAL ASPECT

flexor tendon insertion to distal phalanx

flexor tendon of middle phalanx

short vinculum

short vinculum

long vincula

collateral ligament

LATERAL ASPECT

tendon ■ tendon

the dome-shaped respiratory diaphragm just below the pericardium; it has the appearance of a trifoliate leaf onto which the diaphragmatic muscle fibers converge to insert; the inferior vena cava penetrates the tendon on its way to the right atrium. Also called tendinous center; phrenic center; trefoil tendon.

common t. A tendon that accommodates more than one muscle.

common annular t. A fibrous ring situated within the back of the orbit (eye socket) and attached to the superior, inferior, and medial margins of the optic canal; it serves as origin for the four rectus muscles of the eye. Also called anulus tendineus communis; common tendinous ring; ligament of Zinn.

conjoined t. The fused tendons of two abdominal muscles: the transverse muscle of the abdomen (transversus abdominis) and the internal oblique muscle of the abdomen (obliquus internus abdominis); it inserts onto the crest of the pubic bone and the pectineal line. Also called inguinal falx; conjoint tendon.

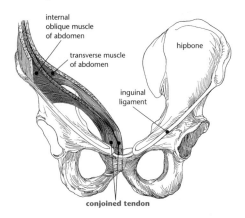

conjoined tendon

conjoint t. See conjoined tendon.

hamstring t. Either of two tendons bounding the popliteal space of the knee; the medial or inner one comprises the tendons of the semimembranous, semitendinous, gracilis and sartorius muscles; the lateral or outer one consists of the tendon of the biceps muscle of the thigh (biceps femoris). Also called hamstring.

intermediate t. A tendon situated between and connecting two bellies of a muscle, such as the bellies of the digastric muscle or the bellies of the omohyoid muscle.

trefoil t. See central tendon of diaphragm.

tendonitis (ten-do-ni′tis) See tendinitis.

teno- Combining form meaning tendon.

tenostosis (ten-os-to′sis) Ossification taking place in a tendon.

tenosynovitis (ten-o-sin-o-vi′tis) Inflammation of the inner lining of a tendon sheath and enclosed tendon; may be associated with systemic disorders (e.g., rheumatoid arthritis, gout, amyloidosis), with elevated blood cholesterol levels, with gonococcal infection (in females), or may be caused by mechanical strain; although simultaneously involving the enclosed tendon, the sheath lining is the site of maximum inflammation. See also tendinitis.

t. crepitans Tenosynovitis that produces a crackling sound upon movement of the affected tendon.

nodular t. A sharply localized tenosynovitis involving usually peripheral joints, considered by some authorities to be a benign tumor, rather than an inflammatory condition, with a tendency to recur after surgical removal.

stenosing t. Tenosynovitis occurring when there is a disproportion between the diameter of a tendon and the space or tunnel in which the tendon glides, causing scarring of the tendon sheath and a flexion contraction (e.g., of a finger).

suppurative t. Tenosynovitis caused by direct invasion by pus-forming bacteria; organisms may gain entry into the tendon sheath cavity through a wound (e.g., when a surgeon accidently punctures the tendon sheath while suturing adjacent structures).

traumatic t. Accumulation of synovial fluid and fibrin in a tendon sheath cavity, which may progress to adhesion formation; most often occurs as an occupational condition (e.g., in the arms of laborers and the wrists of stenographers). Also called traumatic synovitis.

tensor (ten′sor) Tending to make a part tense or firm; applied to muscles (e.g., the tensor tympani muscle that renders the eardrum taut).

teres (te′rēz) Round and elongated; applied to ligaments and muscles.

thenar (the′nar) The fleshy mass of muscles at the base of the thumb.

thoracolumbar (tho-rah-ko-lum′bar) Relating to the thoracic and lumbar regions of the vertebral column.

thorax (tho′raks) The chest; the part of the body between the neck and the diaphragm; the skeletal component consists of twelve thoracic vertebrae posteriorly, the sternum anteriorly,

tendon ■ thorax

and twelve pairs of ribs and costal cartilages connecting them.

thumb (thum) The first digit of the hand.

    gamekeeper's t. Rupture of the ulnar collateral ligament of the metacarpophalangeal joint of the thumb by forcible abduction; if untreated may lead to progressive subluxation.

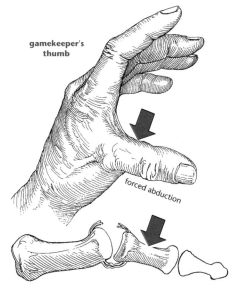

gamekeeper's thumb

forced abduction

    tennis t. Inflammation and calcification of the tendon of the long flexor muscle of the thumb due to activities in which the thumb is subject to great pressure and strain (e.g., in tennis playing).

    trigger t. Condition in which the thumb is arrested in a bent position at the beginning of attempted extension and then suddenly released with an audible click; caused by

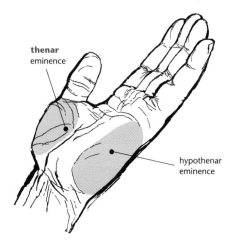

thenar eminence

hypothenar eminence

interference with movement of the tendon within its sheath due to inflammation; commonly associated with osteoarthritis.

thyroarytenoid (thi-ro-ar-ī-te′noid) Relating to both the thyroid and arytenoid cartilages.

thyroepiglottic (thi-ro-ep-ī-glot′ik) Relating to the thyroid cartilage and to the epiglottis.

thyroglossal (thi-ro-glos′al) Relating to the thyroid cartilage or gland and the tongue.

thyrohyoid (thi-ro-hi′oid) Relating to the thyroid cartilage and the hyoid bone, especially their connecting ligaments. Also called hyothyroid.

tibia (tib′e-ah) The larger of the two bones of the leg between the knee and the ankle, medial to the fibula. Popularly called shinbone. See also table of bones in appendix I.

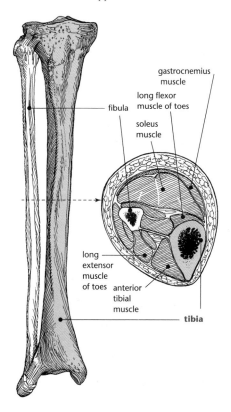

gastrocnemius muscle

long flexor muscle of toes

fibula

soleus muscle

long extensor muscle of toes

anterior tibial muscle

tibia

tibio- Combining form meaning tibia (shinbone).

tibiocalcaneal (tib-e-o-kal-ka′ne-al) Relating to the tibia (shinbone) and the calcaneus (heel bone).

tibiofemoral (tib-e-o-fem′or-al) Relating to the tibia (shinbone) and the femur (thigh bone).

tibiofibular (tib-e-o-fib′u-lar) Relating to the two bones of the leg, tibia and fibula.

thumb ■ tibiofibular

tic (tik) Involuntary, brief, and recurrent twitching of a muscle or a group of muscles, usually involving the face, neck, or shoulders (e.g., needless blinking and shoulder shrugging).

tissue (tish'u) A mass of similar cells and the substance that surrounds them, united to perform a particular function.

    bone t. A hard form of connective tissue that is highly vascular, mineralized, and constantly changing; it consists of cells (osteocytes) embedded in a tough fibrous matrix containing collagen fibers and deposits of mineral salts (calcium phosphate, carbonate, and fluoride); it develops either by transformation of condensed mesenchyme or by replacement of a cartilaginous model. Also called bony tissue; osseous tissue.

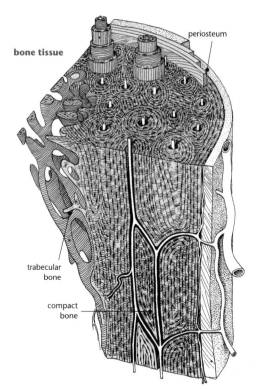

bone tissue

periosteum

trabecular bone

compact bone

    bony t. See bone tissue.

    cancellous t. The loose, latticelike spongy bone containing numerous marrow cavities; found in the interior of all bones, especially towards the articular ends of long bones.

    chondrogenic t. A connective tissue forming the inner layer of the fibrous membrane that covers cartilage (perichondrium), responsible for the production of new cartilage.

    connective t. A general term denoting the principal supporting tissue of the body formed by a considerable proportion of fibrous and ground substance with numerous cell types (fibroblasts, macrophages, plasma cells, neutrophils, eosinophils, lymphocytes, fat cells, etc.) as well as supportive proteins, such as collagen and elastin; it supports and connects various structures throughout the body with the exception of the nervous system; bones, cartilage, fascia, ligaments, and tendons, are some examples of connective tissue. Also called interstitial tissue.

    elastic t. Connective tissue composed chiefly of yellow elastic fibers, giving the tissue elasticity and a yellowish hue; found in some ligaments (e.g., flaval and nuchal ligaments) and in the walls of large arteries and air passages. Also called fibroelastic tissue.

    fibroelastic t. See elastic tissue.

    fibrous t. A dense form of connective tissue containing bundles of closely packed strands of collagenous fibers with little intercellular matrix; found in tendons, ligaments, and aponeuroses.

    interstitial t. See connective tissue.

    muscular t. The substance of a muscle composed of threadlike fibers either striated (skeletal and cardiac) or nonstriated (smooth), which contract upon stimulation.

    myeloid t. The red bone marrow of the ribs, vertebrae and other small bones, which forms both red and white blood cells, consisting of the developmental and adult stages of erythrocytes, granulocytes, and megakaryocytes in a stroma of reticular cells and fibers.

    osseous t. See bone tissue.

    osteogenic t. A fibrous connective tissue comprising the loose inner layer of the membrane covering the surface of bones (periosteum), containing osteoblasts that engage in the formation of bone tissue.

    osteoid t. Bone matrix prior to calcification; uncalcified bone tissue produced by osteoblasts and osteogenic cells, normally found as a thin layer on the advancing surface of developing bone.

    reticular t. The most delicate type of connective tissue, composed of a network of fine reticular cells and reticulin fibers arranged in a mesh to facilitate the free

tic ■ tissue

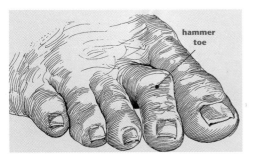

hammer toe

movement of cells and fluids; found in many structures, such as bone marrow.

toe (to) One of the digits of the feet.

   great t. The hallux.

   hammer t. A deformed second toe (usually associated with hallux valgus) in which the second phalanx is permanently flexed and the first phalanx compensates by hyperextending.

   pigeon t.'s See intoe.

tongue (tung) The mobile muscular structure covered with mucous membrane and arising from the floor of the mouth; it serves as the chief organ of taste and aids in chewing, swallowing, and articulation of sounds.

strawberry t. A tongue dotted with enlarged red papillae protruding through a whitish coating; seen in scarlet fever.

tooth (tōōth), pl. teeth Any of the bonelike structures suspended within sockets in the upper and lower jaws by a relatively soft periodontal ligament, which allows slight movement; used to seize, hold, and masticate food; also to assist in articulation of sounds; it is the hardest and chemically most stable tissue in the body, composed of hard dentin surrounding a pulp cavity and covered by enamel on the crown and by cement (cementum) on the root. Because of their durability, teeth are of great forensic importance for identification of otherwise unrecognizable bodies, since their pattern can be compared to dental records of missing persons.

   anterior teeth The teeth situated in the front part of the upper and lower jaws, comprised of the central incisors, lateral incisors and cuspids. Also called labial teeth.

   baby teeth See deciduous teeth.

   canine t. See cuspid.

   dead t. See nonvital tooth.

   deciduous teeth The 20 teeth of the first dentition that generally erupt between the sixth and thirtieth months of life, and after shedding are replaced by permanent teeth; they include four incisors, two cuspids, and four molars in each jaw; the usual times of eruption are: central incisors, six to eight months; lateral incisors, eight to 10 months; first molars, 12 to 16 months; cuspids, 16 to 20 months; second molars, 20 to 30 months;

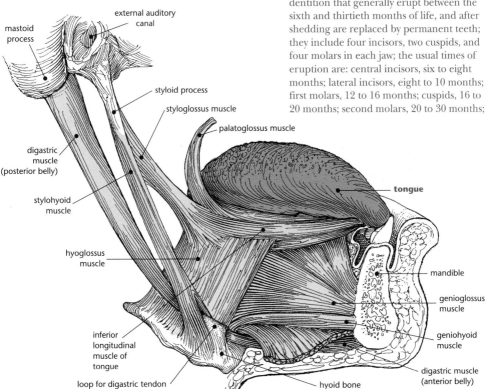

mastoid process

external auditory canal

styloid process

styloglossus muscle

palatoglossus muscle

digastric muscle (posterior belly)

stylohyoid muscle

hyoglossus muscle

tongue

mandible

genioglossus muscle

geniohyoid muscle

inferior longitudinal muscle of tongue

loop for digastric tendon

hyoid bone

digastric muscle (anterior belly)

toe ■ tooth

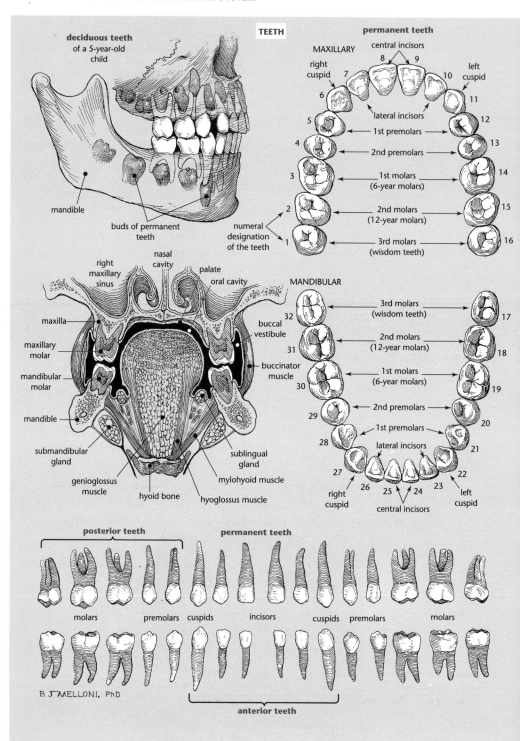

TEETH

deciduous teeth
of a 5-year-old
child

mandible

buds of permanent
teeth

permanent teeth

MAXILLARY

central incisors

right
cuspid

left
cuspid

8   9

7   10

6   11

lateral incisors   12

5   1st premolars

4   2nd premolars   13

3   1st molars   14
                      (6-year molars)
2   2nd molars   15
                      (12-year molars)
1   3rd molars   16
numeral   (wisdom teeth)
designation
of the teeth

right
maxillary
sinus

nasal
cavity

palate

oral cavity

MANDIBULAR

maxilla

maxillary
molar

mandibular
molar

mandible

submandibular
gland

genioglossus
muscle

buccal
vestibule

buccinator
muscle

sublingual
gland

mylohyoid muscle

hyoid bone

hyoglossus muscle

3rd molars
(wisdom teeth)

2nd molars
(12-year molars)

1st molars
(6-year molars)

2nd premolars

1st premolars

lateral incisors

32   17

31   18

30   19

29   20

28   21

27   22

26   25   24   23

central incisors

right
cuspid

left
cuspid

posterior teeth

permanent teeth

molars   premolars cuspids   incisors   cuspids   premolars   molars

B. J. MELLONI, PhD

anterior teeth

tooth ■ tooth

they calcify partly before birth and partly after birth; their roots are progressively resorbed by osteoclasts prior to their being replaced, and as a result the shed or extracted deciduous teeth seem to have short roots. Also called baby teeth; milk teeth; primary teeth.

Hutchinson's teeth Malformed, barrel-shaped permanent incisors with underdeveloped enamel and a notched, narrow edge; occasionally the first molars are also affected and appear dome-shaped, with a pitted occlusal surface. Hutchinson's teeth are considered a sign of congenital syphilis. Also called notched teeth; pegged teeth.

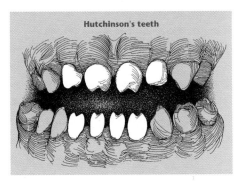

Hutchinson's teeth

impacted t. A tooth that is incapable of erupting completely or even partially, due to its angle of eruption or by being so placed in the jaw as to meet resistance from an adjacent tooth.

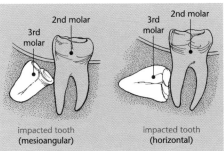

3rd molar · 2nd molar
impacted tooth (mesioangular)

3rd molar · 2nd molar
impacted tooth (horizontal)

labial teeth See anterior teeth.

malacotic teeth Structurally soft teeth that are abnormally susceptible to caries.

mandibular teeth Teeth situated in the lower jaw (mandible).

maxillary teeth Teeth situated in the upper jaw (maxilla).

mottled teeth Teeth characterized by underdevelopment of the enamel and marked by white chalky areas, which in time undergo brown discoloration; usually caused by drinking water containing excessive fluorides during the time of tooth development.

nonvital t. A tooth from which the pulp has been removed or one in which the pulp has died. Also called dead tooth; pulpless tooth.

notched teeth See Hutchinson's teeth.

pegged teeth See Hutchinson's teeth.

permanent teeth The 32 teeth of the second dentition that generally erupt between the ages of six to 21 years, they include four incisors, two cuspids, four bicuspids, and six molars in each jaw; the usual times of eruption are: first molars, six to seven years; central incisors, six to eight years; lateral incisors, seven to nine years; cuspids, nine to 12 years; first and second premolars, 10 to 12 years; second molars, 11 to 13 years; third molars, 17 to 21 years; the cuspid roots are the longest, the first upper molar is the largest tooth, and the lower third molar, which frequently erupts anterosuperiorly, is often impacted against the second molar. Also called succedaneous teeth.

posterior teeth The premolar and molar teeth situated in the back part of the upper and lower jaws. Also called buccal teeth.

premolar teeth The permanent teeth between the cuspid and first molar. See permanent teeth.

primary teeth See deciduous teeth.

protruding teeth Teeth that extend beyond the normal contours of the dental arches; often in an anterior direction.

pulpless t. See nonvital tooth.

sclerotic t. A structurally hard tooth that is resistant to caries.

succedaneous teeth See permanent teeth.

supernumerary t. An accessory natural tooth, in excess of the normal number; most commonly seen in the incisal area.

unerupted t. a) A tooth prior to eruption through the gingiva. b) A tooth that is incapable of erupting through the gingiva.

vital t. A tooth with a living (vital) pulp, in which the nerve and vascular supply are functional.

wisdom t. Third permanent molar; erupts between the ages of 17 and 21 years; so called because it is the last of the permanent teeth to erupt.

torulus (tor'u-lus) A small projection or protuberance.

tooth ■ torulus

torus (to'rus) A protuberance or rounded projection.

> **t. mandibularis** An asymptomatic benign bony projection on the lingual side of the lower jaw between the cuspid and first bicuspid tooth.

> **t. palatinus** A common bony outgrowth in the midline of the hard palate.

> **t. tubarius** A normal ridge posterior to the pharyngeal opening of the auditory tube. Also called eustachian cushion.

trabecula (trah-bek'u-lah), pl. trabec'ulae A connecting anchoring strand made up of connective tissue, bone, or muscle fibers.

> **trabeculae carneae cordis** See fleshy trabeculae of heart.

> **fleshy trabeculae of heart** Irregular muscular projections from most of the inner surface of the ventricles of the heart. Also called trabeculae carneae cordis.

> **septomarginal t.** A thick band of heart muscle usually extending from the interventricular septum to the base of the anterior papillary muscle in the right ventricle; it provides passage for the right branch of the atrioventricular bundle of nerve fibers from the septum to the opposite wall of the ventricle. It may also help in preventing overdistention of the right ventricle. Also called trabecula septomarginalis.

> **t. septomarginalis** See septomarginal trabecula.

trabecular (trah-bek'u-lar) Relating to trabeculae.

trachea (tra'ke-ah) A cartilaginous and membranous tube extending from, and continuous with, the lower part of the larynx to the bronchi.

tracheal (tra'ke-al) Relating to the trachea.

tracheobronchial (tra-ke-o-brong'ke-al) See bronchotracheal.

tracheolaryngeal (tra-ke-o-lah-rin'je-al) See laryngotracheal.

tract (trakt) 1. A series of structures constituting a body system that performs a specialized function. 2. A path.

> **iliotibial t.** A strong, wide, thickened reinforcement of a portion of the fascia lata on the lateral side of the thigh; it extends from the iliac crest of the hipbone and the capsule of the hip joint downward to the lateral condyle of the tibia; it is divided superiorly to receive the greater part of the insertion of the greater gluteal muscle (gluteus maximus) posteriorly and the insertion of the tensor muscle of fascia lata (tensor fasciae latae) anteriorly; the tract protects many of the prominent bony points

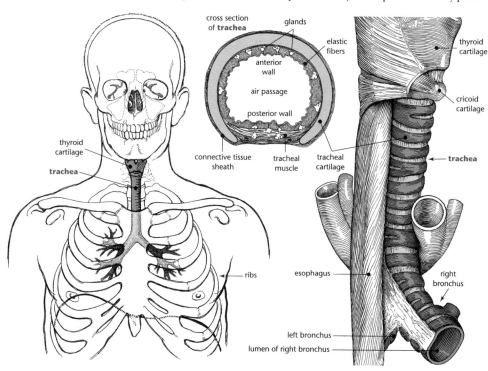

cross section of **trachea**

glands

elastic fibers

anterior wall

air passage

posterior wall

thyroid cartilage

cricoid cartilage

thyroid cartilage

trachea

connective tissue sheath

tracheal muscle

tracheal cartilage

trachea

ribs

esophagus

right bronchus

left bronchus

lumen of right bronchus

torus ■ tract

near the knee joint, such as the condyles of the femur and tibia, and the head of the fibula. Also called iliotibial band.

tragus (tra'gus) The small projection of cartilage in front of, and partly covering, the opening of the external auditory canal.

trans- Prefix meaning across or through.

transiliac (trans-il'e-ak) From one ilium to the other.

transischiac (trans-is'ke-ak) From one ischium (of the hipbone) to the other.

transverse (trans-vers') Passing across the long axis of the body or a structure.

trapezium (trah-pe'ze-um) See table of muscles in appendix II.

triangle (tri'ang-gl) A figure or area formed by connecting three points; a three-cornered area.

  anterior cervical t. A large triangular area of the anterior neck, bounded on top, by the mandible, behind, by the anterior margin of the sternocleidomastoid muscle, and in front, by the midline of the neck. The triangle is subdivided into the muscular, carotid, submental, and digastric triangles.

  carotid t. A small triangular area of the neck, bounded above by the posterior belly of the digastric muscle, behind by the sternocleidomastoid muscle, and below by the superior belly of the omohyoid muscle; it contains the upper part of the common carotid and its bifurcation into the external and internal carotid arteries. It is best seen when the neck is extended and the head slightly rotated contralaterally.

  digastric t. The triangular area bounded above by the mandible and behind, below, and in front, by the posterior and anterior bellies of the digastric muscle; the area contains the submandibular gland. Also called submandibular triangle.

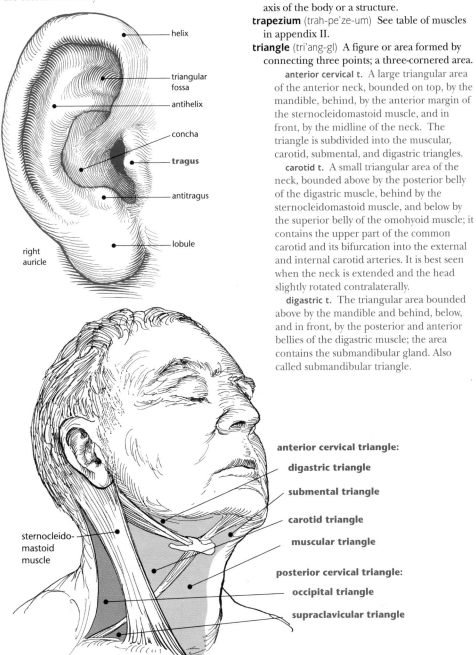

helix
triangular fossa
antihelix
concha
tragus
antitragus
lobule
right auricle

anterior cervical triangle:
  digastric triangle
  submental triangle
  carotid triangle
  muscular triangle
posterior cervical triangle:
  occipital triangle
  supraclavicular triangle

sternocleido-mastoid muscle

tragus ■ triangle

t. of elbow See cubital fossa, under fossa.

femoral t. A triangular area just below the fold of the groin, at the upper and inner part of the thigh; it is bounded above by the inguinal ligament, laterally by the medial border of the sartorius muscle, and medially by the medial border of the long adductor (adductor longus) muscle; the femoral vessels divide the triangle into two parts. Also called Scarpa's triangle.

Grynfelt-Lesshaft t. A triangular area bounded above by the twelfth rib and the serratus posterior inferior muscle, medially by the erector muscle of the spine, and inferolaterally by the internal oblique muscle; it is a weak area that offers little resistance to pressure from within, therefore,

it is a likely site for protrusion of intra-abdominal structures (lumbar hernia). Also called superior lumbar space.

Hesselbach's t. See inguinal triangle.

inguinal t. A triangular area of the anterior abdominal wall bounded below by the medial half of the inguinal ligament, medially by the lower edge of the straight muscle of the abdomen (rectus abdominus), and laterally by a line from the middle of the inguinal ligament to the navel (umbilicus); an important area relating to direct and indirect inguinal hernias. Also called Hesselbach's triangle.

Laimer's t. A triangular area of the upper posterior part of the esophagus, immediately below the cricopharyngeus muscle, in which the posterior wall is variably deficient; it is a likely site for an esophageal diverticulum to occur.

lumbar t. A small triangular area bounded

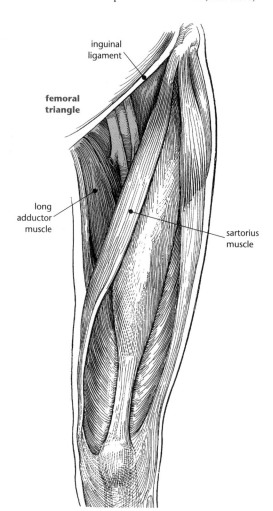

inguinal ligament

femoral triangle

long adductor muscle

sartorius muscle

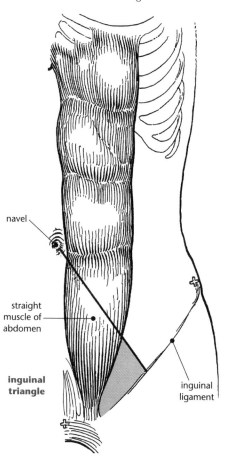

navel

straight muscle of abdomen

inguinal triangle

inguinal ligament

triangle ■ triangle

by the edges of the lateral margin of the latissimus dorsi and the medial margin of the external oblique muscles and the crest of the ilium. Also called inferior lumbar space.

muscular t. A triangular area limited in front by the midline of the neck, from the hyoid bone to the breastbone (sternum), and in the back by the anterior margin of the sternocleidomastoid and the superior belly of the omohyoid muscle; it is the largest subdivision of the anterior cervical triangle.

occipital t. The triangular area of the posterior neck formed by the sternocleidomastoid, trapezius, and omohyoid muscles; the larger division of the posterior cervical triangle.

posterior cervical t. A triangular area of the posterior neck, bounded, in front, by the posterior margin of the sternocleidomastoid muscle, behind, by the anterior margin of the trapezius muscle, below by the clavicle. The inferior belly of the omohyoid muscle divides the triangle into an upper occipital triangle and a lower supraclavicular triangle.

Scarpa's t. See femoral triangle.

subclavian t. See supraclavicular triangle.

submandibular t. See digastric triangle.

submental t. Triangular region bounded laterally by the anterior belly of the digastric muscle, medially by the midline of the neck from the hyoid bone to the chin (mental symphysis), and below, by the hyoid bone. Also called suprahyoid triangle.

supraclavicular t. The small triangular area of the neck, bounded by the sternocleidomastoid muscle, the inferior belly of the omohyoid muscle and by the clavicle; the smaller division of the posterior cervical triangle. Also called subclavian triangle.

suprahyoid t. See submental triangle.

Ward's t. A triangular area in the neck of the femur near the hip joint, seen on x-ray film and characterized by diminished density in the trabecular pattern; it represents a relatively weak area that is vulnerable to fracture. It is one of the areas commonly assessed by densitometry to estimate the extent of osteoporosis.

triceps (tri'seps) Having three sites of origin (e.g., the triceps muscle). See also table of muscles in appendix II.

triquetral (tri-kwe'tral) 1. Relating to a triangular structure. 2. See table of bones in appendix I.

trochanter (tro-kan'ter) One of two prominences (greater and lesser) on the upper end of the

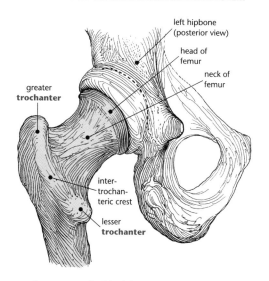

femur, near the hip joint.

trochanteric (tro-kan-ter'ik) Relating to a trochanter.

trochlea (trok'le-ah) 1. Any pulley-like structure. 2. The fibrous loop in the orbit (eye socket) through which passes the tendon of the superior oblique muscle of the eyeball.

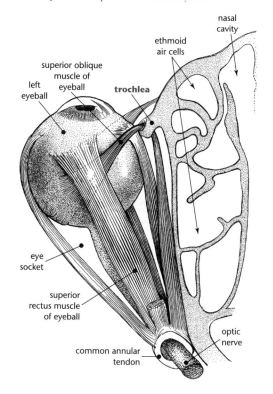

t. of humerus The pulley-shaped, grooved, condylar surface at the lower end of the humerus; it articulates with the trochlear notch of the ulna.

peroneal t. A small elevation on the lateral side of the calcaneus (heel bone), about 2 cm below the lateral malleolus; it separates the tendon of the long peroneal muscle (peroneus longus) from the tendon of the short peroneal muscle (peroneus brevis). Also called peroneal spine of calcaneus.

t. of talus The rounded, superior surface of the talus that articulates with the distal ends of the tibia and fibula in the ankle joint.

trochoid (tro'koid) Permitting rotation, as a pivot; applied to certain articulations.

tubercle (too'ber-kl) A rounded elevation on a structure, such as a bone.

adductor t. of femur A small projection on the medial surface of the lower part of the femur, situated on the upper part of the medial condyle, which provides attachment to the tendon of the great adductor (adductor magnus) muscle; it is an important surgical landmark and can be easily palpated.

anterior t. of atlas A median conical protuberance on the front of the anterior arch of the atlas (first cervical vertebra); it provides attachment to the anterior longitudinal ligament.

anterior t. of calcaneus A small rounded tubercle on the bottom of the front part of the calcaneus (heel bone); it marks the distal limit of the attachment of the long plantar ligament.

auricular t. A small elevation on the ear frequently seen on the inner edge of the helix. Also called tubercle of Darwin.

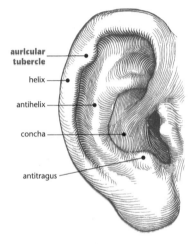

carotid t. The large anterior tubercle on either side of the sixth cervical vertebra; the common carotid artery lies anteriorly to it and can be compressed against it.

conoid t. A prominent elevation on the bottom surface of the lateral part of the clavicle that gives attachment to the conoid ligament.

corniculate t. The elevation on either side of the larynx produced by the underlying corniculate cartilage of the posterior part of the aryepiglottic fold of mucous membrane.

costal t. See tubercle of rib.

t. of Darwin See auricular tubercle.

genial t.'s Small bony elevations on the lower part of the inner surface of the chin (mental protuberance); they provide attachment for the geniohyoid and genioglossus muscles. Also called mental spines.

greater t. of humerus A large bony prominence on the lateral side of the upper end of the arm bone (humerus), to which the supraspinatus, infraspinatus, and teres minor muscles are attached; it is the most lateral bony prominence of the shoulder region and responsible for the rounded contour of the shoulder. Also called greater tuberosity of humerus.

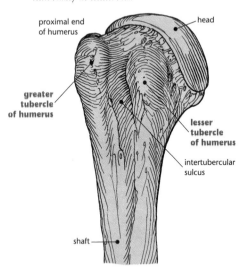

t. of iliac crest A prominence on the outer lip of the iliac crest of the hipbone, approximately 5 cm above and behind the anterior superior iliac spine.

infraglenoid t. A roughened prominence just below the glenoid fossa of the scapula; it

trochoid ■ tubercle

provides attachment for the tendon of the long head of the triceps muscle of the arm (triceps brachii muscle).

intercondylar t. One of two bony tubercles (lateral and medial) of the eminence on the intercondylar area of the uppermost part of the tibia.

lesser t. of humerus A bony prominence on the anterior surface of the humerus just beyond its anatomic neck, near the shoulder joint; it provides attachment for the subscapular muscle; its lateral edge forms the medial border of the intertubercular sulcus. Also called lesser tuberosity of humerus.

marginal t. of zygomatic bone See tubercle of zygomatic bone.

nuchal t. The prominent elevation formed by the tip of the spinous process of the seventh cervical vertebra, clearly seen and easily palpated at the lower end of the nuchal furrow at the back of the neck.

pharyngeal t.
See pharyngeal spine, under spine.

posterior t. of atlas A median conical protuberance on the back of the posterior arch of the atlas (first cervical vertebra); it represents a rudimentary spinous process and provides attachment to the nuchal ligament.

pterygoid t. See pterygoid tuberosity of mandible, under tuberosity.

pubic t. A small tubercle at the lateral end of the pubic crest, on either side, about 2 cm from the pubic symphysis; it provides attachment to the tendons of the straight muscle of the abdomen (rectus abdominis muscle) and the pyramidal muscle. Also called pubic spine.

t. of radius
See radial tuberosity, under tuberosity.

t. of rib A knoblike eminence on the posterior surface of a rib at the junction of its neck and shaft; it articulates with the transverse process of the corresponding thoracic vertebra. Also called costal tubercle.

t. of root of the zygoma A bony protuberance on the inferior border of the zygomatic process of the temporal bone, to which are attached fibers of the lateral ligament of the temporomandibular joint.

scalene t. A small area of elevated roughness on the inner border of the upper surface of the first rib, separating the groove for the subclavian artery from the groove for the subclavian vein; it provides attachment to the tendon of the anterior scalene muscle.

t. of sella turcica The slight transverse ridge in front of the pituitary (hypophyseal) fossa at the base of the skull.

supraglenoid t. An elevated roughened area immediately above the glenoid fossa of the scapula; it provides attachment to the tendon of the biceps muscle of the arm (biceps brachii).

t. of tibia See tibial tuberosity, under tuberosity.

t. of zygomatic bone A small, rounded bony projection from the temporal border of the frontal process of the zygomatic bone just below the frontozygomatic suture; it can be felt through the skin. Also called marginal tubercle of zygomatic bone.

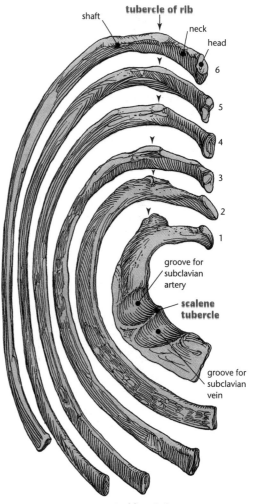

upper aspect of first 6 ribs

tubercle ■ tubercle

tuberosity (too-bĕ-ros'ĭ-te) A rounded protuberance from the surface of a bone or cartilage.

calcaneal t. The prominent posterior plantar extremity of the calcaneus that forms the projection of the heel; it bears lateral and medial processess.

deltoid t. of humerus A linear, raised area on the lateral surface of the middle part of the humerus to which the deltoid muscle is attached. Also called deltoid eminence; deltoid crest; deltoid ridge.

gluteal t. of femur A broad, rough, vertical ridge on the posterior aspect of the upper end of the shaft of the femur; it extends from the base of the greater trochanter to the lateral lip of the linea aspera; it affords insertion to the lower part of the greatest gluteal muscle (gluteus maximus) and the pubic part of the great adductor muscle (adductor magnus). Also called gluteal ridge of femur; gluteal crest.

greater t. of humerus See greater tubercle of humerus, under tubercle.

iliac t. A rough, everted prominence on the medial aspect of the ilium between the posterior part of the iliac crest and the auricular surface; it affords attachment to the posterior sacroiliac ligament.

ischial t. The enlarged rough lower part of the ischium of the hipbone; divided by a transverse ridge into an upper and lower area; the upper part provides attachment for the hamstring muscles and the inferior gemellus muscle; the lower part (on which the body rests in the sitting position) affords attachment to the great adductor (adductor magnus) muscle and the sacrotuberous ligament.

lesser t. of humerus See lesser tubercle of humerus, under tubercle.

pterygoid t. of mandible A roughened surface on the inner side of the angle of the mandible for the insertion of the medial pterygoid muscle. Also called pterygoid tubercle.

radial t. A broad bony prominence on the medial surface of the radius just below its neck, which affords attachment to the biceps muscle of the arm (biceps brachii). Also called tuberosity of radius; tubercle of radius.

t. of radius See radial tuberosity.

sacral t. The roughened area on the back of the sacrum between the lateral sacral crest and the auricular surface; it affords attachment to the sacroiliac ligaments.

t. of tibia See tibial tuberosity.

tibial t. A broad triangular projection on the front of the upper end of the tibia; the upper portion of the tuberosity provides attachment for the ligament of the patella and the lower portion is associated with the infrapatellar bursa. Also called tuberosity of tibia; tubercle of tibia.

t. of ulna A bony prominence on the anterior aspect of the upper end of the ulna between the coronoid process and the shaft of the bone; it affords attachment to the brachial muscle (brachialis).

turbinate (tur'bĭ-nāt) A shell-shaped anatomic structure.

inferior t. See inferior concha, under concha.

middle t. See middle concha, under concha.

sphenoid t. See sphenoid concha, under concha.

superior t. See superior concha, under concha.

twitching (twich'ing) The occurrence of brief skeletal muscle contractions or a single spasmodic contraction of a muscle fiber.

fascicular t. Twitching of bundles of skeletal muscle fibers or large groups of muscle fibers.

tympanic (tim-pan'ik) 1. Relating to the middle ear chamber and eardrum. 2. Resonant.

tympanosquamosal (tim-pah-no-skwah-mo'sal) Relating to the tympanic and squamous parts of the temporal bone.

tympanum (tim'pah-num) The middle ear chamber and the tympanic **membrane** (eardrum) combined.

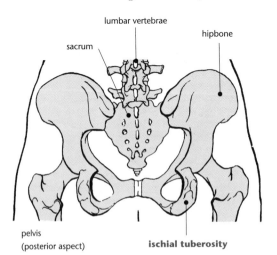

lumbar vertebrae

hipbone

sacrum

pelvis
(posterior aspect)

ischial tuberosity

tuberosity ■ tympanum

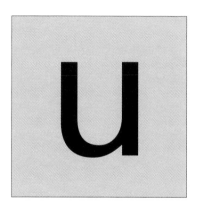

ulna (ul'nah) The larger of the two bones of the forearm, extending from the elbow to the wrist, on the opposite side of the thumb. Popularly called elbow bone. See also table of bones in appendix I.

ulnar (ul'nar) Relating to the ulna.

ulnocarpal (ul-no-kar'pal) Relating to the ulna and the carpus, or denoting the ulnar aspect of the wrist.

ulnoradial (ul-no-ra'de-al) Relating to the two bones of the forearm, ulna and radius.

uncinate (un'sĭ-nāt) Hook-shaped or hooklike.

uniarticular (u-ne-ar-tik'u-lar) Relating to a single joint; monarticular.

union (ūn'yun) The process of growing or joining together.

> **faulty u.** Condition in which tissues have united in an improper position.
>
> **fibrous u.** Formation of a fibrous callus on a bone at the site of a fracture without development of bone tissue.
>
> **vicious u.** A faulty union that results in deformity.

unipennate (u-nĭ-pen'āt) Feather-shaped on one side only; applied to a muscle that has a tendon on one side. Also called demipenniform; semipenniform.

unstriated (un-stri'āt-ed) Lacking stripes or striations; applied to smooth muscles.

uvula (u'vu-lah) A fleshy mass resembling a grape.

> **palatine u.** The grape-like process that hangs from the middle of the posterior border of the soft palate, just above the root of the tongue; composed of the uvula muscle and connective tissue.

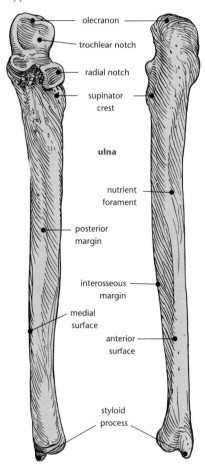

olecranon
trochlear notch
radial notch
supinator crest

ulna

nutrient foramen
posterior margin
interosseous margin
medial surface
anterior surface
styloid process

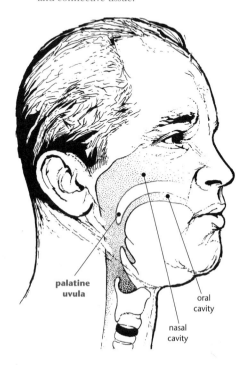

palatine uvula

oral cavity
nasal cavity

ulna ■ uvula

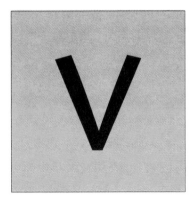

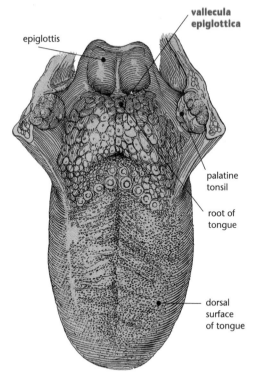

epiglottis

vallecula
epiglottica

palatine
tonsil

root of
tongue

dorsal
surface
of tongue

valgus (val'gus) Bent outward; away from the central line of the body; said of a deformed part, as in hallux valgus.

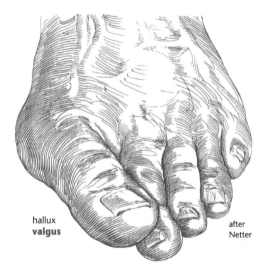

hallux
valgus

after
Netter

vallecula (vah-lek'u-lah) A small groove or depression on the surface of a part.

    v. epiglottica A depression between the epiglottis and the root of the tongue on either side of the median glosso-epiglottic fold.

valve (valv) A fold of the lining membrane within a tubular structure or hollow organ, so placed as to permit passage of a body fluid in one direction only.

    ileocecal v. A valve between the small and large intestines, at the junction of the ileum and cecum; it regulates the flow of intestinal contents and prevents their backward flow. Also called ileocecal sphincter.

varus (va'rus) Bent inward, toward the central line of the body; said of a deformed part, as in genu varus.

vastus (vas'tus) Large, vast. See also table of muscles in appendix II.

ventrad (ven'trad) Toward the ventral or anterior aspect of the body.

ventral (ven'tral) Relating to the ventral or anterior aspect of the body.

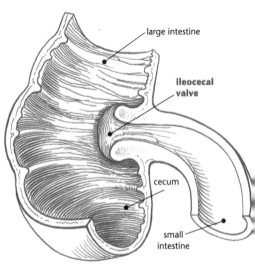

large intestine

**ileocecal
valve**

cecum

small
intestine

valgus ■ ventral

vertebra (ver'tĕ-brah), pl. ver'tebrae One of the 33 bones forming the spinal column; they are divided into 7 cervical, 12 thoracic, 5 lumbar, 5 sacral, and 4 coccygeal vertebrae; the bones are joined together by fibrocartilaginous disks. See also table of bones in appendix I.

vertebral (ver'te-bral) Relating to a vertebra or the vertebrae.

vertebrocostal (ver-tĕ-bro-kos'tal) Relating to a vertebra and a rib or a vertebra and a costal cartilage.

vertebrosacral (ver-tĕ-bro-sa'kral) Relating to the vertebrae, usually the lumbar vertebrae, and the sacrum.

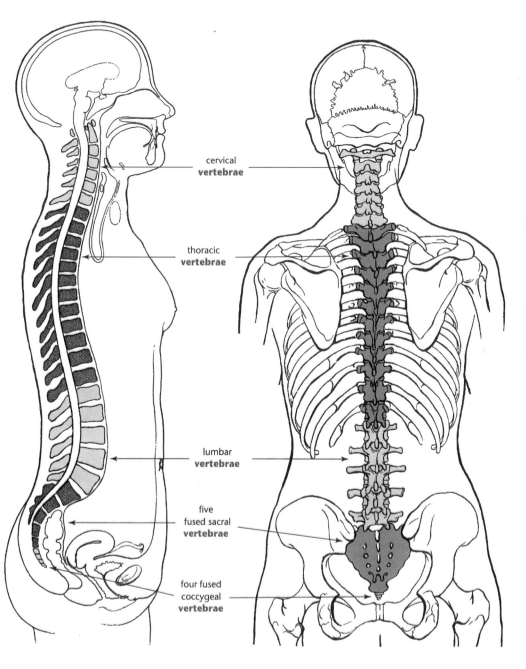

cervical **vertebrae**

thoracic **vertebrae**

lumbar **vertebrae**

five fused sacral **vertebrae**

four fused coccygeal **vertebrae**

vertebra ■ vertebrosacral

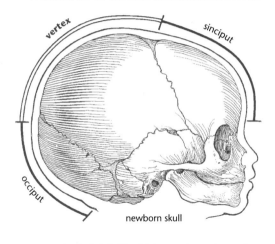

newborn skull

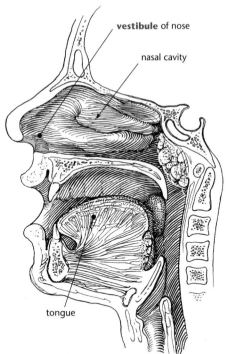

vertex (ver'teks) 1. The highest point at the vault of the skull. 2. The crown of the fetal head.

vestibular (ves-tib'u-lar) Relating to a vestibule, especially of the inner ear where balance functions are governed.

vestibule (ves'tĭ-būl) A small cavity or chamber at the entrance of a canal.

> **buccal v.** The vestibule of the mouth between the cheeks and the gums.

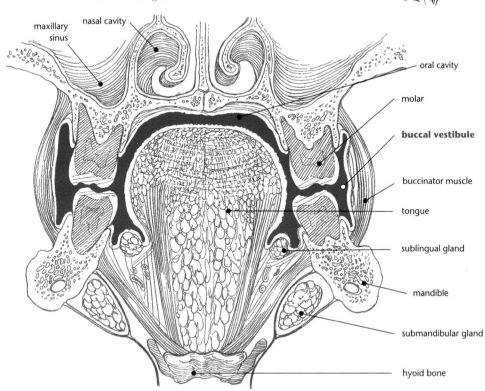

vertex ■ vestibule

v. of ear The oval cavity in the bony labyrinth of the inner ear; it communicates with the cochlea anteriorly and the semicircular canals posteriorly.

labial v. The vestibule of the mouth between the lips and the gums.

v. of nose
The space just inside the nostrils.

vinculum (ving'ku-lum) A frenulum or restrictive bandlike structure.

vola (vo'lah) Latin for the palm of the hand or the sole of the foot.

volar (vo'lar) Relating to the palm of the hand or the sole of the foot.

vomer (vo'mer) A thin, flat bone forming the lower and back portions of the nasal septum. See also table of bones in appendix I.

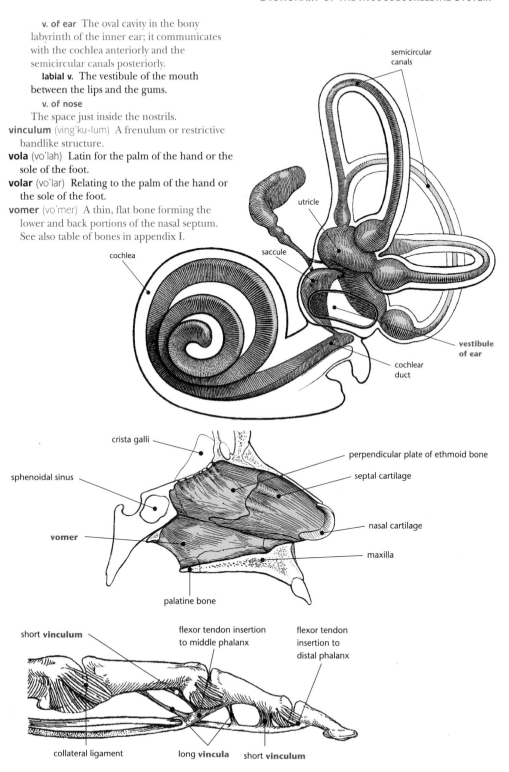

vinculum ■ vomer

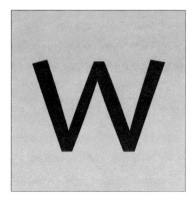

water-on-the-knee Colloquialism for accumulation of fluid within or around the knee joint, usually caused by bursitis.

window (win'do) An opening in any partition-like anatomic structure or membrane.

    cochlear w. See round window.

    oval w. An oval opening between the middle ear chamber and the vestibule of the inner ear; it is covered by the footplate of the stapes which is fixed to the margin of the opening by the annular ligament. Also called vestibular window; fenestra of vestibule; fenestra ovalis.

    round w. A round opening in the medial wall of the middle ear chamber leading to the scala tympani of the cochlea; it is covered by the secondary tympanic membrane. Also called cochlear window; fenestra of cochlea; fenestra rotunda.

    vestibular w. See oval window.

wing (wing) A flattened, laterally projecting anatomic process bearing a fancied resemblance to a wing of a bird.

    w. of ilium The upper, flattened, wing-like expansion of the hipbone.

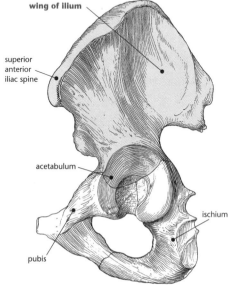

wing of ilium

superior anterior iliac spine

acetabulum

ischium

pubis

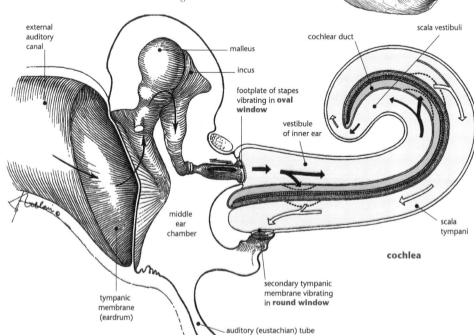

external auditory canal

malleus

incus

footplate of stapes vibrating in **oval window**

vestibule of inner ear

cochlear duct

scala vestibuli

middle ear chamber

scala tympani

cochlea

secondary tympanic membrane vibrating in **round window**

tympanic membrane (eardrum)

auditory (eustachian) tube

water-on-the-knee ■ wing

greater w. of sphenoid bone The larger of two processes that project laterally from the body of the sphenoid bone at the base of the skull; it forms part of the floor of the middle cranial fossa, the lateral wall of the orbit and of the temporal and infratemporal fossa. Also called major wing of sphenoid bone.

lesser w. of sphenoid bone The smaller of two processes that project laterally from the body of the sphenoid bone at the base of the skull; it forms part of the floor of the anterior cranial fossa and the roof of the orbit; it is separated from the greater wing of the sphenoid bone by the superior orbital fissure. Also called small wing of

sphenoid bone.

major w. of sphenoid bone See greater wing of sphenoid bone.

small w. of sphenoid bone See lesser wing of sphenoid bone.

wrist (rist) The carpal bones and adjoining structures between the forearm and the hand. See also table of bones in appendix I.

gymnast's w. Prominence of the head of the ulna at the wrist, with pain and limited range of motion and, sometimes, abnormalities of the growth plates of the radius and ulna; caused by repetitive compression of the bones during gymnastic exercises (e.g., handstands).

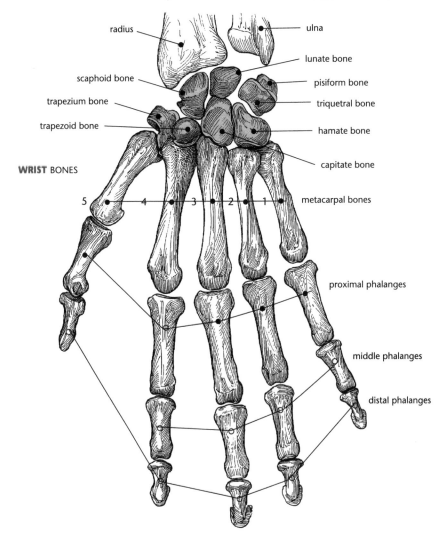

radius — ulna
lunate bone
scaphoid bone — pisiform bone
trapezium bone — triquetral bone
trapezoid bone — hamate bone
capitate bone
WRIST BONES
5   4   3   2   1   metacarpal bones
proximal phalanges
middle phalanges
distal phalanges

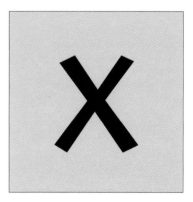

xipho- Combining form denoting a relationship to the xiphoid process of the sternum.

xiphoid (zif'oid) Shaped like a sword; applied especially to the xiphoid process. See under process.

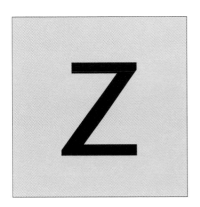

zone (zōn) An area with differentiating characteristics; especially an encircling region distinguished from adjacent parts.

    orbital z. of hip joint The deep, circularly arranged fibers of the articular capsule of the hip joint.

zygoma (zi-go'mah) 1. See zygomatic arch, under arch. 2. Term sometimes applies to the zygomatic bone. See also table of bones in appendix I.

zygomatic (zi-go-mat'ik) Relating to the zygomatic bone (cheek bone).

APPENDIX I

BONE	LOCATION	DESCRIPTION	ARTICULATIONS
ankle b.	see talus		
anvil b.	see incus		
astragalus	see talus		
atlas *atlas*	neck	first cervical vertebra	occipital (above), axis (below)
axis epistropheus *axis*	neck	second cervical vertebra	atlas (above), 3rd cervical vertebra (below)
backbones	see vertebrae		
calcaneus heel b. *calcaneus*	foot	largest of the tarsal b.'s situated at back of foot, forming heel; somewhat cuboidal	talus (above), cuboid (in front)
capitate b. magnum b. *os capitatum*	wrist	largest of carpal b.'s, occupies center of wrist	2nd, 3rd, and 4th metacarpal b.'s; lunate, scaphoid, trapezoid, and hamate b.'s
carpal b.'s wrist b.'s *ossa carpi*	wrist	eight in number, arranged in two rows: scaphoid, lunate, triquetral, and pisiform (proximal); trapezium, trapezoid, capitate, and hamate (distal)	

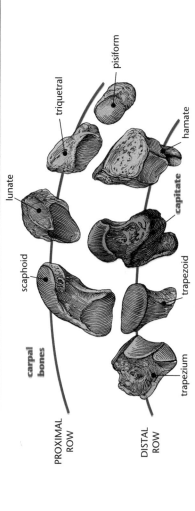

carpal bones

PROXIMAL ROW

DISTAL ROW

scaphoid

lunate

triquetral

pisiform

trapezium

trapezoid

capitate

hamate

BONE	LOCATION	DESCRIPTION	ARTICULATIONS
cheekbone	see zygomatic bone		
clavicle collarbone *clavicula*	shoulder	long curved b. placed nearly horizontally above 1st rib	sternum, scapula, cartilage of 1st rib
coccyx tail b. *os coccygis*	lower back	from 3 to 5 triangular rudimentary vertebrae with only the first not fused	sacrum
concha, inferior nasal inferior turbinate b. *concha nasalis inferior*	skull	thin, irregular, scrolled-shaped b. extending horizontally along lateral wall of nasal cavity	ethmoid, maxilla, palatine b.'s
cuboid *os cuboideum*	foot	pyramidal b. on lateral side of foot, proximal to 4th and 5th metatarsal b.'s	calcaneus, lateral cuneiform, 4th and 5th metatarsal b.'s, navicular
cuneiform b., intermediate second cuneiform b. *os cuneiforme intermedium*	foot	wedge-shaped; smallest of the three cuneiforms, positioned between medial and lateral ones	navicular, medial cuneiform, lateral cuneiform, 2nd metatarsal
cuneiform b., lateral external cuneiform b. *os cuneiforme laterale*	foot	intermediate-sized cuneiform located in center of front row of tarsal b.'s	navicular, intermediate cuneiform, cuboid, 2nd, 3rd, and 4th metatarsals

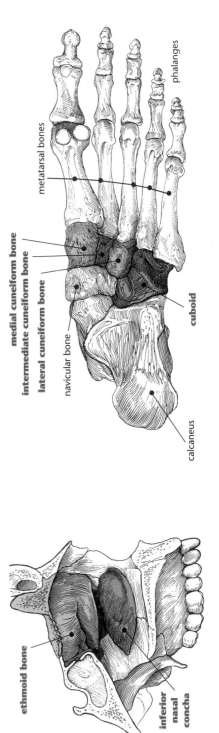

phalanges

metatarsal bones

medial cuneiform bone
intermediate cuneiform bone
lateral cuneiform bone

navicular bone

cuboid

calcaneus

ethmoid bone

inferior nasal concha

Term		Region	Description	Articulates with
cuneiform b., medial internal cuneiform b. *os cuneiforme mediale*		foot	largest of the three cuneiforms, at medial side of foot between navicular and 1st metatarsal	navicular, intermediate cuneiform, 1st and 2nd metatarsals
elbow b.		see ulna		
ethmoid b. *os ethmoidale*		skull	unpaired, T-shaped b. forming part of nasal septum and roof of nasal cavity; curled processes form superior and middle conchae	sphenoid, frontal, both nasal, lacrimal, and palatine b.'s; maxillae, inferior nasal concha, vomer
fabella *fabella*		knee	sesamoid b. in lateral head of gastrocnemius muscle behind lateral condyle of femur	femur
femur thigh b. *femur*		thigh	longest and heaviest b. in body, situated between the hip and knee	hipbone, patella, tibia

Figure labels: frontal bone, frontal sinus, zygomatic bone, inferior nasal concha, maxillary molar, crista galli, **ethmoid bone**, hard palate, orbit, maxillary sinus, nasal cavity

BONE	LOCATION	DESCRIPTION	ARTICULATIONS
fibula splint b. *fibula*	leg	lateral b. of leg	tibia, talus
flank b.	see ilium		
frontal b. Forehead b. *os frontale*	skull	flat b. forming anterior part of skull	ethmoid, sphenoid, maxillae, and both nasal, parietal, lacrimal, and zygomatic b.'s
greater multangular b.	see trapezium bone		
hamate b. unciform b. *os hamatum*	wrist	most medial b. of distal row of carpals; distinguished by hook-like process (hamulus) that projects from its palmar surface	lunate, triquetral, capitate, 4th and 5th metacarpals
hammer b.	see malleus		
hipbone innominate b. *os coxae*	pelvis and hip	large, broad, irregularly shaped b. that forms greater part of pelvis; consists of three parts: ilium, ischium, and pubis	femur, sacrum, with its fellow of opposite side at pubic symphysis
humerus arm b. *humerus*	arm	longest and largest b. of upper limb, situated between shoulder and elbow	scapula, radius, and ulna
hyoid b. lingual b. *os hyoideum*	neck	U-shaped b. in front of neck between mandible and larynx	suspended from tips of skull's styloid processes by ligaments
ilium flank b. *os ilium*	pelvis	broad expanded upper part of the hipbone, divisible into a body and an ala	sacrum, femur, ischium, pubis
incus anvil b. *incus*	middle ear chamber	middle b. of auditory ossicles	malleus, stapes
inferior turbinate b.	see concha, inferior		
innominate b.	see hipbone		
ischium *os ischii*	pelvis	inferior and dorsal part of the hipbone, divisible into a body and a ramus	femur, ilium, pubis
lacrimal b. *os lacrimale*	skull	smallest and most fragile b. of the face; resembles a fingernail and is situated in medial wall of orbit	ethmoid, frontal, maxilla, inferior nasal concha

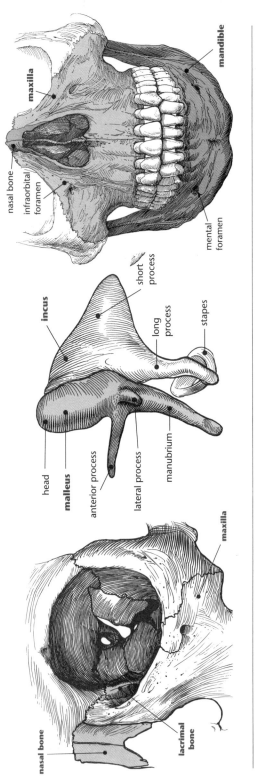

nasal bone
infraorbital foramen
maxilla
mandible
mental foramen

incus
short process
long process
stapes
head
malleus
anterior process
lateral process
manubrium

nasal bone
lacrimal bone
maxilla

lesser multangular b.	see trapezoid bone		
lunate b. semilunar b. *os lunatum*	wrist	in center of proximal row of carpus between scaphoid and triquetral b.'s	radius, capitate, hamate, triquetral, scaphoid
malar b.	see zygomatic bone		
malleus hammer b. *malleus*	middle ear chamber	most lateral b. of ossicles, somewhat resembling a hammer and consisting of a head, neck, and three processes	tympanic membrane and incus
mandible lower jaw b. *mandibula*	lower portion of face	horseshoe-shaped b containing the lower teeth; strongest b. of face	mandibular fossa of both temporal b.'s
maxilla maxillary b. *maxilla*	middle portion of face	largest b. of the face except the mandible; contains the upper teeth; encloses the maxillary sinus	frontal, ethmoid, nasal, zygomatic, lacrimal, vomer, inferior nasal concha, other maxilla
metacarpus metacarpal b.'s *ossa metacarpalia*	hand, between wrist and fingers	five slender b.'s of the hand proper, each consisting of a body and two extremities (head and base), and numbered from 1st to 5th starting from the thumb side	base of first metacarpal with trapezium, base of other metacarpals with each other and with distal row of carpal b.'s, heads with corresponding phalanges

BONE	LOCATION	DESCRIPTION	ARTICULATIONS
metatarsus metatarsal b.'s *os metatarsalia*	foot between distal row of tarsal b.'s and first phalanges of toes	five slender b.'s of the foot proper, each consisting of a body and two extremities (head and base), and numbered from 1st to 5th starting from the big toe side	distal tarsal b.'s, bases with each other, heads with corresponding phalanges
multangular b., greater	see trapezium bone		
multangular b., lesser	see trapezoid bone		
nasal b. *os nasale*	middle of face	one of two paired b.'s positioned side-by-side to form bridge of nose	frontal, ethmoid, opposite nasal, maxilla
navicular b. navicular b. of foot scaphoid b. of foot *os naviculare*	foot	situated at medial side of tarsus between talus and cuneiform b.'s	talus, three cuneiforms, occasionally with cuboid
navicular b. of hand	see scaphoid bone		
occipital b. *os occipitale*	skull	unpaired saucer-shaped b. forming posterior part of base of cranium pierced by the foramen magnum	both parietals and temporals; sphenoid, atlas
palatine b. palate b. *os palatinum*	skull	one of two, somewhat L-shaped paired b.'s, the two forming the posterior part of hard palate, part of floor and lateral wall of nasal cavity, and part of floor of orbit	sphenoid, ethmoid, maxilla, vomer, opposite palatine, inferior nasal concha
parietal b. *os parietale*	skull	paired b.'s between frontal and occipital b.'s forming sides and roof of cranium	opposite parietal, frontal, occipital, temporal, sphenoid
patella kneecap *patella*	knee	flat, rounded, triangular b. (sesamoid), situated in front of knee joint	femur
pelvis	a bony ring resembling a basin, composed of two hipbones, sacrum, and coccyx		
phalanages of foot *ossa digitorum pedis*	foot	miniature long b.'s, two in great toe and three in each of other toes	proximal row of phalanges with corresponding metatarsal b.'s and middle phalanges; middle phalanges with proximal and distal phalanges; ungual phalanges with mid phalanges
phalanges of hand *ossa digitorum manus*	hand	miniature long b.'s, two in thumb and three in each of other fingers	proximal row of phalanges with corresponding metacarpal b.'s and middle phalanges; middle phalanges

with proximal and distal phalanges; ungual phalanges with mid phalanges

pisiform b. *os pisiforme*	wrist	most medial of proximal row of carpus; smallest carpal b.	triquetral
pubis *os pubis*	pelvis	anterior lower portion of hipbone	ilium, ischium, femur
radius *radius*	forearm, between elbow and wrist	lateral b. of forearm; proximal end is small and forms small part of elbow; distal end is large and forms large part of wrist joint	humerus, ulna, lunate, scaphoid
ribs *os costale*	chest	12 pairs of thin, narrow, arch-shaped b.'s forming posterior and lateral walls of chest	all posteriorly with vertebral column; upper seven pairs anteriorly with sternum, through intervention of costal cartilages; lower five pairs anteriorly with costal cartilages; lowest two pairs free at ventral extremities (floating)

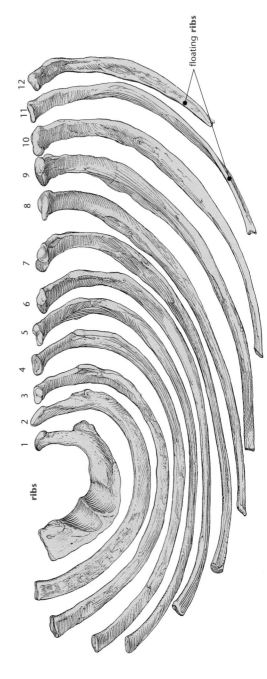

ribs

floating **ribs**

1 2 3 4 5 6 7 8 9 10 11 12

Illustrations: pelvis (anterior view) with labels **sacrum**, right hipbone, coccyx; scapula (posterior view) with label **scapula**; ossicles of the ear with labels malleus, incus, **stapes**.

BONE	LOCATION	DESCRIPTION	ARTICULATIONS
sacrum *os sacrum*	lower back	large triangular b. formed by fusion of five vertebrae, and situated at dorsal part of pelvis	above with last lumbar vertebra, at each side with ilium, below with coccyx
scaphoid b. scaphoid b. of hand navicular b. of hand *os scaphoideum*	wrist	largest b. of proximal row of carpus located at thumb side	radius, trapezium, trapezoid, capitate, lunate
scaphoid b. of foot	see navicular bone		
scapula shoulder blade *scapula*	shoulder	large, flat, triangular b. forming dorsal part of shoulder girdle	clavicle, humerus
semilunar b.	see lunate bone		
sesamoid b.'s *ossa sesamoidea*	extremities, usually within tendons	small rounded b.'s embedded in certain tendons; some constant ones include	none

271

shinbone	see tibia		
sphenoid b. *os sphenoidale*	base of skull	unpaired, irregularly shaped b. forming anterior part of base of skull and portions of cranial, orbital, and nasal cavities	vomer, ethmoid, frontal, both parietals, temporals, zygomatics, and palatines; also articulates with tuberosity of maxilla
stapes stirrup *stapes*	middle ear chamber	most medial b. of auditory ossicles, somewhat resembling a stirrup	incus, oval window
stirrup b.	see stapes		
sternum breastbone *sternum*	chest	elongated, flattened, dagger-shaped b. forming ventral wall of thorax; consists of three parts: manubrium, body, xiphoid process	both clavicles and first seven pairs of costal cartilages
sutural b.'s wormian b.'s *ossa saturarum*	skull	irregular, isolated b.'s occasionally found along cranial sutures, especially the lambdoid suture	usually occipital and parietal b.'s
talus ankle b. astragalus *talus*	ankle	second largest of the tarsal b.'s; supports tibia and rests on calcaneus	tibia, fibula, calcaneus, navicular

those in the tendons of quadriceps muscle of thigh, short flexor muscle of big toe, long peroneal muscle, anterior and posterior tibial muscles, and greater psoas muscle; the patella (kneecap) is the largest sesamoid b.

Sternum figure labels: manubrium, body, xiphoid process, **sternum**

Foot figure labels: **tibia**, **talus**, navicular bone, cuneiform bone, metatarsal bone, phalanges, calcaneus

BONE	LOCATION	DESCRIPTION	ARTICULATIONS
temporal b. *os temporale*	skull	irregularly shaped b. consisting of three parts: squamous, petrous, and tympanic; forms part of side and base of cranium	occipital. parietal. zygomatic. sphenoid. mandible

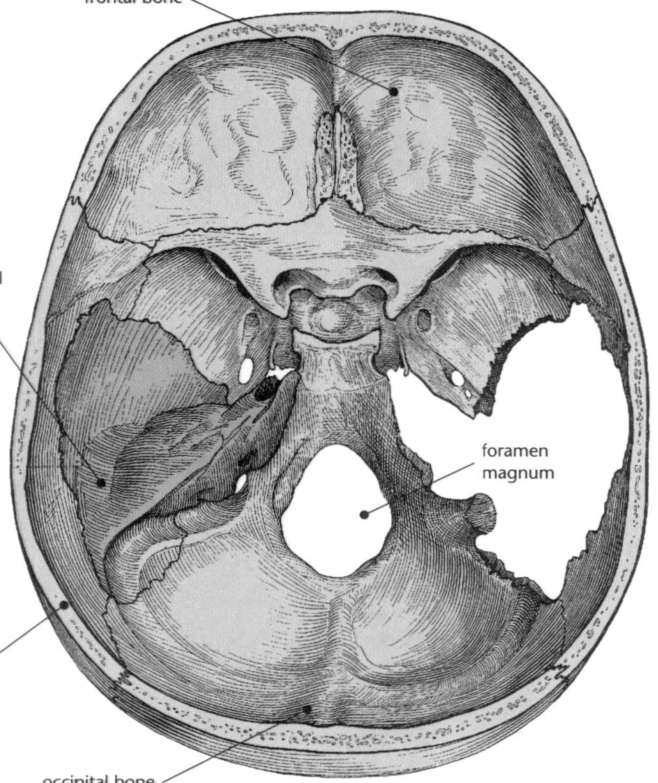

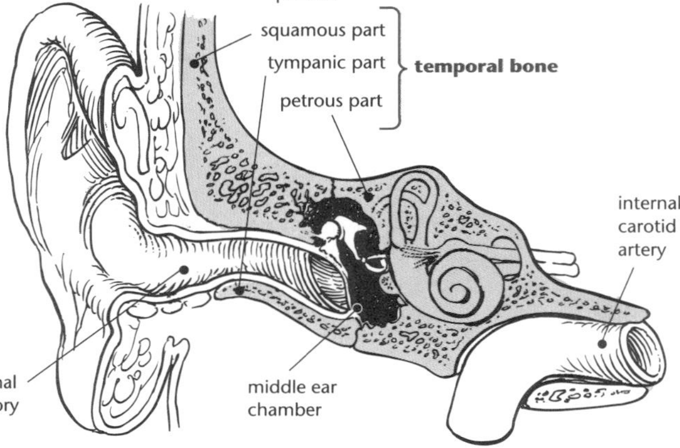

temporal bone
(lateral aspect)

postglenoid tubercle

external auditory canal

mastoid foramen

mastoid process

styloid process

mandibular fossa

articular tubercle

zygomatic process

temporal bone

squamous part

tympanic part

petrous part

internal carotid artery

middle ear chamber

external auditory canal

frontal bone

foramen magnum

temporal bone

parietal bone

occipital bone

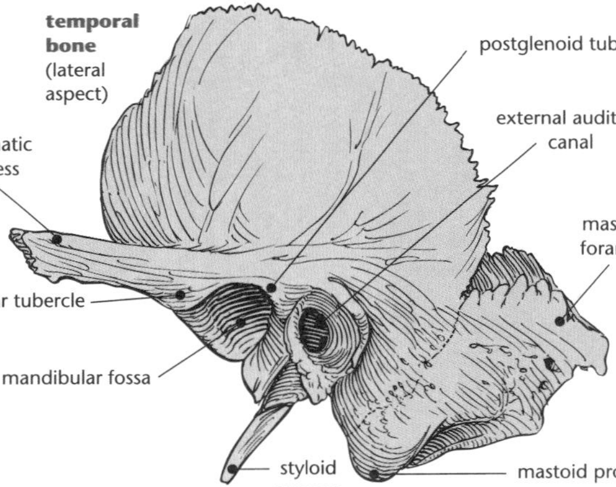

273

Term	Location	Description	Articulations
tibia shinbone *tibia*	leg	situated at medial side of leg between ankle and knee joints; second largest b. in the body	above with femur and fibula; below with fibula and talus
trapezium b. greater multangular b. *os trapezium*	wrist	most lateral of four b.'s of distal row of carpus	scaphoid, 1st and 2nd metacarpals, trapezoid
trapezoid b. lesser multangular b. *os trapezoideum*	wrist	smallest b. in distal row of carpus	scaphoid, 2nd metacarpal, capitate, trapezium
triquetral b. triangular b. *os triquetrum*	wrist	pyramidal shape; second from little finger side of proximal row of carpus	lunate, pisiform, hamate
triangular b.	see triquetral b.		
turbinate b., inferior	see concha, inferior nasal		
turbinate b., middle	not a separate bone: see ethmoid bone		
turbinate b., superior	not a separate bone: see ethmoid bone		
ulna elbow b. *ulna*	forearm	medial b. of forearm; lies parallel with radius	humerus, radius
unciform b.	see hamate bone		
vertebrae, cervical backbones *vertebrae cervicales*	back of neck	seven segments of vertebral column; smallest of the true vertebrae; possess a foramen in each transverse process	1st vertebra with skull, all others with adjoining vertebrae
vertebrae, lumbar backbones *vertebrae lumbales*	lower back	five segments of vertebral column; largest b.'s of movable part of vertebral column	with adjoining vertebrae; 5th lumbar vertebra with sacrum
vertebrae, thoracic backbones *vertebrae thoracicae*	back	12 segments of vertebral column; possess facets on the sides of all the bodies and first ten also have facets on the transverse processes	with adjoining vertebrae, heads of ribs, tubercles of ribs (except 11th and 12th)
vomer *vomer*	skull	thin, flat b. forming posterior and inferior part of nasal septum	ethmoid, sphenoid, both maxillae, both palatines; also articulates with septal cartilage of nose
wormian b.'s	see sutural bones		
zygomatic b. malar b. cheekbone *os zygomaticum*	skull	forms prominence of cheek and lower lateral aspects of orbit	frontal, sphenoid, temporal, maxilla

APPENDIX II

MUSCLE	ORIGIN	INSERTION	ACTION
abductor m. of big toe *m. abductor hallucis*	calcaneus, plantar aponeurosis	proximal phalanx of big toe (joined by short flexor m. of big toe)	abducts and aids in flexion of big toe
abductor m. of little finger *m. abductor digiti minimi manus*	pisiform bone, tendon of ulnar flexor muscle of wrist	proximal phalanx of 5th digit	abducts little finger
abductor m. of little toe *m. abductor digiti minimi pedis*	lateral tubercle of calcaneus, plantar aponeurosis	proximal phalanx of little toe	abducts and flexes little toe
abductor m. of thumb, long *m. abductor pollicis longus*	posterior surface of ulna, middle third of radius	1st metacarpal bone	abducts and extends thumb
abductor m. of thumb, short *m. abductor pollicis brevis*	flexor retinaculum of hand, scaphoid and trapezium	proximal phalanx of thumb	abducts and aids in flexion of thumb
adductor m., great *m. adductor magnus*	adductor part: inferior ramus of pubis, ramus of ischium; extensor part: ischial tuberosity	adductor part: linea aspera of femur; extensor part: adductor tubercle of femur	adducts, flexes, and rotates thigh medially
adductor m., long *m. adductor longus*	pubis, below pubic crest	linea aspera of femur	adducts, flexes, and rotates thigh medially
adductor m., smallest *m. adductor minimus*	the proximal portion of the great adductor muscle when it forms a distinct muscle		
adductor m., short *m. adductor brevis*	pubis, below origin of the long adductor muscle	upper part of linea aspera of femur	adducts, flexes, and rotates thigh laterally
adductor m. of big toe *m. adductor hallucis*	oblique head: bases of middle three metatarsal bones; transverse head: metatarsophalangeal ligaments of lateral three toes	proximal phalanx of big toe (joined by flexor m. of big toe)	oblique head: adducts and flexes big toe; transverse head: supports transverse arch, adducts big toe
adductor m. of thumb *m. adductor pollicis*	oblique head: capitate, 2nd and 3rd metacarpal bones; transverse head: 3rd metacarpal bone	proximal phalanx of thumb; medial sesamoid bone	adducts and aids in apposition of thumb
anconeus m. *m. aconeus*	back of lateral condyle of humerus	olecranon process, posterior surface of ulna	extends forearm, adducts ulna in pronation of wrist
antitragus m. *m. antitragicus*	outer surface of antitragus of ear	caudate process of helix and antihelix	thought to be vestigial
arrector m.'s of hair *mm. arrectores pilorum*	dermis	hair follicles	elevates hairs of skin; aids in discharging sebum

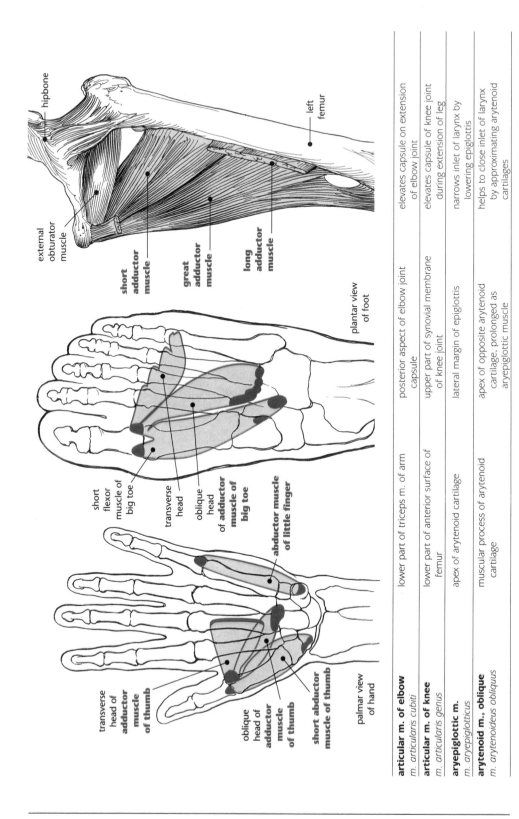

hipbone

left femur

external obturator muscle

short adductor muscle

great adductor muscle

long adductor muscle

plantar view of foot

short flexor muscle of big toe

transverse head

oblique head of adductor muscle of big toe

abductor muscle of little finger

transverse head of adductor muscle of thumb

oblique head of adductor muscle of thumb

short abductor muscle of thumb

palmar view of hand

articular m. of elbow *m. articularis cubiti*	lower part of triceps m. of arm	posterior aspect of elbow joint capsule	elevates capsule on extension of elbow joint
articular m. of knee *m. articularis genus*	lower part of anterior surface of femur	upper part of synovial membrane of knee joint	elevates capsule of knee joint during extension of leg
aryepiglottic m. *m. aryepiglotticus*	apex of arytenoid cartilage	lateral margin of epiglottis	narrows inlet of larynx by lowering epiglottis
arytenoid m., oblique *m. arytenoideus obliquus*	muscular process of arytenoid cartilage	apex of opposite arytenoid cartilage, prolonged as aryepiglottic muscle	helps to close inlet of larynx by approximating arytenoid cartilages

MUSCLE	ORIGIN	INSERTION	ACTION
arytenoid m., transverse (only unpaired muscle of larynx) *m. arytenoideus transversus*	posterior surface of arytenoid cartilage	posterior surface of opposite arytenoid cartilage	approximates arytenoid cartilages; constricts entrance to larynx during swallowing
auricular m., anterior *m. auricularis anterior*	superficial temporal fascia	cartilage of ear	feeble forward movement of auricle
auricular m., posterior *m. auricularis posterior*	mastoid process	cartilage of ear	feeble backward movement of auricle
auricular m., superior *m. auricularis superior*	temporal fascia; epicranial aponeurosis	cartilage of ear	feeble elevation of auricle
auricular m., transverse *m. auricularis transversus*	upper surface of auricle	circumference of auricle	retracts helix
biceps m. of arm *m. biceps brachii*	long head: supraglenoid tubercle of scapula; short head: apex of coracoid process	tuberosity of radius; posterior border of ulna through bicipital aponeurosis	flexes forearm and arm; supinates hand
biceps m. of thigh *m. biceps femoris*	long head: ischial tuberosity; short head: linea aspera and second supracondylar ridge of femur	head of fibula, lateral condyle of tibia	flexes knee, rotates leg laterally; long head extends thigh
brachial m. *m. brachialis*	anterior surface of distal two-thirds of humerus	coronoid process of ulna	flexes forearm
brachioradial m. *m. brachioradialis*	lateral supracondylar ridge and intermuscular septum of humerus	lower end of radius	flexes forearm
bronchoesophageal m. *m. bronchoesophageus*	muscle fibers arising from wall of left bronchus	musculature of esophagus	reinforces esophagus
buccinator m. *m. buccinator*	pterygomandibular raphe, alveolar processes of jaws	orbicular m. (*orbicularis oris*) at angle of mouth	retracts angle of mouth by compressing cheek
bulbocavernous m. *m. bulbospongiosus*	female: central tendon of perineum; male: median raphe over bulb of penis, central tendon of perineum	female: dorsum of clitoris, uro-genital diaphragm; male: corpus spongiosum, root of penis	female: compresses vaginal orifice; male: compresses urethra, assists in ejaculation
canine m.	see levator muscle of angle of mouth		
ceratocricoid m. *m. ceratocricoideus*	lower margin of cricoid cartilage	inferior cornu (horn) of thyroid cartilage	helps posterior cricoarytenoid muscle separate vocal cords
chin m. *m. mentalis*	incisive fossa of mandible	skin of chin	raises and protrudes lower lip
chondroglossus m. *m. chondroglossus*	lesser cornu (horn) and body of hyoid bone	side of tongue	depresses tongue

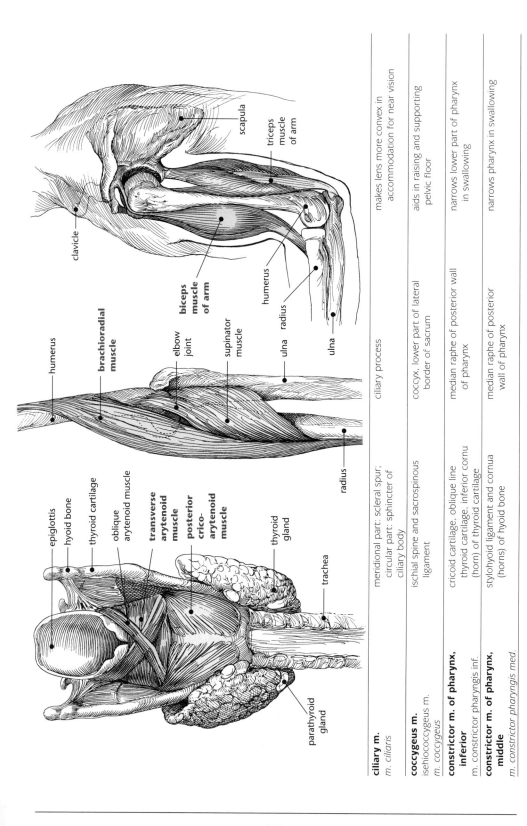

ciliary m. m. ciliaris	meridional part: scleral spur; circular part: sphincter of ciliary body	ciliary process	makes lens more convex in accommodation for near vision
coccygeus m. ischiococcygeus m. m. coccygeus	ischial spine and sacrospinous ligament	coccyx, lower part of lateral border of sacrum	aids in raising and supporting pelvic floor
constrictor m. of pharynx, inferior m. constrictor pharyngis inf.	cricoid cartilage, oblique line thyroid cartilage, inferior cornu (horn) of thyroid cartilage	median raphe of posterior wall of pharynx	narrows lower part of pharynx in swallowing
constrictor m. of pharynx, middle m. constrictor pharyngis med.	stylohyoid ligament and cornua (horns) of hyoid bone	median raphe of posterior wall of pharynx	narrows pharynx in swallowing

MUSCLE	ORIGIN	INSERTION	ACTION
constrictor m. of pharynx, superior *m. constrictor pharyngis sup.*	medial pterygoid plate, pterygoid hamulus, pterygomandibular raphe, mandible, side of tongue	median raphe of posterior wall of pharynx; pharyngeal tubercle of skull	narrows pharynx in swallowing
coracobrachial m. *m. coracobrachialis*	coracoid process of scapula (shoulder blade)	midway along inner side of humerus	flexes, adducts arm
corrugator. m *m. corrugator*	brow ridge of frontal bone	skin of eyebrow	draws eyebrows together, wrinkles forehead
cremaster m. *m. cremaster*	inferior border of internal oblique abdominal muscle	spermatic cord	in male: elevates testis; in female: encircles round lig.
cricoarytenoid m., lateral *m. cricoarytenoideus lateralis*	upper margin of arch of cricoid cartilage	muscular process of arytenoid cartilage	approximates vocal cords so they meet in midline for phonation
cricoarytenoid m., posterior *cricoarytenoideus post.*	posterior surface of lamina of cricoid cartilage	muscular process of arytenoid cartilage	separates vocal cords, opening the glottis
cricothyroid m. *m. cricothyroideus*	anterior surface of arch of cricoid cartilage	lamina and inferior cornu (horn) of thyroid cartilage	lengthens, stretches, and tenses vocal cords
deltoid m. *m. deltoideus*	lateral third of clavicle, acromion, and spine of scapula	deltoid tuberosity of shaft of humerus	abductor of arm, aids in flexion, extension and lateral rotation of arm
depressor m., superciliary *m. depressor supercilii*	orbicular fibers of the eye; medial palpebral ligament	skin of eyebrow	pulls eyebrow downward
depressor m. of angle of mouth triangular m. *m. depressor anguli oris*	oblique line of mandible	angle of mouth	pulls corner of mouth downward
depressor m. of lower lip quadrate m. of lower lip *m. depressor labii inferior*	mandible adjacent to mental foramen	skin of lower lip	draws lower lip downward and somewhat laterally
depressor m. of nasal septum *m. depressor septi nasi*	incisive fossa of maxilla, over roots of incisor teeth	ala and septum of nose	widens the nostrils in deep inspiration
detrusor m. of urinary bladder *m. detrusor vesicae*	wall of urinary bladder, consisting of three layers of nonstriated muscular fibers		empties urinary bladder
diaphragm diaphragmatic m. *diaphragma*	xiphoid process, six lower costal cartilages, four lower ribs, lumbar vertebrae, arcuate ligaments	central tendon of diaphragm	increases capacity of thorax in inspiration (main muscle of respiration)
diaphragm m., pelvic	composed of the coccygeus and levator ani muscles sheathed in a superior and inferior layer of fascia		forms floor to support pelvic viscera
digastric m. *m. digastricus*	digastric notch at mastoid process; mandible near symphysis	tendon bound to hyoid bone by fascia	raises hyoid bone and base of tongue, lowers mandible

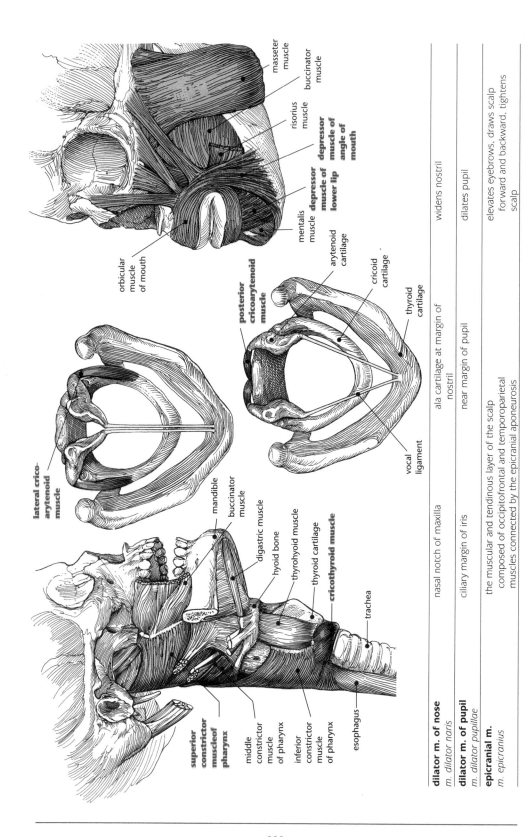

masseter muscle

buccinator muscle

risorius muscle

depressor muscle of angle of mouth

depressor muscle of lower lip

mentalis muscle

orbicular muscle of mouth

arytenoid cartilage

cricoid cartilage

thyroid cartilage

posterior cricoarytenoid muscle

vocal ligament

lateral cricoarytenoid muscle

mandible

buccinator muscle

digastric muscle

hyoid bone

thyrohyoid muscle

thyroid cartilage

cricothyroid muscle

trachea

superior constrictor muscle of pharynx

middle constrictor muscle of pharynx

inferior constrictor muscle of pharynx

esophagus

dilator m. of nose *m. dilator naris*	nasal notch of maxilla	widens nostril
dilator m. of pupil *m. dilator pupillae*	ciliary margin of iris ala cartilage at margin of nostril near margin of pupil	dilates pupil
epicranial m. *m. epicranius*	the muscular and tendinous layer of the scalp composed of occipitofrontal and temporoparietal muscles connected by the epicranial aponeurosis	elevates eyebrows, draws scalp forward and backward, tightens scalp

MUSCLE	ORIGIN	INSERTION	ACTION
erector m. of penis	see ischiocavernous muscle		
erector m. of spine *m. erector spinae*	deep muscle arising from the broad and thick tendon attached to the middle crest of sacrum, spinous processes of lumbar and 11th and 12th thoracic vertebrae, and back part of the iliac crest; it splits in the upper lumbar region into three columns of muscles: iliocostal (lateral division), longissimus (intermediate division), and spinal (medial division)		
extensor m. of fingers *m. extensor digitorum*	lateral epicondyle of humerus	phalanges of digits 2 to 5, via dorsal digital expansion	extends fingers, hand, and forearm
extensor m. of big toe, long *m. extensor hallucis longus*	middle of fibula, interosseous membrane	distal phalanx of big toe	extends big toe, dorsiflexes foot
extensor m. of big toe, short *m. extensor hallucis brevis*	dorsal surface of calcaneus	base of proximal phalanx of big toe	dorsiflexes big toe
extensor m. of index finger *m. extensor indicis*	posterior surface of ulna, interosseous membrane	extensor expansion of index finger	extends index finger and hand
extensor m. of little finger *m. extensor digiti minimi manus*	lateral epicondyle of humerus	extensor expansion of little finger	extends little finger
extensor m. of thumb, long *m. extensor pollicis longus*	middle third of ulna, adjacent interosseous membrane	distal phalanx of thumb	extends distal phalanx of thumb, abducts hand
extensor m. of thumb, short *m. extensor pollicis brevis*	middle third of radius, interosseous membrane	proximal phalanx of thumb	extends thumb and abducts hand
extensor m. of toes, long *m. extensor digitorum longus pedis*	lateral condyle of tibia, upper three-fourths of fibula, interosseous membrane	extensor expansion of four lateral toes (by four slips)	extends toes and dorsiflexes foot
extensor m. of toes, short *m. extensor digitorum brevis pedis*	dorsal surface of calcaneus	extensor tendons of 2nd, 3rd, and 4th toes	extends toes
extensor m. of wrist, long radial *m. extensor carpi radialis longus*	lateral supracondylar ridge of humerus	2nd metacarpal bone	extends wrist; adducts hand
extensor m. of wrist, short radial *m. extensor carpi radialis brevis*	lateral epicondyle of humerus, radial collateral ligament of elbow joint	3rd metacarpal bone	extends wrist; abducts hand
extensor m. of wrist, ulnar *m. extensor carpi ulnaris*	humeral head: lateral epicondyle of humerus; ulnar head: posterior border of ulna	5th metacarpal bone	extends wrist; adducts hand
fibular m.	see peroneal muscle		
flexor m. of fingers, deep *m. flexor digitorum profundus manus*	proximal three-fourths of ulna and adjacent interosseous membrane	distal phalanges of fingers	flexes terminal phalanges; lateral four digits; aids in flexing wrist

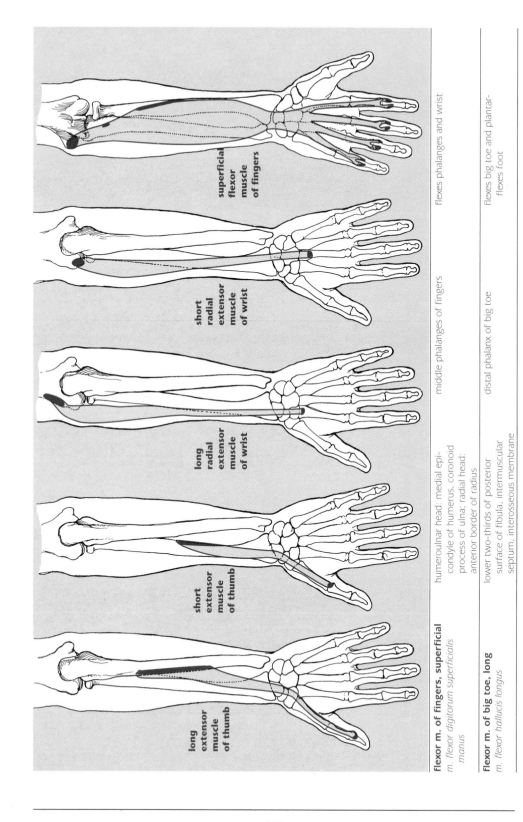

long extensor muscle of thumb

short extensor muscle of thumb

long radial extensor muscle of wrist

short radial extensor muscle of wrist

superficial flexor muscle of fingers

flexor m. of fingers, superficial *m. flexor digitorum superficialis manus*	humeroulnar head: medial epicondyle of humerus, coronoid process of ulna; radial head: anterior border of radius	middle phalanges of fingers		flexes phalanges and wrist
flexor m. of big toe, long *m. flexor hallucis longus*	lower two-thirds of posterior surface of fibula, intermuscular septum, interosseous membrane	distal phalanx of big toe		flexes big toe and plantar-flexes foot

MUSCLE	ORIGIN	INSERTION	ACTION
flexor m. of big toe, short *m. flexor hallucis brevis*	cuboid and lateral cuneiform bones	both sides of proximal phalanx of big toe	flexes big toe
flexor m. of little finger, short *m. flexor digiti minimi brevis manus*	hook of hamate, flexor retinaculum	proximal phalanx of little finger	flexes proximal phalanx of little finger
flexor m. of little toe, short *m. flexor digiti minimi brevis pedis*	base of 5th metatarsal and plantar fascia	lateral surface of proximal phalanx of little toe	flexes little toe
flexor m. of thumb, long *m. flexor pollicis longus*	radius, adjacent interosseous membrane, coronoid process of ulna	distal phalanx of thumb	flexes thumb
flexor m. of thumb, short *m. flexor pollicis brevis*	trapezium, trapezoid, and capitate bones of wrist	proximal phalanx of thumb	flexes thumb
flexor m. of toes, long *m. flexor digitorum longus pedis*	middle half of tibia	distal phalanges of lateral four toes (by four tendons)	flexes 2nd to 5th toes and plantarflexes foot
flexor m. of toes, short *m. flexor digitorum brevis pedis*	tuberosity of calcaneus and plantar fascia	middle phalanges of four lateral toes	flexes four lateral toes
flexor m. of wrist, radial *m. flexor carpi radialis*	medial epicondyle of humerus; antibrachial fascia	bases of 2nd and 3rd metacarpal bones	flexes wrist; aids in pronation and abduction of hand
flexor m. of wrist, ulnar *m. flexor carpi ulnaris*	humeral head: medial epicondyle of humerus; ulnar head: olecranon and posterior border of ulna	pisiform, hamate, and 5th metacarpal bones; flexor retinaculum	flexes wrist; adducts hand
frontal b.	see occipitofrontal muscle		
gastrocnemius m. *m. gastrocnemius*	medial head: popliteal surface of femur, upper part of medial condyle of femur; lateral head: lateral condyle of femur	calcaneus via calcaneal tendon (tendo calcaneus), in common with soleus muscle	flexes leg and plantarflexes foot
gemellus m., inferior *m. gemellus inferior*	lower margin of lesser sciatic notch	greater trochanter via internal obturator tendon	rotates thigh laterally
gemellus m., superior *m. gemellus superior*	spine of ischium	greater trochanter via internal obturator tendon	rotates thigh laterally; abducts flexed thigh
genioglossus m. *m. genioglossus*	mental spine (genial tubercle) of the mandible	ventral surface of tongue and body of hyoid bone	protrudes, retracts, and depresses tongue, elevates hyoid bone
geniohyoid m. *m. geniohyoideus*	mental spine (genial tubercle) of the mandible	body of hyoid bone	elevates hyoid bone and draws it forward

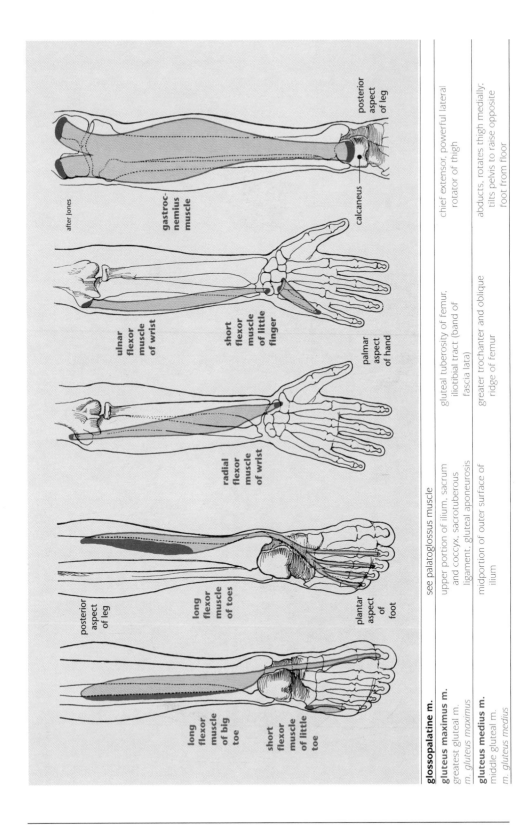

after Jones

glossopalatine m.	*see palatoglossus muscle*		
gluteus maximus m. greatest gluteal m. *m. gluteus maximus*	upper portion of ilium, sacrum and coccyx, sacrotuberous ligament, gluteal aponeurosis	gluteal tuberosity of femur, iliotibial tract (band of fascia lata)	chief extensor, powerful lateral rotator of thigh
gluteus medius m. middle gluteal m. *m. gluteus medius*	midportion of outer surface of ilium	greater trochanter and oblique ridge of femur	abducts, rotates thigh medially; tilts pelvis to raise opposite foot from floor

MUSCLE	ORIGIN	INSERTION	ACTION
gluteus minimus m. least gluteal m. *m. gluteus minimus*	lower portion of outer surface of ilium	greater trochanter of femur, capsule of hip joint	abducts, rotates thigh medially
gracilis m. *m. gracilis*	lower half of pubis	medial side of upper part of tibia	adducts thigh, flexes and rotates leg medially
helix m., smaller *m. helicis minor*	anterior rim of helix	crux of helix	thought to be vestigial

Muscle	Origin	Insertion	Action
hyoglossal m. hyoglossus m. *m. hyoglossus*	body and greater cornu (horn) of hyoid bone	side of tongue	retracts, depresses tongue
iliac m. *m. iliacus*	iliac fossa, lateral aspect of sacrum	greater psoas tendon, lesser trochanter of femur	flexes thigh
iliococcygeal m. *m. iliococcygeus*	ischial spine and arching tendon over internal obturator muscle	coccyx and perineal body between tip of coccyx and anal canal	supports pelvic viscera
iliocostal m. *m. iliocostalis*	the lateral division of erector m. of spine composed of three parts: iliocostal m. of loins, iliocostal m. of neck, iliocostal m. of thorax		extends vertebral column and assists in lateral movements of trunk
iliocostal m. of loins *m. iliocostalis lumborum*	iliac crest and thoracolumbar fascia	transverse processes of lumbar vertebrae, angles of lower seven ribs	extends lumbar vertebral column and flexes it laterally
iliocostal m. of neck *m. iliocostalis cervicis*	angles of 3rd, 4th, 5th, and 6th ribs	transverse processes of 4th, 5th, and 6th cervical vertebrae	extends cervical vertebral column and flexes it laterally
iliocostal m. of thorax *m. iliocostalis thoracis*	lower six ribs, medial to the angles of the ribs	angles of upper six ribs, transverse process of 7th cervical vertebra	extends thoracic vertebral column and flexes it laterally
iliopsoas m. *m. iliopsoas*	a compound m. consisting of the iliac and greater psoas m.'s, which join to form the iliopsoas tendon; it inserts onto the lesser trochanter of femur		
incisive m.'s of lower lip *mm. incisivi labii inferior*	portion of orbicular m. of mouth (orbicularis oris)	angle of mouth	make vestibule of mouth shallow; aid in articulation
incisive m.'s of upper lip *mm. incisivi labii superior*	portion of orbicular m. of mouth (orbicularis oris)	angle of mouth	make vestibule of mouth shallow; aid in articulation
infrahyoid m.'s *mm. infrahyoidei*	the ribbon-like muscles below the hyoid bone including the omohyoid, sternohyoid, sternothyroid, and thyrohyoid muscles		
infraspinous m. *m. infraspinatus*	infraspinous fossa of scapula	midportion of greater tubercle of humerus	rotates arm laterally
intercostal m.'s, external *mm. intercostales externi*	inferior border of rib	superior border of rib below origin	draw ribs together
intercostal m.'s, innermost *mm. intercostales intimi*	superior border of rib	inferior border of rib above origin	draw ribs together
intercostal m.'s, internal *mm. intercostales interni*	inferior border of rib; costal cartilage	superior border of rib below origin, costal cartilage	draw ribs together
interosseous m.'s palmar (three in number) *mm. interossei palmares*	medial side of 2nd metacarpal, lateral side of 4th and 5th metacarpals	base of proximal phalanx in line with its origin	adduct 2nd, 4th, and 5th fingers; aid in flexing proximal phalanges

MUSCLE	ORIGIN	INSERTION	ACTION
interosseous m.'s, plantar (three in number) *mm. interossei plantares*	medial side of 3rd. 4th, and 5th metatarsals	medial side of proximal phalanges of 3rd, 4th, and 5th toes	adduct three lateral toes toward 2nd toe; flex toes
interosseous m.'s of foot, dorsal (four in number) *mm. interossei dorsales pedis*	adjacent sides of metatarsals	proximal phalanges of both sides of 2nd toe, lateral side of 3rd and 4th toes	abduct lateral toes, move 2nd toe from side to side; flex proximal phalanges
interosseous m.'s of hand, dorsal (four in number) *mm. interossei dorsales manus*	adjacent sides of metacarpals	extensor tendons of 2nd, 3rd, and 4th fingers	abduct 2nd, 3rd, and 4th fingers, spread fingers, flex proximal phalanges

first cervical vertebra

fourth cervical vertebra

levator muscle of scapula

posterior surface of scapula

deltoid muscle

trapezius muscle

latissimus dorsi muscle

thoracolumbar fascia

scapula

iliac crest

dorsal interosseous muscles of hand

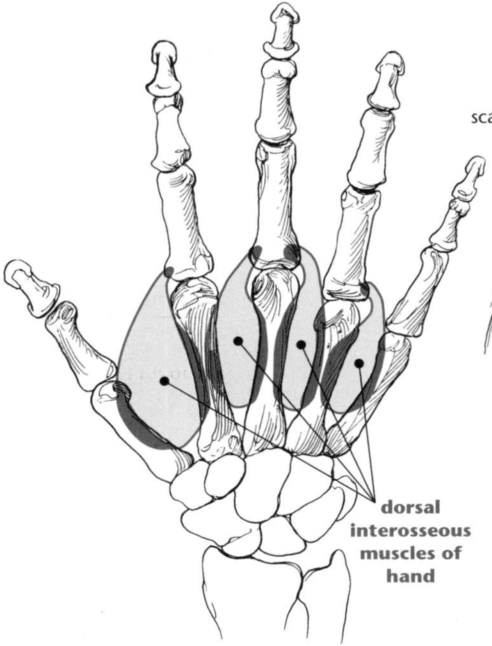

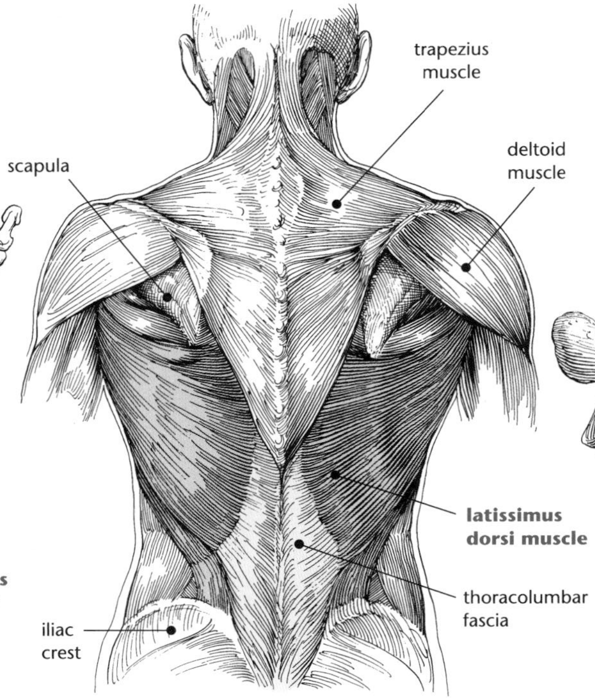

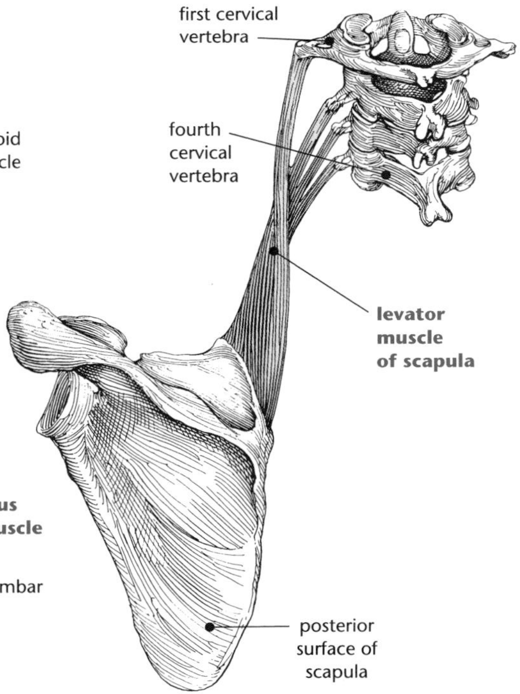

Muscle	Origin	Insertion	Action
interspinal m.'s *mm. interspinales*	short muscles between the spinous processes of contiguous vertebrae on either side of the interspinous ligament		extend vertebral column
intertransverse m.'s *mm. intertransversarii*	small paired muscles between the transverse processes of contiguous vertebrae		aid in maintaining erect posture by extension, lateral flexion, and rotation of the body
ischiocavernous m. *m. ischiocavernosus*	ramus of ischium adjacent to crus of penis or clitoris	crus near pubic symphysis	maintains erection of penis or clitoris
ischiococcygeus m.	see coccygeus muscle		
latissimus dorsi m. *m. latissimus dorsi*	spinous processes of vertebrae T7 to S3, thoracolumbar fascia, iliac crest, lower four ribs, inferior angle of scapula	floor of intertubercular groove of humerus	adducts, extends, and medially rotates arm
levator ani m. *m. levator ani*	the main m. of the pelvic floor within the lesser pelvis; comprised of pubococcygeal, iliococcygeal, and puborectal m.'s, as well as the levator m. of prostate in the male		supports pelvic viscera and separates it from the perineum; constricts lower end of rectum and vagina
levator m. of angle of mouth canine m. *m. levator anguli oris*	maxilla next to cuspid fossa, just below infraorbital foramen	corner of mouth	raises angle of mouth
levator m. of soft palate *m. levator veli palatini*	apex of petrous part of temporal bone and undersurface of cartilaginous part of auditory tube	aponeurosis of soft palate	raises soft palate in swallowing; aids in opening orifice of auditory tube
levator m. of prostate *m. levator prostatae*	pubic symphysis	fascia of prostate	elevates and compresses prostate
levator m.'s of ribs *mm. levatores costarum*	transverse processes of 7th cervical and first eleven thoracic vertebrae	angle of rib below	aid in raising ribs; extend vertebral column
levator m. of scapula *m. levator scapulae*	transverse processes of first four cervical vertebrae	vertebral (medial) border of scapula	raises scapula; aids in rotating neck
levator m. of thyroid gland *m. levator glandulae thyroideae*	isthmus or pyramidal lobe of thyroid gland	body of hyoid bone	stabilizes thyroid gland
levator m. of upper eyelid *m. levator palpebrae superior*	roof of orbital cavity above optic canal	skin and tarsal plate of upper eyelid, and superior fornix of conjunctiva	raises upper eyelid
levator m. of upper lip quadrate m. of upper lip *m. levator labii superior*	maxilla and zygomatic bone above level of infraorbital foramen	muscular substance of upper lip and margin of nostril	raises upper lip, dilates nostril

MUSCLE	ORIGIN	INSERTION	ACTION
levator m. of upper lip and ala of nose *m. levator labii superior alaeque nasi*	frontal process of maxilla	skin of upper lip, ala of nose	raises upper lip, dilates nostril
long m. of head *...m. longus capitis*	transverse processes of 3rd to 6th cervical vertebrae	basal part of occipital bone	flexes head
...ng m. of neck *...longus colli*	superior oblique part: anterior tubercle of transverse processes of 3rd, 4th, and 5th cervical vertebrae;	superior oblique part: antero-lateral surface of tubercle on anterior arch of 1st vertebra (atlas);	bends neck forward and slightly rotates cervical portion of vertebral column

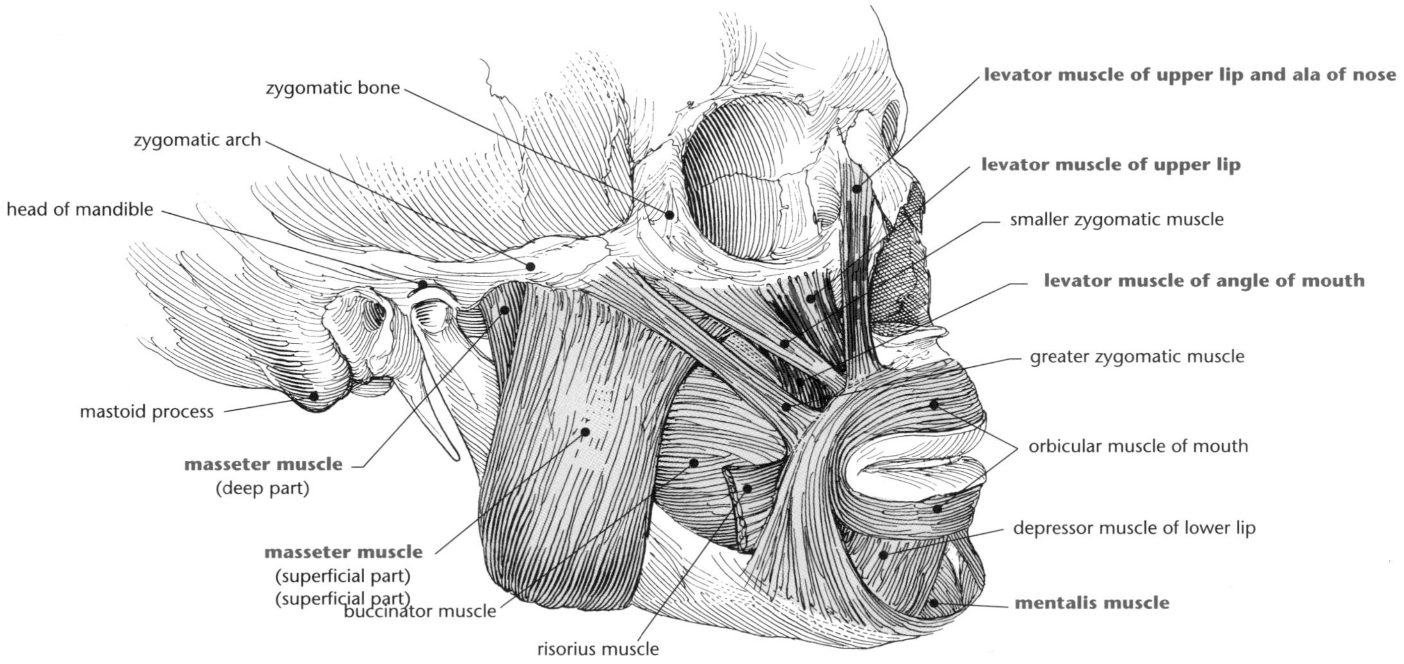

Diagram labels:

levator muscle of upper lip and ala of nose

levator muscle of upper lip

smaller zygomatic muscle

levator muscle of angle of mouth

greater zygomatic muscle

orbicular muscle of mouth

depressor muscle of lower lip

mentalis muscle

zygomatic bone

zygomatic arch

head of mandible

mastoid process

masseter muscle (deep part)

masseter muscle (superficial part)

(superficial part)

buccinator muscle

risorius muscle

Muscle	Origin	Insertion	Action
...ssimus m. of head ...elomastoid m. longissimus capitis	inferior oblique part: front of bodies of first two or three thoracic vertebrae; vertical part: front of bodies of first three thoracic and last three cervical vertebrae	inferior oblique part: anterior tubercle of transverse processes of 5th & 6th cervical vertebrae; vertical part: front of bodies of 2nd, 3rd, and 4th cervical vertebrae mastoid process of temporal bone	draws head backward, rotates head
longissimus m. of neck m. longissimus cervicis	transverse processes of 1st to 6th thoracic vertebrae	transverse processes of 2nd through 6th cervical vertebrae	bends vertebral column backward and laterally
longissimus m. of thorax longissimus dorsi m. m. longissimus thoracis	thoracolumbar fascia, transverse processes of lower six thoracic and first two lumbar vertebrae	transverse processes of lumbar and thoracic vertebrae, inferior border of lower ribs	bends vertebral column backward and laterally
longitudinal m. of tongue, inferior m. longitudinalis inferior linguae	undersurface of tongue at base	tip of tongue	acts to alter shape of tongue
longitudinal m. of tongue, superior m. longitudinalis superior linguae	submucosa and median septum of tongue	margins of tongue	acts to alter shape of tongue
lumbrical m.'s of foot (four in number) mm. lumbricales pedis	tendons of long flexor m.'s of toes	medial side of proximal phalanges and extensor tendon of four lateral toes	flex proximal, extend middle and distal phalanges
lumbrical m.'s of hand (four In number) mm. lumbricales manus	tendons of deep flexor m.'s of fingers	extensor tendons of four lateral fingers	flex proximal, extend middle and distal phalanges
masseter m. m. masseter	superficial part: zygomatic process and arch; deep part: zygomatic arch	superficial part: ramus and angle of lower jaw; deep part: upper half of ramus, coronoid process of lower jaw	closes mouth, clenches teeth (muscle of mastication)
mentalis m. m. levator menti	incisor fossa of mandible	skin of chin	raises and protrudes lower lip
multifidus m. m. multifidus	sacrum and transverse processes of lumbar, thoracic, and lower cervical vertebrae	spinous processes of lumbar, thoracic, and lower cervical vertebrae	extends, rotates vertebral column; maintains posture
m. of Treitz	see suspensory muscle of duodenum		

290

MUSCLE	ORIGIN	INSERTION	ACTION
mylohyoid m. *m. mylohyoideus*	mylohyoid line of mandible	median raphe and hyoid bone	elevates floor of mouth, tongue, hyoid bone, and larynx; depresses mandible
nasal m. *m. nasalis*	maxilla adjacent to cuspid and incisor teeth	side of nose above nostril	draws margin of nostril toward septum
oblique m. of abdomen, external *m. obliquus externus abdominis*	inferior border of lower eight ribs	anterior half of crest of ilium, linea alba through rectus sheath, inguinal ligament	flexes and rotates vertebral column, tenses abdominal wall; aids defecation and micturition
oblique m. of abdomen, internal *m. obliquus internus abdominis*	iliac crest, thoracolumbar fascia, inguinal ligament	lower three or four costal cartilages, linea alba by conjoint tendon to pubis	flexes and rotates vertebral column, tenses abdominal wall
oblique m. of auricle *m. obliquus auriculae*	eminence of concha on medial surface of auricular cartilage	convexity of helix	thought to be vestigial
oblique m. of eyeball, inferior *m. obliquus inferior bulbi*	floor of orbital cavity at anterior margin	between insertion of superior and lateral recti	rotates eyeball upward and outward
oblique m. of eyeball, superior *m. obliquus superior bulbi*	lesser wing of sphenoid bone above the optic canal	after passing through a fibrous pulley, reverses direction to insert on sclera, deep to superior rectus m.	rotates eyeball downward and outward
oblique m. of head, inferior *m. obliquus capitis inferior*	spine of 2nd vertebra (axis)	transverse process of 1st vertebra (atlas)	rotates head laterally
oblique m. of head, superior *m. obliquus capitis superior*	transverse process of first vertebra (atlas)	outer third of curved, lower line of the occipital bone	rotates head laterally; bends head backward
obturator m., external *m. obturatorius externus*	external margin of obturator foramen of pelvis, obturator membrane	trochanteric fossa of femur	flexes and rotates thigh laterally
obturator m., internal *m. obturatorius internus*	pelvic surface of hipbone and internal margin of obturator foramen, obturator membrane	greater trochanter of femur	abducts and laterally rotates thigh
occipital m.	see occipitofrontal muscle		
occipitofrontal m. *m. occipitofrontalis*	frontal part: epicranial aponeurosis; occipital part: highest nuchal line of occipital bone	frontal part: skin of eyebrow, root of nose; occipital part: epicranial aponeurosis	frontal part: elevates eyebrow, wrinkles forehead; occipital part: draws scalp backward
omohyoid m. *m. omohyoideus*	medial tip of suprascapular notch on upper scapula	lower border of body of hyoid bone	depresses and retracts hyoid bone

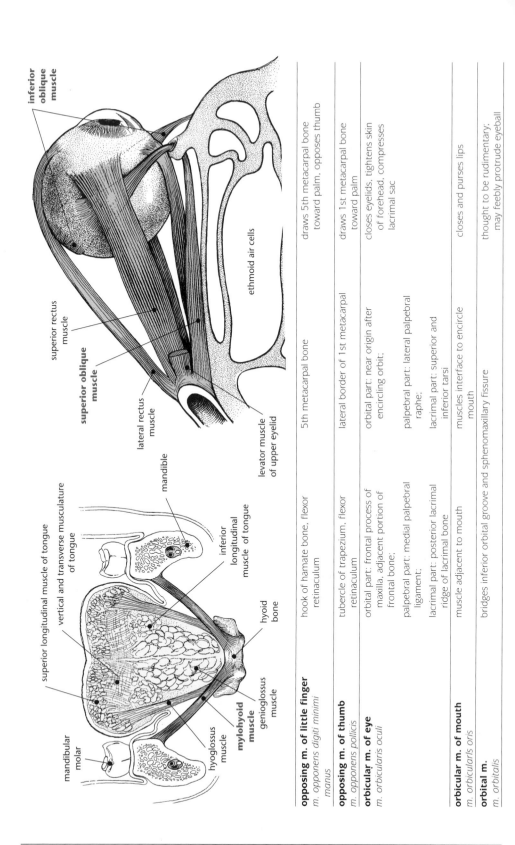

opposing m. of little finger *m. opponens digiti minimi manus*	hook of hamate bone, flexor retinaculum	5th metacarpal bone	draws 5th metacarpal bone toward palm, opposes thumb
opposing m. of thumb *m. opponens pollicis*	tubercle of trapezium, flexor retinaculum	lateral border of 1st metacarpal	draws 1st metacarpal bone toward palm
orbicular m. of eye *m. orbicularis oculi*	orbital part: frontal process of maxilla, adjacent portion of frontal bone; palpebral part: medial palpebral ligament; lacrimal part: posterior lacrimal ridge of lacrimal bone	orbital part: near origin after encircling orbit; palpebral part: lateral palpebral raphe; lacrimal part: superior and inferior tarsi	closes eyelids, tightens skin of forehead, compresses lacrimal sac
orbicular m. of mouth *m. orbicularis oris*	muscle adjacent to mouth	muscles interface to encircle mouth	closes and purses lips
orbital m. *m. orbitalis*	bridges inferior orbital groove and sphenomaxillary fissure		thought to be rudimentary; may feebly protrude eyeball

MUSCLE	ORIGIN	INSERTION	ACTION
palatoglossus m. glossopalatine m. *m. palatoglossus*	undersurface of soft palate	dorsum and side of tongue	elevates back of tongue and narrows fauces
palatopharyngeal m. *m. palatopharyngeus*	soft palate; back of hard palate	posterior wall of thyroid cartilage and wall of pharynx	elevates pharynx and shortens it during act of swallowing; narrows fauces
palmar m., long *m. palmaris longus*	medial epicondyle of humerus	flexor retinaculum, palmar aponeurosis	flexes hand
palmar m., short *m. palmaris brevis*	flexor retinaculum; medial side of palmar aponeurosis	skin of palm over hypothenar eminence	aids in deepening hollow of palm, wrinkles skin of palm
pectinate m.'s *mm. pectinati*	a number of muscular columns projecting from the inner walls of the atria of the heart		contract in systole the right atrium of the heart
pectineal m. *m. pectineus*	pectineal line of pubis	pectineal line of femur between lesser trochanter and linea aspera	adducts and aids in flexion of of thigh
pectoral m., greater *m. pectoralis major*	medial half of clavicle, sternum and costal cartilages; aponeurosis of external oblique m. of abdomen; 6th rib	lateral lip of intertubercular groove of humerus	flexes, adducts, and rotates arm medially
pectoral m., smaller *m. pectoralis minor*	anterior aspect of 3rd through 5th ribs, near costal cartilages	coracoid process of scapula	draws scapula downward, elevates ribs
pectoralis major m.	see pectoral muscle, greater		
pectoralis minor m.	see pectoral muscle, smaller		
peroneal m., long fibular m.. long *m. peroneus longus*	upper two-thirds of fibula; crural septum	1st metatarsal bone, medial cuneiform bone	aids in plantar flexion, everts foot; helps maintain transverse arch of foot
peroneal m., short fibular m.. short *m. peroneus brevis*	lower two-thirds of fibula; crural septum	tuberosity of 5th metatarsal bone	aids in plantar flexion; everts foot; aids in preventing over-inversion of foot
peroneal m., third *m. peroneus tertius*	distal third of fibula; crural fascia	fascia of 5th metatarsal bone, on dorsum of foot	dorsiflexes and everts foot
piriform m. *m. piriformis*	internal aspect of sacrum, sacrotuberous ligament	upper portion of greater trochanter of femur	rotates thigh laterally
plantar m. *m. plantaris*	supracondylar line just above lateral condyle of femur; oblique popliteal ligament	posterior part of calcaneus (along with calcaneal tendon)	plantar flexion of foot

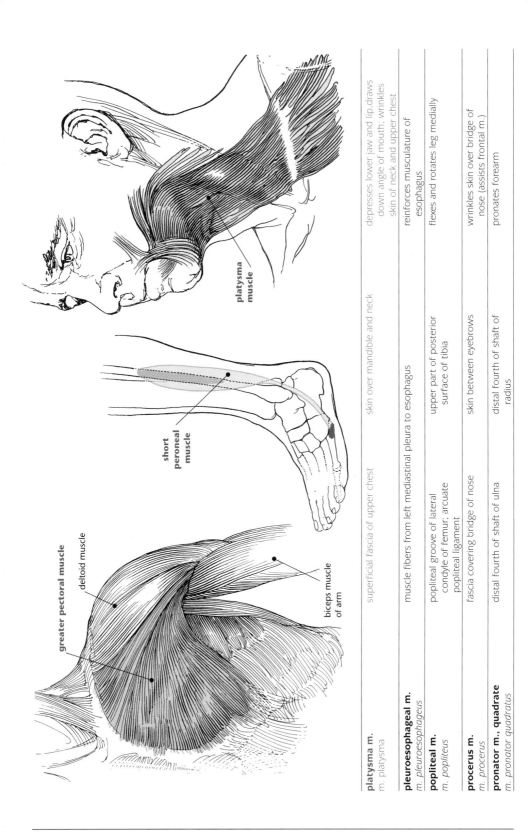

platysma m. m. platysma	superficial fascia of upper chest	skin over mandible and neck	depresses lower jaw and lip; draws down angle of mouth; wrinkles skin of neck and upper chest
pleuroesophageal m. m. pleuroesophageus	muscle fibers from left mediastinal pleura to esophagus		reinforces musculature of esophagus
popliteal m. m. popliteus	popliteal groove of lateral condyle of femur; arcuate popliteal ligament	upper part of posterior surface of tibia	flexes and rotates leg medially
procerus m. m. procerus	fascia covering bridge of nose	skin between eyebrows	wrinkles skin over bridge of nose (assists frontal m.)
pronator m., quadrate m. pronator quadratus	distal fourth of shaft of ulna	distal fourth of shaft of radius	pronates forearm

greater pectoral muscle

deltoid muscle

biceps muscle of arm

short peroneal muscle

platysma muscle

MUSCLE	ORIGIN	INSERTION	ACTION
pronator m., round *m. pronator teres*	humeral part: medial epicondyle of humerus; ulnar part: coronoid process of ulna	lateral aspect of radius at point of maximum convexity	pronates and flexes forearm
psoas m., greater *m. psoas major*	transverse processes and bodies of lumbar vertebrae; body of 12th thoracic vertebra	lesser trochanter of femur	flexes and medially rotates thigh
psoas m., smaller *m. psoas minor*	bodies of last thoracic and 1st lumbar vertebra	pectineal line of hipbone	flexes vertebral column
pterygoid m., lateral external pterygoid m. *m. pterygoideus lateralis*	lateral pterygoid plate and greater wing of sphenoid bone	condyle of mandible, capsule of temporomandibular joint	opens mouth and protrudes mandible
pterygoid m., medial internal pterygoid m. *m. pterygoideus medialis*	maxillary tuberosity and lateral pterygoid plate, tubercle of palatine bone	medial surface of ramus and angle of mandible	closes mouth, protrudes mandible and moves it side to side

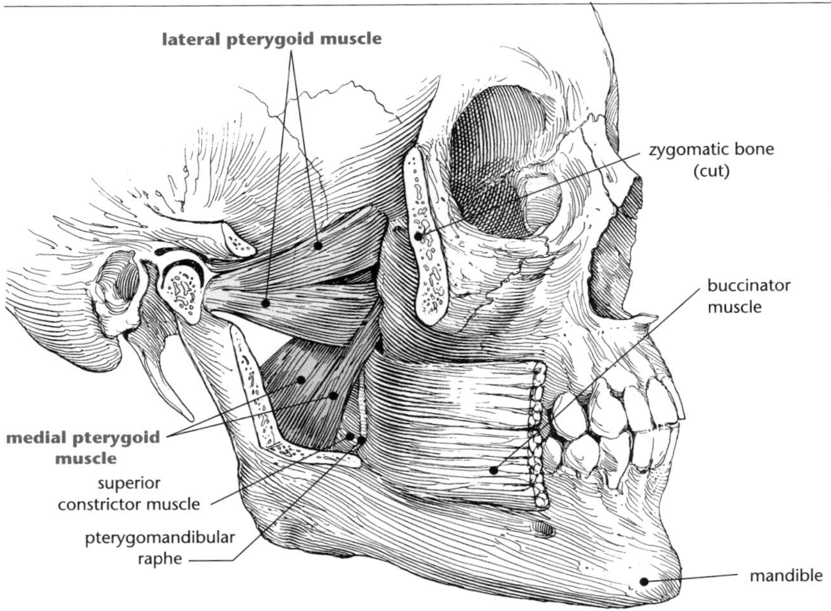

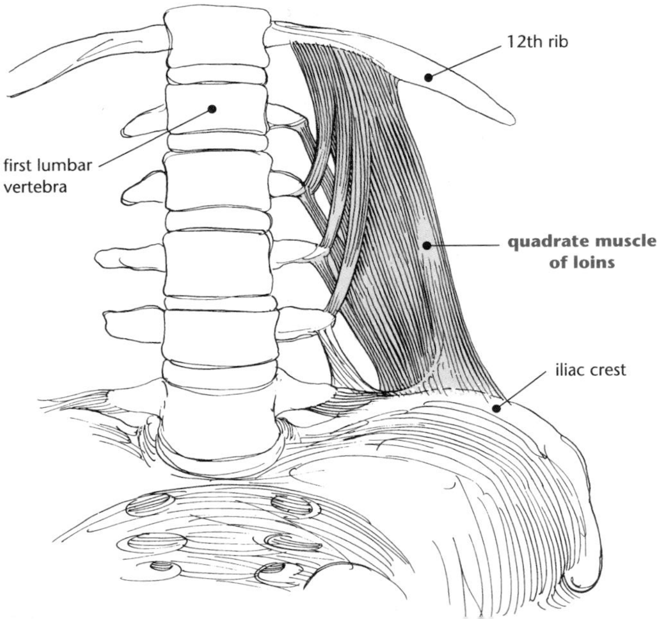

quadrate muscle of loins

12th rib

iliac crest

first lumbar vertebra

zygomatic bone (cut)

buccinator muscle

mandible

lateral pterygoid muscle

medial pterygoid muscle

superior constrictor muscle

pterygomandibular raphe

Muscle	Origin	Insertion	Action
pubococcygeal m. *m. pubococcygeus*	back of pubis and obturator fascia	coccyx and perineal body	supports pelvic floor
puborectal m. *m. puborectalis*	back of pubis and pubic symphysis	interdigitates to form a sling which passes behind rectum	holds anal canal at right angle to rectum
pubovaginal m. *m. pubovaginalis*	part of levator ani muscle in the female		
pubovesical m. *m. pubovesicalis*	posterior surface of body of pubis	female: around fundus of bladder to front of vagina; male: around fundus of bladder to prostate	strengthens musculature of urinary bladder; secures base of bladder
pyramidal m. *m. pyramidalis*	pubis and pubic symphysis	linea alba	tenses abdominal wall
quadrate m. of loins *m. quadratus lumborum*	iliac crest, transverse processes of lumbar vertebrae, iliolumbar ligament	12th rib, transverse processes of upper lumbar vertebrae	draws rib cage downward, bends vertebral column laterally
quadrate m. of lower lip *m. quadratus labii inferior*	see depressor muscle of lower lip		
quadrate m. of sole accessory flexor m. *m. quadratus plantae*	calcaneus and plantar fascia	tendons of long flexor m. of toes (m. flexor digitorum longus)	aids in flexing all toes except the big toe
quadrate m. of thigh *m. quadratus femoris*	proximal part of external border of tuberosity of ischium	proximal part of linea quad-rata (line extending vertically and distally from inter-trochanteric crest of femur)	rotates thigh laterally
quadrate m. of upper lip	see levator muscle of upper lip		
quadratus lumborum m.	see quadrate muscle of loins		
quadriceps m. of thigh *m. quadriceps femoris*	the four-headed fleshy mass that covers the front and sides of the femur, consisting of the rectus m. of thigh (m. rectus femoris), lateral vastus m. (m. vastus lateralis), medial vastus m. (m. vastus medialis), and intermediate vastus m. (m. vastus intermedius)		great extensor m. of leg
rectococcygeus m. *m. rectococcygeus*	smooth muscle fibers in the pelvic fascia between the coccyx and rectum		secures rectum
rectourethral m. *m. rectourethralis*	smooth muscle fibers in the pelvic fascia between the rectum and membranous urethra of male		secures urethra
rectouterine m. *m. rectouterinus*	bundle of smooth muscle fibers in pelvic fascia between rectum and cervix of uterus		secures uterus
rectus m. of abdomen *m. rectus abdominis*	pubic crest; pubic symphysis	xiphoid process, 5th to 7th costal cartilages	tenses abdominal wall; draws thorax downward; flexes vertebral column

MUSCLE	ORIGIN	INSERTION	ACTION
rectus m. of eyeball, inferior *m. rectus inferior bulbi*	common tendon ring around optic canal	lower part of sclera posterior to corneoscleral junction	rotates eyeball downward and somewhat medially
rectus m. of eyeball, lateral *m. rectus lateralis bulbi*	common tendon ring around optic canal; orbital surface of greater wing of sphenoid	lateral part of sclera posterior to corneoscleral junction	rotates eyeball laterally
rectus m. of eyeball, medial *m. rectus medialis bulbi*	common tendon ring around optic canal	medial part of sclera posterior to corneoscleral junction	rotates eyeball medially
rectus m. of eyeball, superior *m. rectus superior bulbi*	common tendon ring around optic canal	top part of sclera posterior to corneoscleral junction	rotates eyeball upward and somewhat medially

trapezius muscle

deltoid muscle

smaller rhomboid muscle

greater rhomboid muscle

scapula

humerus

medial rectus muscle of eyeball

superior oblique muscle of eyeball

inferior oblique muscle of eyeball

lateral rectus muscle of eyeball

superior rectus muscle of eyeball

inferior rectus muscle of eyeball

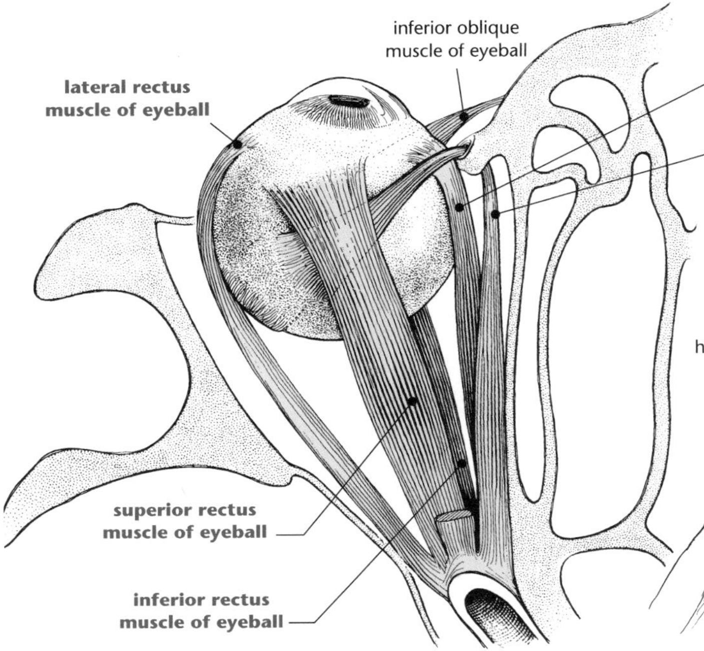

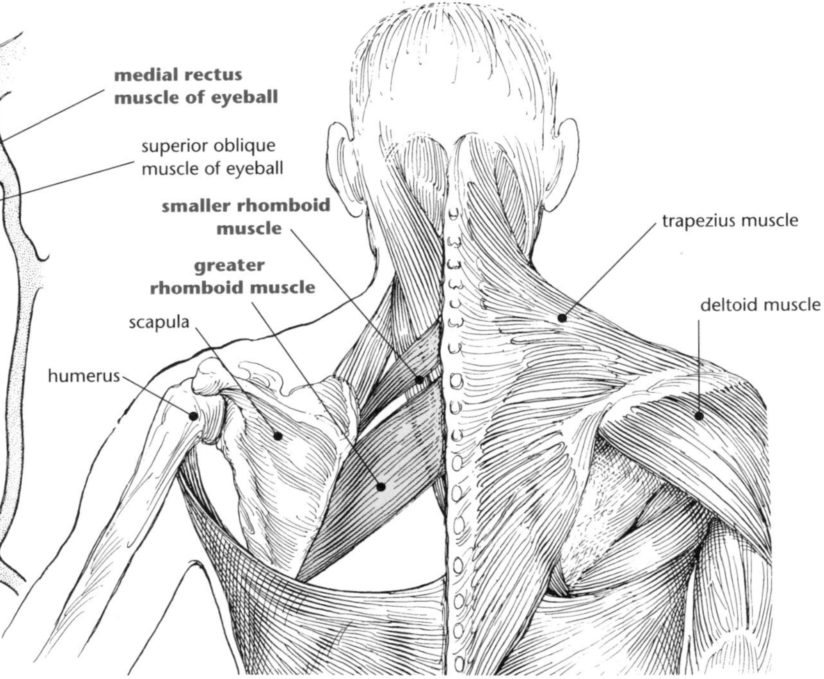

rectus m. of head, anterior *m. rectus capitis anterior*	lateral portion of 1st vertebra (atlas)	flexes and supports head
rectus m. of head, lateral *m. rectus capitis lateralis*	transverse process of 1st vertebra (atlas)	aids in lateral movement of head; supports head
rectus m. of head, greater posterior *m. rectus capitis post. major*	spinous process of 2nd vertebra (axis)	extends head
rectus m. of head, smaller posterior *m. rectus capitis post. minor*	posterior tubercle of 1st vertebra (atlas)	extends head
rectus m. of thigh *m. rectus femoris*	anterior inferior iliac spine, rim of acetabulum	extends leg and flexes thigh
rhomboid m., greater *m. rhomboideus major*	spinous processes of 2nd to 5th thoracic vertebrae	adducts and laterally rotates scapula
rhomboid m., smaller *m. rhomboideus minor*	spinous processes of 7th cervical and 1st thoracic vertebrae and lower part of nuchal ligament	adducts and laterally rotates scapula
risorius m. *m. risorius*	fascia over masseter muscle; platysma muscle	retracts angle of mouth
rotator m.'s *m. rotatores*	transverse processes of all vertebrae below second cervical	extend and rotate the vertebral column toward opposite side
sacrococcygeus m., dorsal *m. sacrococcygeus dorsalis*	a muscular slip from the dorsal aspect of the sacrum to the coccyx	protects sacrococcygeal joint
sacrococcygeus m., ventral *m. sacrococcygeus ventralis*	a muscular slip from the ventral aspect of the sacrum to the coccyx	protects sacrococcygeal joint
sacrospinal m.	see erector muscle of spine	
salpingopharyngeal m. *m. salpingopharyngeus*	cartilage of auditory tube near nasopharyngeal orifice	elevates nasopharynx
sartorius m. *m. sartorius*	anterior superior iliac spine	flexes thigh and leg; rotates thigh laterally
scalene m., anterior *m. scalenus anterior*	transverse processes of 3rd to 6th cervical vertebrae	raises 1st rib, stabilizes or inclines neck to the side
scalene m., middle *m. scalenus medius*	transverse processes of first six cervical vertebrae	raises 1st rib, stabilizes or inclines neck to the side
scalene m., posterior *m. scalenus posterior*	transverse processes of 5th to 7th cervical vertebrae	raises 2nd rib, stabilizes or inclines neck to the side

MUSCLE	ORIGIN	INSERTION	ACTION
scalene m., smallest *m. scalenus minimus*	occasional extra muscle fibers or slip of posterior scalene muscle		tenses dome of pleura
semimembranous m. *m. semimembranosus*	tuberosity of ischium	medial condyle of tibia; oblique popliteal ligament	extends thigh, flexes and rotates leg medially
semispinal m. of head *m. semispinalis capitis*	transverse processes of six upper thoracic and four lower cervical vertebrae	occipital bone between superior and inferior nuchal lines	rotates head and draws it backward
semispinal m. of neck *m. semispinalis cervicis*	transverse processes of upper six thoracic vertebrae	spinous processes of 2nd to 6th cervical vertebrae	extends and rotates vertebral column
semispinal m. of thorax *m. semispinalis thoracis*	transverse processes of lower six thoracic vertebrae	spinous processes of upper six thoracic and lower two cervical vertebrae	extends and rotates vertebral column
semitendinous m. *m. semitendinosus*	tuberosity of ischium (in common with biceps m. of thigh)	upper part of tibia near tibial tuberosity	flexes and rotates leg medially, extends thigh
serratus m., anterior *m. serratus anterior*	lateral surface of eight or nine uppermost ribs	anterior surface of vertebral border of scapula	draws scapula forward and laterally, rotates scapula in raising arm
serratus m., inferior posterior *m. serratus posterior inferior*	spinous processes of last two thoracic and first two or three lumbar vertebrae; supraspinal ligament	inferior borders of the lowest four ribs, slightly beyond their angles	draws the ribs outward and downward (counteracting the inward pull of the diaphragm)
serratus m., superior posterior *m. serratus posterior superior*	caudal part of nuchal ligament, spinous processes of the 7th cervical and first two or three thoracic vertebrae; supraspinal ligament	upper borders of the 2nd, 3rd, 4th, and 5th ribs, slightly beyond their angles	raises the ribs
soleus m. *m. soleus*	upper third of fibula, soleal line of tibia, tendinous arch	calcaneus by calcaneal tendon (tendo calcaneus)	plantarflexes foot
sphincter m. of anus, external *m. sphincter ani externus*	tip of coccyx, anococcygeal ligament	central tendon of perineum, skin	closes anal canal and anus
sphincter m. of anus, internal *m. sphincter ani internus*	1 cm thick muscular ring surrounding approximately 2.5 cm of the upper part of the anal canal, about 6 mm from the orifice of the anus		aids in occlusion of anal orifice and expulsion of feces
sphincter m. of bile duct *m. sphincter choledochus*	circular muscle around the lower part of the bile duct within the wall of the duodenum (part of the sphincter muscle of hepatopancreatic ampulla)		constricts lower part of bile duct
sphincter m. of hepatopancreatic ampulla	circular muscle around the terminal part of the main pancreatic duct and bile duct, including the duodenal ampulla		constricts both lower part of bile duct and main

sphincter of Oddi *m. sphincter ampullae hepatopancreaticae*	(papilla of Vater)	pancreatic duct
sphincter m. of pupil *m. sphincter pupillae*	circular fibers of the iris arranged in a narrow band about 1 mm in width	constricts pupil
sphincter m. of pylorus *m. sphincter pylori*	thick muscular ring at the end of the stomach, near opening into duodenum	acts as valve to close pyloric lumen
sphincter m. of urethra external urethral sphincter m. *m. sphincter urethrae*	fibers interdigitate around urethra ramus of pubis	compresses urethra
sphincter m. of urinary bladder *m. sphincter vesicae urinariae*	thick muscular ring toward the lower part of bladder around internal urethral orifice	acts as valve to close internal urethral orifice

superior posterior serratus muscle

scapula

vertebrae

inferior posterior serratus muscle

anterior serratus muscle

clavicle

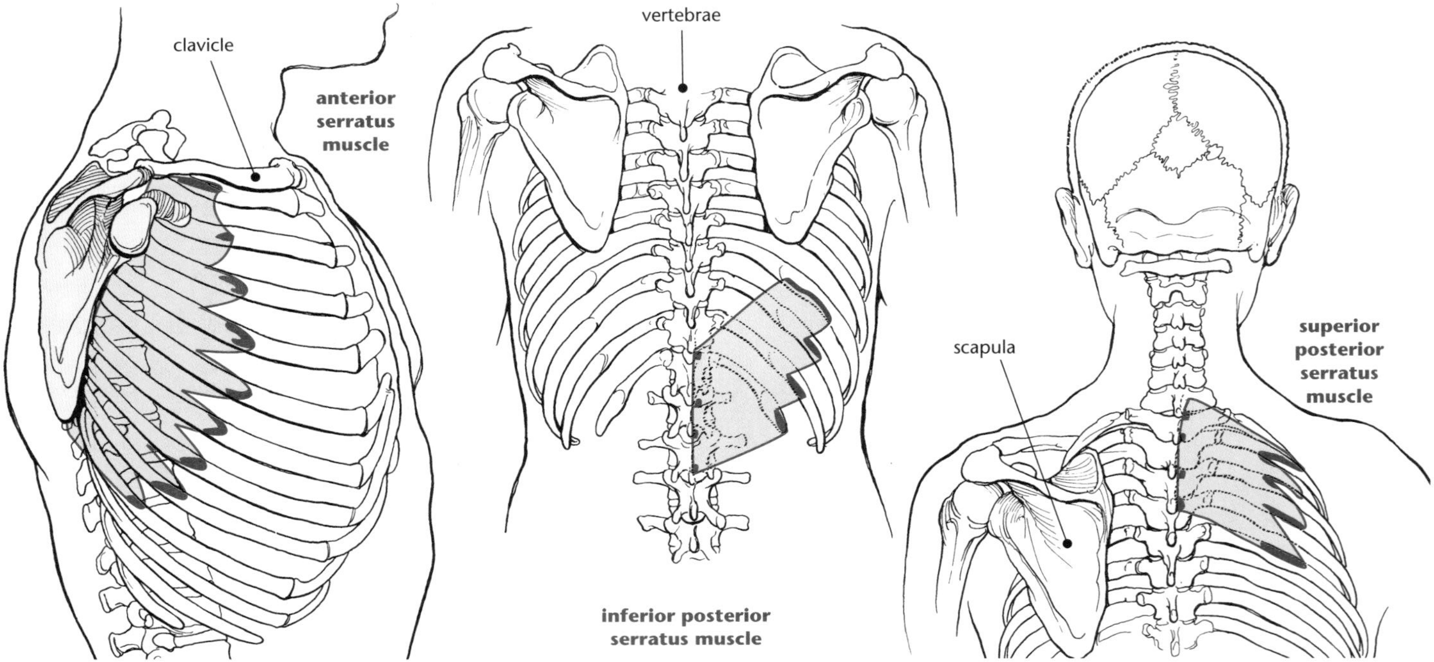

MUSCLE	ORIGIN	INSERTION	ACTION
sphincter m. of vagina *m. sphincter vaginae*	pubic symphysis	interdigitates around and inter-laces into vaginal barrel	constricts vaginal orifice
sphincter of Oddi	see sphincter muscle of hepatopancreatic ampulla		
spinal m. of head biventer cervicis m. *m. spinalis capitis*	spinous processes of 6th cervical to 2nd thoracic vertebrae	occipital bone between superior and inferior nuchal lines	extends head
spinal m. of neck *m. spinalis cervicis*	spinous processes of 7th cervical to 2nd thoracic vertebrae	spinous processes of 2nd, 3rd, and 4th cervical vertebrae	extends vertebral column

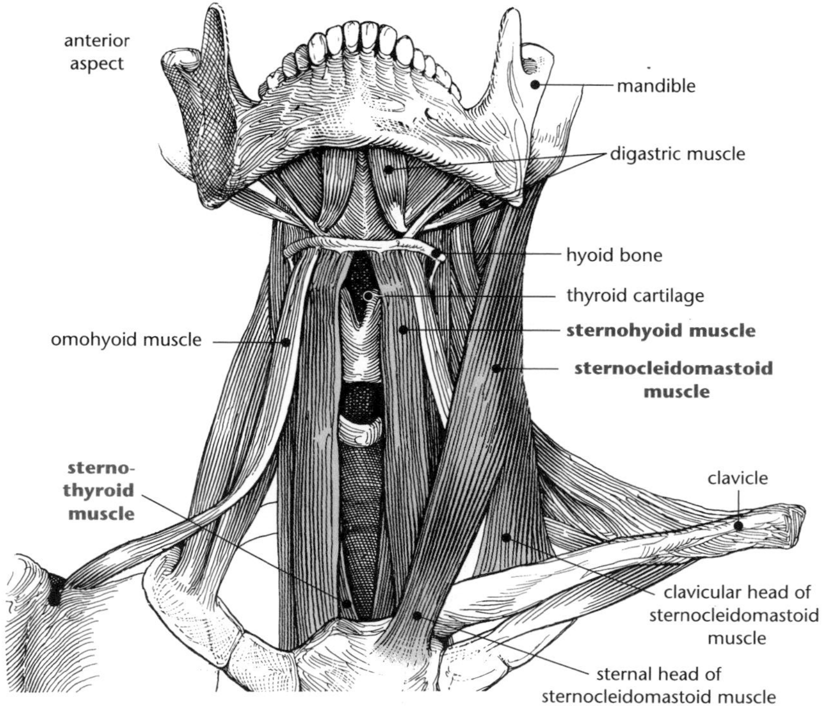

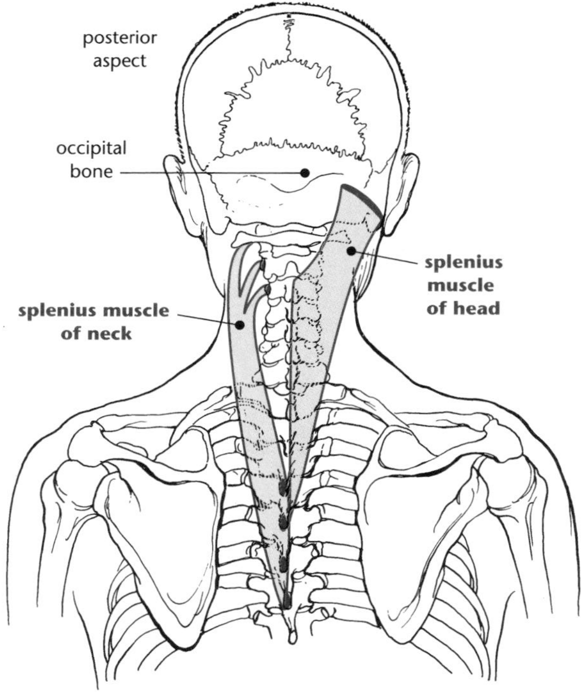

posterior aspect

splenius muscle of head

occipital bone

splenius muscle of neck

anterior aspect

mandible

digastric muscle

hyoid bone

thyroid cartilage

sternohyoid muscle

sternocleidomastoid muscle

clavicle

clavicular head of sternocleidomastoid muscle

sternal head of sternocleidomastoid muscle

omohyoid muscle

sterno-thyroid muscle

Muscle	Origin/Insertion	Action
spinal m. of thorax *m. spinalis thoracis*	spinous processes of upper two lumbar and lower two thoracic vertebrae	spinous processes of 2nd to 7th thoracic vertebrae	extends vertebral column
splenius m. of head *m. splenius capitis*	spinous processes of upper thoracic vertebrae; nuchal ligament	mastoid process and superior nuchal line	inclines and rotates head
splenius m. of neck splenius colli m. *m. splenius cervicis*	spinous processes of 3rd to 6th thoracic vertebrae; nuchal ligament	posterior tubercles of the transverse processes of upper two or three cervical vertebrae	extends head and neck; turns head toward the same side
stapedius m. *m. stapedius*	bony canal in pyramidal eminence on posterior wall of middle ear	posterior surface of neck of stapes	dampens excessive vibrations of stapes by tilting baseplate
sternal m. *m. sternalis*	small superficial muscular band at sternal end of greater pectoral muscle (m. pectoralis major), parallel with the margin of sternum		protects sternum
sternocleidomastoid m. *m. sternocleidomastoideus*	sternal head: anterior surface of manubrium; clavicular head: medial third of clavicle	mastoid process, superior nuchal line of occipital bone	rotates and extends head. flexes vertebral column
sternocostal m.	see transverse muscle of thorax		
sternohyoid m. *m. sternohyoideus*	medial end of clavicle, first costal cartilage, posterior surface of manubrium	lower border of body of hyoid bone	depresses hyoid bone and larynx from elevated position during swallowing
sternothyroid m. *m. sternothyroideus*	dorsal surface of upper part of sternum and medial edge of first costal cartilage	oblique line on lamina of thyroid cartilage	draws thyroid cartilage downward from elevated position during swallowing
styloglossus m. *m. styloglossus*	lower end of styloid process.	longitudinal part: side of tongue near dorsal surface: oblique part: over hyoglossus m.	raises and retracts tongue
stylohyoid m. *m. stylohyoideus*	posterior and lateral surfaces of styloid process near base	hyoid bone at junction of greater cornu (horn) and body	draws hyoid bone upward and backward
stylopharyngeus m. *m. stylopharyngeus*	root of styloid process of temporal bone	borders of thyroid cartilage, wall of pharynx	elevates and opens pharynx
subclavius m. *m. subclavius*	junction of 1st rib and costal cartilages	lower surface of clavicle	depresses lateral end of clavicle
subcostal m.'s *mm. subcostales*	inner surface of lower ribs near their angles	lower inner surface of 2nd to 3rd rib below rib of origin	draw adjacent ribs together; depresses lower ribs
subscapular m. *m. subscapularis*	subscapular fossa	lesser tubercle of humerus	rotates arm medially
supinator m. *m. supinator*	lateral epicondyle of humerus, supinator crest of ulna	upper third of radius	supinates the forearm by rotating radius

MUSCLE	ORIGIN	INSERTION	ACTION
suprahyoid m.'s *mm. suprahyoidei*	group of muscles attached to the upper part of the hyoid bone from the skull, including the digastric, stylohyoid, mylohyoid, and geniohyoid muscles		elevates hyoid bone
supraspinous m. *m. supraspinatus*	supraspinous fossa	superior aspect of greater tubercle of humerus	abducts arm
suspensory m. of duodenum ligament of Treitz suspensory lig. of duodenum *m. suspensorius duodeni*	connective tissue around celiac artery and right crus of diaphragm	superior border of duodeno-jejunal junction, part of ascending duodenum	acts as suspensory ligament of duodenum
tarsal m., inferior *m. tarsalis inferior*	aponeurosis of inferior rectus muscle of eyeball	lower border of tarsal plate of lower eyelid	widens palpebral fissure by depressing lower eyelid
tarsal m., superior *m. tarsalis superior*	aponeurosis of levator muscle of upper eyelid	upper border of tarsus plate of upper eyelid	widens palpebral fissure by raising upper eyelid
temporal m. *m. temporalis*	temporal fossa on side of cranium	coronoid process of mandible	closes mouth, clenches teeth, retracts lower jaw
temporoparietal m. *m. temporoparietalis*	temporal fascia above ear	frontal part of epicranial aponeurosis	tightens scalp
tensor m. of fascia lata *m. tensor fasciae latae*	iliac crest, anterior superior iliac spine, fascia lata	iliotibial tract of fascia lata	extends knee with lateral rotation of leg
tensor m. of soft palate *m. tensor veli palatini*	spine of sphenoid, scaphoid, fossa of pterygoid process, cartilage and membrane of the auditory tube	midline of aponeurosis of soft palate; wall of auditory tube	elevates palate and opens auditory tube
tensor m. of tympanum tensor m. of tympanic membrane *m. tensor tympani*	cartilaginous part of auditory tube and adjoining part of great wing of sphenoid bone	manubrium of malleus near its root	draws tympanic membrane medially, thus increasing its tension
teres major m. *m. teres major*	inferior lateral border of scapula	crest of lesser tubercle of humerus	adducts and rotates arm medially
teres minor m. *m. teres minor*	lateral border of scapula	inferior aspect of greater tubercle of humerus	rotates arm laterally, and weakly adducts it
thyroarytenoid m. *m. thyroarytenoideus*	inside of thyroid cartilage	lateral surface of arytenoid cartilage	aids in closure of laryngeal inlet, relaxes vocal ligament
thyroepiglottic m. *m. thyroepiglotticus*	inside of thyroid cartilage	margin of epiglottis	depresses the epiglottis, widens inlet of larynx
thyrohyoid m. *m. thyrohyoideus*	oblique line of thyroid cartilage	greater cornu (horn) of hyoid bone	elevates larynx, depresses hyoid bone

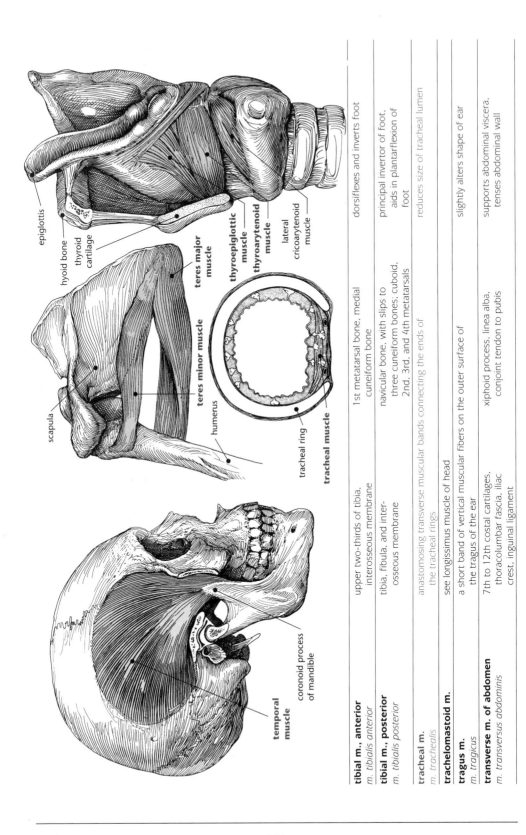

epiglottis
hyoid bone
thyroid cartilage
thyroepiglottic muscle
thyroarytenoid muscle
lateral cricoarytenoid muscle

teres major muscle
teres minor muscle
scapula
humerus
tracheal ring
tracheal muscle

temporal muscle
coronoid process of mandible

Muscle	Origin	Insertion	Action
tibial m., anterior *m. tibialis anterior*	upper two-thirds of tibia, interosseous membrane	1st metatarsal bone, medial cuneiform bone	dorsiflexes and inverts foot
tibial m., posterior *m. tibialis posterior*	tibia, fibula, and interosseous membrane	navicular bone, with slips to three cuneiform bones; cuboid, 2nd, 3rd, and 4th metatarsals	principal invertor of foot, aids in plantarflexion of foot
tracheal m. *m. trachealis*	anastomosing transverse muscular bands connecting the ends of the tracheal rings		reduces size of tracheal lumen
trachelomastoid m.	see longissimus muscle of head		
tragus m. *m. tragicus*	a short band of vertical muscular fibers on the outer surface of the tragus of the ear		slightly alters shape of ear
transverse m. of abdomen *m. transversus abdominis*	7th to 12th costal cartilages, thoracolumbar fascia, iliac crest, inguinal ligament	xiphoid process, linea alba, conjoint tendon to pubis	supports abdominal viscera, tenses abdominal wall

MUSCLE	ORIGIN	INSERTION	ACTION
transverse m. of auricle	see auricular muscle, transverse		
transverse m. of chin *m. transversus menti*	superficial muscular fibers of depressor muscle of angle of mouth which turn back and cross to the opposite side below the chin		aids in drawing angle of mouth downward
transverse m. of nape *m. transversus nuchae*	an occasional muscle passing between the tendons of the trapezius and sternocleidomastoid muscles		moves scalp feebly
transverse m. of perineum, deep *m. transversus perinei profundus*	inferior ramus of ischium	central tendon of perineum, external anal sphincter	supports pelvic viscera
transverse m. of perineum, superficial *m. transversus perinei superficialis*	ramus of ischium near tuberosity	central tendon of perineum	supports pelvic viscera
transverse m. of thorax sternocostal m. *m. transversus thoracis*	xiphoid process, posterior surface of lower part of sternum, adjacent costal cartilages	2nd to 6th costal cartilages (inner surface)	narrows chest, draws costal cartilages downward
transverse m. of tongue *m. transversus linguae*	median fibrous septum of tongue	submucous fibrous tissue at sides of tongue	narrows and elongates tongue
trapezius m. *m. trapezius*		superior part: posterior border of lateral third of clavicle; middle part: medial margin of acromion, superior lip of posterior border of scapular spine; inferior part: tubercle at apex of medial end of scapular spine	elevates, rotates, and retracts scapula (shoulder blade)

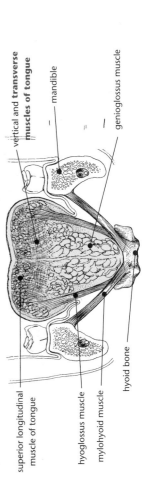

vertical and **transverse muscles of tongue**

mandible

genioglossus muscle

superior longitudinal muscle of tongue

hyoglossus muscle

mylohyoid muscle

hyoid bone

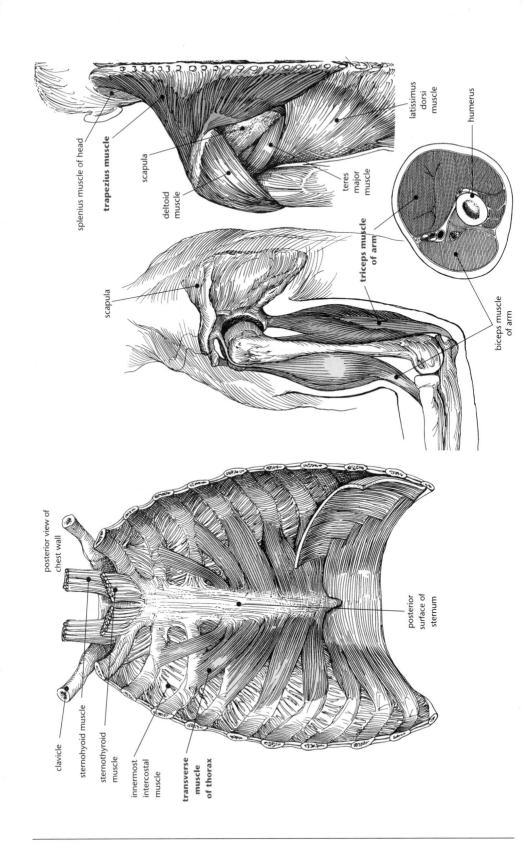

splenius muscle of head

trapezius muscle

scapula

deltoid muscle

teres major muscle

latissimus dorsi muscle

humerus

scapula

triceps muscle of arm

biceps muscle of arm

posterior view of chest wall

posterior surface of sternum

clavicle

sternohyoid muscle

sternothyroid muscle

innermost intercostal muscle

transverse muscle of thorax

MUSCLE	ORIGIN	INSERTION	ACTION
triangular m.	see depressor muscle of angle of mouth		
triceps m. of arm *m. triceps brachii*	long head: infraglenoid tubercle of scapula; lateral head: proximal humerus; medial head: distal half of humerus	posterior part of superior surface of olecranon process of ulna; adjacent deep fascia; articular capsule of elbow joint	main extensor of forearm
triceps of calf *m. triceps surae*	combined gastrocnemius and soleus muscles; its tendon of insertion is the calcaneal tendon		plantarflexes foot
uvula m. *m. uvulae*	palatine aponeurosis & posterior nasal spine of palatine bone	mucous membrane and connective tissue of uvula	elevates uvula
vastus m., intermediate *m. vastus intermedius*	anterior and lateral surface of upper two-thirds of femur	common tendon of quadriceps m. of thigh, patella	extends leg
vastus m., lateral *m. vastus lateralis*	lateral aspect of upper part of femur	common tendon of quadriceps m. of thigh, patella	extends leg
vastus m., medial *m. vastus medialis*	medial aspect of femur	common tendon of quadriceps m. of thigh, patella	extends leg
vertical m. of tongue *m. verticalis linguae*	dorsal fascia of tongue	undersurface of tongue	aids in mastication, swallowing, and speech by altering shape of tongue
vocal m. *m. vocalis*	inner surface of thyroid cartilage near midline	vocal process of arytenoid cartilage	adjusts tension of vocal cords
zygomatic m., greater *m. zygomaticus major*	zygomatic arch	angle of mouth	draws upper lip upward and laterally
zygomatic m., smaller *m. zygomaticus minor*	malar surface of zygomatic bone	upper lip	aids in forming nasolabial furrow (muscle of facial expression)

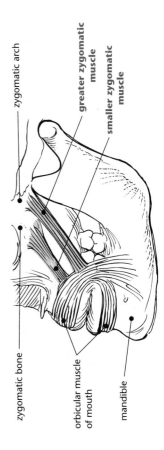

zygomatic bone

orbicular muscle of mouth

mandible

zygomatic arch

greater zygomatic muscle

smaller zygomatic muscle

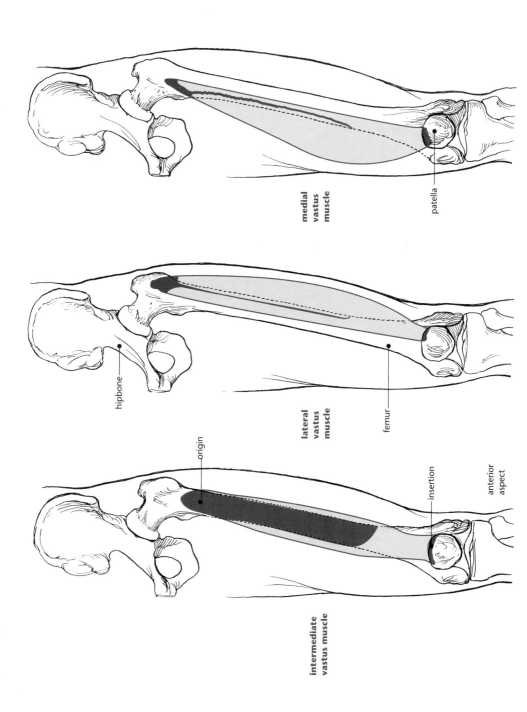

medial vastus muscle

patella

hipbone

lateral vastus muscle

femur

origin

insertion

anterior aspect

intermediate vastus muscle